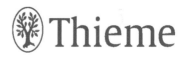

Cervical Spine Deformity Surgery

Christopher P. Ames, MD
Professor
Clinical Neurological Surgery and Orthopaedic Surgery
University of California, San Francisco
Director of Spinal Deformity Surgery
UCSF Medical Center
San Francisco, California, USA

K. Daniel Riew, MD
Professor of Orthopedic Surgery, Columbia University
Chief, Cervical Spine Surgery & Co-Director, Spine Division
Co-Director, Columbia University Spine Fellowship
Department of Orthopedic Surgery
Columbia University/ New York Presbyterian Hospital
New York, New York, USA

Justin S. Smith, MD, PhD
Harrison Distinguished Professor
Chief of Spine Division
Department of Neurosurgery
University of Virginia
Charlottesville, Virginia, USA

Kuniyoshi Abumi, MD
Director
Sapporo Orthopaedic Hospital-Centre for Spinal Disorders
Professor Emeritus
Hokkaido University
Sapporo, Japan

137 illustrations

Thieme
New York • Stuttgart • Delhi • Rio de Janeiro

Executive Editor: Timothy Hiscock
Managing Editor: Sarah Landis
Director, Editorial Services: Mary Jo Casey
Production Editor: Torsten Scheihagen
International Production Director: Andreas Schabert
Editorial Director: Sue Hodgson
International Marketing Director: Fiona Henderson
International Sales Director: Louisa Turrell
Director of Institutional Sales: Adam Bernacki
Senior Vice President and Chief Operating Officer: Sarah Vanderbilt
President: Brian D. Scanlan

Library of Congress Cataloging-in-Publication Data

Names: Ames, Christopher P., editor. | Riew, K. Daniel, editor. |
    Smith, Justin S., editor. | Abumi, Kuniyoshi, 1948- editor.
Title: Cervical spine deformity surgery / [edited by]
    Christopher P. Ames, K. Daniel Riew, Justin S. Smith,
    Kuniyoshi Abumi.
Description: New York : Thieme, [2019] | Includes bibliographical
    references.
Identifiers: LCCN 2019017956| ISBN 9781626239012 (hardcover) |
    ISBN 9781626239029 (eISBN)
Subjects: | MESH: Cervical Vertebrae–surgery | Spinal
    Diseases–surgery
Classification: LCC RD768 | NLM WE 727 | DDC 617.4/71–dc23
    LC record available at https://lccn.loc.gov/2019017956

© 2019 Thieme Medical Publishers, Inc.
Thieme Publishers New York
333 Seventh Avenue, New York, NY 10001 USA
+1 800 782 3488, customerservice@thieme.com

Thieme Publishers Stuttgart
Rüdigerstrasse 14, 70469 Stuttgart, Germany
+49 [0]711 8931 421, customerservice@thieme.de

Thieme Publishers Delhi
A-12, Second Floor, Sector-2, Noida-201301
Uttar Pradesh, India
+91 120 45 566 00, customerservice@thieme.in

Thieme Publishers Rio de Janeiro,
Thieme Publicações Ltda.
Edifício Rodolpho de Paoli, 25º andar
Av. Nilo Peçanha, 50 – Sala 2508
Rio de Janeiro 20020-906 Brasil
+55 21 3172 2297 / +55 21 3172-1896
www.thiemerevinter.com.br

Cover design: Thieme Publishing Group
Typesetting by DiTech Process Solutions

Printed in Germany by CPI books, Leck   5 4 3 2 1

ISBN 978-1-62623-901-2

Also available as an e-book:
eISBN 978-1-62623-902-9

Important note: Medicine is an ever-changing science undergoing continual development. Research and clinical experience are continually expanding our knowledge, in particular our knowledge of proper treatment and drug therapy. Insofar as this book mentions any dosage or application, readers may rest assured that the authors, editors, and publishers have made every effort to ensure that such references are in accordance with **the state of knowledge at the time of production of the book.**

Nevertheless, this does not involve, imply, or express any guarantee or responsibility on the part of the publishers in respect to any dosage instructions and forms of applications stated in the book. **Every user is requested to examine carefully** the manufacturers' leaflets accompanying each drug and to check, if necessary in consultation with a physician or specialist, whether the dosage schedules mentioned therein or the contraindications stated by the manufacturers differ from the statements made in the present book. Such examination is particularly important with drugs that are either rarely used or have been newly released on the market. Every dosage schedule or every form of application used is entirely at the user's own risk and responsibility. The authors and publishers request every user to report to the publishers any discrepancies or inaccuracies noticed. If errors in this work are found after publication, errata will be posted at www.thieme.com on the product description page.

Some of the product names, patents, and registered designs referred to in this book are in fact registered trademarks or proprietary names even though specific reference to this fact is not always made in the text. Therefore, the appearance of a name without designation as proprietary is not to be construed as a representation by the publisher that it is in the public domain.

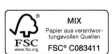

I dedicate this work to my children Pearson, Sebastian, and Scarlett who have always provided love and balance in my life. I would also like to acknowledge my residents, fellows, and mentees who have stimulated me with their questions and impressed me with their dedication to the care of our complex patients. Finally, I want to express my tremendous gratitude to my patients who have taught me the most in caring for them and provided an example to me of true courage.

–Christopher P. Ames

I dedicate this to my wife, Mary, without whose love and constant support I would not be where I am today, as well as our 3 grown children, Brad, Grant, and Julia. They are the light of our lives, and nothing in this world would be worthwhile without their love, health, and happiness.

–K. Daniel Riew

I would like to extend my gratitude to my mentors who provided me with not only the knowledge base and principles to care for patients with spinal deformities, but also helped to ignite the passion to help move the field forward.

–Justin S. Smith

I dedicate this work to my wife, Noriko. Without her understanding to sacrifice our family time, my complex work of cervical spinal surgery would not have progressed as it has. I would also like to express appreciation for my fellows and colleagues who have provided me with important ideas and always encouraged me to continue my difficult work.

–Kuniyoshi Abumi

Contents

Foreword

Cervical Spine Deformity Surgery, edited by Christopher Ames, Daniel Riew, Justin Smith, and Kuniyoshi Abumi, is a work of monumental proportions. The field of cervical deformity surgery is evolving and expanding rapidly. This field has lagged behind its thoracic and lumbar deformity surgery counterpart, predominantly as a result of a focus on complex thoracolumbar deformities in prior decades. Now, with more surgeons focusing on the cervical spine, the field of cervical spine deformity surgery has blossomed. The knowledge base is equally rapidly expanding. Hence, a book that incorporates the newest information regarding the fundamentals and techniques that are unique to the cervical spine is both timely and much needed.

Cervical Spine Deformity Surgery presents the relevant material in an incredibly organized manner. This book provides all one needs to know, and then some, regarding cervical spine deformity surgery—from the basics to the very complex. The book begins with discussions on anatomy, patho-etiology, imaging, sagittal balance, natural history, disability assessment, etc., followed by discussions on the wide variety of nuances associated with the decision-making process and surgical strategy determination. The book then concludes with discussions regarding complications, surgical nuances, etc.

Overall, this book is jam-packed with information and extremely well illustrated. It is up to date and perhaps even a bit futuristic, considering all the bases that have been covered. It serves as both a reference and a comprehensive primer. Of extreme importance, the editors and the authors are all at the very top of the field—representing a who's who of spine surgery, if you will. This book should be on the shelf of all providers and researchers dealing with cervical spine deformities.

I close by emphasizing the extraordinary worth of this book. It is a comprehensive and complete treatise on the subject, elegant in its presentation. Credit this, in part, to the high-quality standards associated with the publisher, Thieme. Finally, this book presents many complex concepts and techniques in a way that makes the complex seem simple. The editors and authors are to be heartily congratulated for a job very well done.

Edward C. Benzel, MD
Emeritus Chairman of Neurosurgery
Neurological Institute
Cleveland Clinic
Cleveland, Ohio, USA

Preface

Although cervical spinal deformity can have profound impacts, including pain, disability, and neurologic compromise, considerably less progress has been made in the study of these conditions compared with the more common, well-recognized thoracolumbar deformities. Early studies of cervical deformity focused on small series of patients who underwent procedures that were considered high-risk with resulting substantial morbidity. More recent advances in anesthesia and critical care, surgical techniques, and spinal instrumentation have led to a renewed interest in the surgical treatment of these often complex, high-risk deformities.

Despite the growing interest in providing surgical treatment for cervical deformity patients, there remain few resources that detail its modern clinical assessment, radiographic evaluation, and surgical treatment approaches. Much of this knowledge is experiencing a rapid evolution and is currently spread across the experts in the field with no single reference source. It is against this backdrop that this text was conceived as a concise source of current cervical deformity knowledge compiled from the literature and recognized experts in the field.

The text begins with a background on the marked health impact of cervical deformity and a primer on the clinical and radiographic assessment of these patients. Subsequent chapters detail surgical planning to address these conditions, including the range of osteotomies for correction and technique nuances from the experts. Importantly, multiple chapters address surgical and medical complications associated with these procedures and discuss risk stratification of these often-frail patients. Among the final chapters is a focused discussion of ongoing efforts to create a clinically meaningful comprehensive classification of cervical deformity.

The field of cervical deformity surgery is undergoing rapid advancements, with the ultimate goal of improving the health state and quality of life of those affected. The Editors are deeply grateful to the experts who have contributed to this text and hope that the readers find this work useful as they endeavor to care for their cervical deformity patients.

Christopher P. Ames, MD
K. Daniel Riew, MD
Justin S. Smith, MD, PhD
Kuniyoshi Abumi, MD

Contributors

Kuniyoshi Abumi, MD
Director
Sapporo Orthopaedic Hospital-Centre for Spinal Disorders
Professor Emeritus
Hokkaido University
Sapporo, Japan

Christopher P. Ames, MD
Professor
Clinical Neurological Surgery and Orthopaedic Surgery
University of California, San Francisco
Director of Spinal Deformity Surgery
UCSF Medical Center
San Francisco, California, USA

Philippe Bancel, MD
Orthopaedic Surgeon
Spine Department
Arago Institut
Paris, France

Shay Bess, MD
Denver International Spine Center
Presbyterian St. Luke's Hospital and Rocky Mountain
    Hospital for Children
Denver, Colorado, USA

Brandon B. Carlson, MD, MPH
Assistant Professor
Department of Orthopedic Surgery
Marc A. Asher, MD Comprehensive Spine Center
University of Kansas Medical Center
Kansas City, Kansas, USA

Winward Choy, MD
Resident
Department of Neurosurgery
University of California, San Francisco
San Francisco, California, USA

Bhargav D. Desai, MD
Resident
Department of Neurosurgery
University of Virginia
Charlottesville, Virginia, USA

Ananth S. Eleswarapu, MD
Assistant Professor
Department of Orthopaedic Surgery
University of Miami
Miami, Florida, USA

Juanita Garces, MD
Assistant Professor
Department of Neurosurgery
St. Mary's Medical Center
Huntington, West Virginia, USA

Jae Taek Hong, MD, PhD
Professor
Department of Neurosurgery
Eunpyeong St. Mary's Hospital
Catholic University of Korea
Seoul, South Korea

Sravisht Iyer, MD
Assistant Attending
Spine Surgery
Hospital for Special Surgery
New York, New York, USA

Deeptee Jain, MD
Spine Surgery Fellow
Department of Orthopaedic Surgery
New York University
New York, New York, USA

Hyung Suk Juh, MD
Clinical Fellow
Department of Orthopedic Surgery
Kyung Hee University
Seoul, South Korea

Khaled M. Kebaish, MD
Division Chief, Orthopaedic Spine Surgery
Professor of Orthopaedic Surgery
Department of Orthopaedic Surgery
The Johns Hopkins University
Baltimore, Maryland, USA

Cheung Kue Kim, MD, PhD
Clinical Fellow
Department of Orthopedic Surgery
Kyung Hee University
Seoul, South Korea

Han Jo Kim, MD
Associate Professor of Orthopaedic Surgery
Director of Spine Fellowship
Hospital for Special Surgery
New York, New York, USA

Ki-Tack Kim, MD, PhD
Professor
Orthopedic Surgery
Kyung Hee University
Seoul, South Korea

Yong-Chan Kim, MD, PhD
Professor
Department of Orthopedic Surgery
Kyung Hee University
Seoul, South Korea

Eric Klineberg, MD
Professor & Vice Chair of Administration
Co-Director of the UCD Spine Center
Adult and Pediatric Spinal Surgery
Department of Orthopaedic Surgery
University of California, Davis
Sacramento, California, USA

Heiko Koller, MD
Professor
Department of Neurosurgery
Technical University Munich (TUM)
Klinikum Rechts der Isar
Munich, Bavaria, Germany

Virginie Lafage, PhD
Senior Director Spine Research
Spine Service
Hospital for Special Surgery
New York, New York, USA

Darryl Lau, MD
Chief Resident
Department of Neurological Surgery
University of California, San Francisco
San Francisco, California, USA

Sang Hun Lee, MD, PhD
Assistant Professor
Department of Orthopedic Surgery
Johns Hopkins University
Baltimore, Maryland, USA

Marcus D. Mazur, MD
Assistant Professor
Department of Neurosurgery
University of Utah
Salt Lake City, Utah, USA

Emily K. Miller, MD
Resident
Department of Physical Medicine and Rehabilitation
Stanford University
Palo Alto, California, USA

Jeffrey P. Mullin, MD, MBA
Assistant Professor
Department of Neurosurgery
University at Buffalo
Buffalo, New York, USA

Cecilia L. Dalle Ore, MD
Resident
Department of Neurological Surgery
University of California, San Francisco
San Francisco, California, USA

Joshua M. Pahys, MD
Clinical Adjunct Associate Professor
Department of Orthopaedic Surgery
Sidney Kimmel College of Medicine at Thomas Jefferson
    University
Shriners Hospitals for Children
Philadelphia, Pennsylvania, USA

Tejbir S. Pannu, MD, MS
Spine Research Fellow
Orthopedic Surgery-Spine Service
Hospital for Special Surgery, Weill Cornell Medical College
New York, New York, USA

Peter G. Passias, MD, MS
Associate Professor of Orthopaedic and Neurosurgery
NYU School of Medicine
New York, New York, USA

Themistocles S. Protopsaltis, MD
Chief, Division of Spine Surgery
Associate Professor of Orthopaedic Surgery and
    Neurosurgery
Department of Orthopedic Surgery
NYU Langone Health
New York, New York, USA

Tina Raman, MD
Assistant Professor, Spine Surgery
Department of Orthopaedic Surgery
NYU Langone Orthopaedic Hospital
New York, New York, USA

K. Daniel Riew, MD
Professor of Orthopedic Surgery, Columbia University
Chief, Cervical Spine Surgery & Co-Director,
   Spine Division
Co-Director, Columbia University Spine Fellowship
Department of Orthopedic Surgery
Columbia University/ New York Presbyterian Hospital
New York, New York, USA

Flynn Andrew Rowan, MD
Assistant Professor
Department of Orthopedics
Indiana University
Indianapolis, Indiana, USA

Amanda N. Sacino, MD, PhD
Resident
Department of Neurosurgery
Johns Hopkins Hospital
Baltimore, Maryland, USA

Amer F. Samdani, MD
Chief of Surgery
Shriners Hospitals for Children
Philadelphia, Pennsylvania, USA

Frank J. Schwab, MD
Professor
Department of Orthopaedic Surgery
Weil Cornell Medical College
New York, New York, USA

Anand H. Segar, MBChB, DPhil(Oxon), FRACS
Spine Fellow
Department of Orthopedic Surgery
NYU Langone Orthopedic Hospital, NYU Langone Health
New York, New York, USA

Christopher I. Shaffrey, MD
Chief
Spine Division
Departments of Orthopaedic Surgery and Neurosurgery
Duke University
Durham, North Carolina, USA

Justin S. Smith, MD, PhD
Harrison Distinguished Professor
Chief of Spine Division
Department of Neurosurgery
University of Virginia
Charlottesville, Virginia, USA

Paul D. Sponseller, MD
Sponseller Professor and Head, Pediatric Orthopaedics
Johns Hopkins Medical Institutions
Baltimore, Maryland, USA

Nicholas D. Stekas, MS
Clinical Researcher
Department of Orthopedic Surgery
NYU Langone Orthopedic Hospital
New York, New York, USA

Lee A. Tan, MD
Assistant Professor
Department of Neurosurgery
UCSF Medical Center
San Francisco, California, USA

Davis G. Taylor, MD
Resident
Department of Neurosurgery
University of Virginia
Charlottesville, Virginia, USA

Vincent C. Traynelis, MD
Professor and Vice Chair
Department of Neurosurgery
Rush University Medical Center
Chicago, Illinois, USA

Corinna C. Zygourakis, MD
Assistant Professor
Department of Neurosurgery
Stanford University School of Medicine
Stanford, California, USA

1 Adult Cervical Spinal Deformity and Comparative Impact on Health

Juanita Garces, Davis G. Taylor, Bhargav D. Desai, Christopher I. Shaffrey, Christopher P. Ames, Shay Bess, and Justin S. Smith

Abstract

Cervical spinal deformity is a complex pathological entity composed of various musculoskeletal deformities and associated disease processes, the end state of which may result in significant negative effects on health-related quality of life (HRQOL), including pain, disability, and neurologic deficit. Patient-reported outcome measures (PROMs) can be used to compare cervical deformity within itself as well as to population-based general health and to other chronic disease states. Measurements of HRQOL can be used to assess overall health quality based on an established set of parameters such as mobility, self-care, usual activities, pain/discomfort, and anxiety/depression. Based on standardized measures of HRQOL, patients with symptomatic adult cervical spinal deformity have demonstrated significant declines in HRQOL, similar to deformities of the thoracolumbar spine. This chapter summarizes the effects of cervical deformity on HRQOL with disease-specific measures including disability, neck pain, radiculopathy, and myelopathy, as well as population-based general health measures.

Keywords: health-related quality of life, cervical deformity, comparative impact on health, Euro-QOL five dimensions, disability, health impact

1.1 Introduction

In recent years, increasing evidence has demonstrated correlations of thoracolumbar spinal parameters and global alignment with health-related quality of life (HRQOL). Similarly, increasing attention has been given to adult cervical spinal deformity (ACSD) with regard to regional and overall spinal alignment, functional disability, and HRQOL.[1,2]

The normal cervical spine has the essential purpose of transmitting axial load from the cranium, allowing normal head and neck movement and maintaining horizontal gaze while providing the necessary bony protection of the cervical spinal cord. Although the causes of ACSD are multifactorial and range from iatrogenic to degenerative processes, they can ultimately result in a deviation from the normal cervical alignment with significant detriment to HRQOL. Cervical deformity can be associated with neck pain, radiculopathy, myelopathy, changes in head position and horizontal gaze, dysphagia, and obstructive respiratory states.[3] These disease manifestations have been shown to play a significant role in the functional capabilities of ACSD patients and to negatively impact overall quality of life, comparable to other chronic general health disease states based on the Euro-QOL five dimensions (EQ-5D) scale and the modified Japanese orthopedic association (mJOA) score.[4,5,6,7] This chapter will review ACSD and its disease-specific and general health measures and summarize data that compare the health state of ACSD patients with a normative population, as well as with other chronic disease states.[8]

1.2 Cervical Deformity and Disease-Specific Measures

Over the past decade, significant attention has been given to the impact of sagittal alignment on pain and functional disability among patients with thoracolumbar disease.[9] The regional parameters most often used to define sagittal alignment of the cervical spine include C2–C7 sagittal vertical axis (SVA) and cervical lordosis measured by C2–C7 Cobb angle (▶ Fig. 1.1). It has also been recognized that assessment of cervical alignment, especially in the setting of deformity, may benefit from a broader assessment of spinopelvic alignment, including measures of thoracic kyphosis, lumbar lordosis, C7–S1 SVA, pelvic tilt, and the pelvic incidence to lumbar lordosis (PI–LL) mismatch.[10,11,12,13,14,15,16,17]

Among patients with poor thoracolumbar sagittal alignment, compensatory measures may be required to maintain upright posture and horizontal gaze. The cervical spine has demonstrated a wide range of normal curvatures (▶ Table 1.1) with reciprocal changes occurring in response to global alignment and surgical correction of C2–C7 SVA.[18,19,20,21,22,23,24] Better understanding of the relationships between global spinal alignment and the cervical spine has been increasingly of interest in the management of spinal deformity.[25] However, a uniform classification system of cervical deformity has been lacking among practitioners, leading to variability in reporting. A recent report by Ames et al proposed a comprehensive classification for cervical deformity that includes a major deformity descriptor with five modifiers (C2–C7 SVA, horizontal gaze, T1 slope minus C2–C7 lordosis, mJOA myelopathy score, and the Scoliosis Research Society-Schwab adult thoracolumbar deformity classification modifiers).[8]

Multiple PROMs have been developed over the years that can be applied to cervical deformity as a means of quantifying the clinical manifestations of the disease. The mJOA score is the most commonly used standardized measure for the assessment of cervical myelopathy and can be used to assess the severity of myelopathy that may be associated with cervical deformity.[27] The mJOA is a questionnaire typically completed by the physician that provides assessment of the motor dysfunction in the upper and lower extremities, sensory function in the upper extremities, and bladder function.

In addition to axial neck pain, cervical deformity may be associated with foraminal stenosis or other processes resulting in cervical radiculopathy.[28] Patients with cervical radiculopathy may suffer from functional disabilities related to the use of the afflicted extremity and arm pain, with up to 38% of patients with cervical radiculopathy falling into a "poor" category based

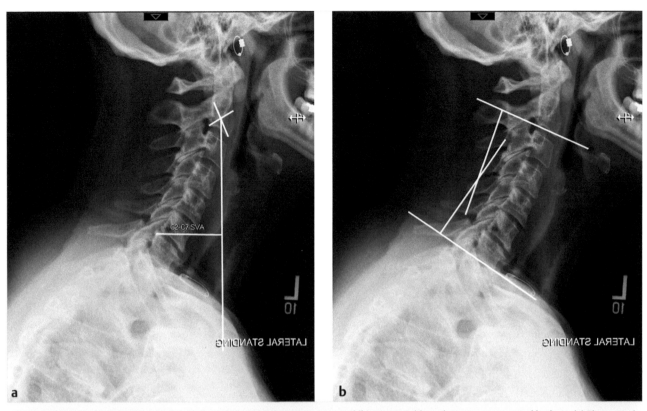

Fig. 1.1 Example of **(a)** C2–C7 sagittal vertical axis (C2–C7 SVA) measurement and **(b)** C2–C7 Cobb angle to measure cervical lordosis. **(a)** The vertical line is a plumb line dropped from the center of the C2 body. The horizontal line represents the C2–C7 SVA as the measurement from the C2 plumb line to the posterior-superior corner of the C7 body. **(b)** The C2–C7 Cobb angle is used to assess cervical lordosis and is measured by obtaining a line parallel to the inferior endplate of C2 and another line parallel to the inferior endplate of C7. Perpendicular lines are drawn from each of these lines, and their intersecting angle *a* is the Cobb angle.

Table 1.1 Normal cervical segmental angles and sagittal vertical axis (SVA) in asymptomatic adults

A. Normal cervical segmental angles		
	Level	Angle (mean ± SD)
	C0–1	2.1 ± 5.0
	C1–2	-32.2 ± 7.0
	C2–3	-1.9 ± 5.2
	C3–4	-1.5 ± 5.0
	C4–5	-0.6 ± 4.4
	C5–6	-1.1 ± 5.1
	C6–7	-4.5 ± 4.3
Totals	C2–7	-9.6
	C1–7	-41.8
Negative sign indicates lordosis		
B. Normal SVA values		
	From C2	Mean ± SD (mm)
	to C7	15.6 ± 11.2
	to sacrum	13.2 ± 29.5

Source: Data from Hardacker et al.[26]

on work ability index.[29,30] The Visual Analog Scale (VAS) and Neck Disability Index (NDI) scores are other standardized measures that can be used to assess neck pain and disability associated with neck pathology, respectively.[31] ▸ Fig. 1.2 summarizes the relationship between NDI score and C2–C7 SVA in a series of patients treated with posterior instrumented arthrodesis and demonstrates an overall positive correlation between C2–C7 SVA and NDI score.[25]

Underlying cervical deformity can also be a negative contributor to the quality of life for patients with degenerative cervical spine disease. In a recent publication by Bakhsheshian et al, patients with increased kyphotic deformities and other evidence of cervical spine deformities were noted to have higher incidence of cervical spondylotic myelopathy compared to normal population-based controls.[32] Tang et al concluded that a C2–C7 SVA greater than 40 mm was associated with at least moderate disability based on the NDI.[33] In a recent study from Ailon et al, the authors assessed 55 ACSD patients presenting for surgical treatment as part of a multicenter prospective study.[34] Compared with preoperative baseline HRQOL assessments, 1 year following surgery, ACSD patients had significant improvement in NDI (from 50.5 to 38.0, $p < 0.001$), neck pain numeric rating scale score VAS (from 6.9 to 4.3, $p < 0.001$), EQ-5D index (from 0.51 to 0.66, $p < 0.001$), and EQ-5D subscores: mobility (from 1.9 to 1.7, $p = 0.019$), usual activities (from 2.2 to 1.9, $p = 0.007$), pain/discomfort (from 2.4 to 2.1, $p < 0.001$), and anxiety/depression (from 1.8 to 1.5, $p = 0.014$).

1.3 Cervical Deformity and Population-Based General Health

General measures of HRQOL can enable comparison of disease impact relative to a normative population and can enable comparison of the impact of ACSD with the impact of other chronic disease states. One commonly used measure that allows comparison between disease states, the EQ-5D, provides an objective quantification of a patient's functional capabilities based on the categories of mobility, self-care, usual activities of daily living, anxiety and depression, and pain and discomfort.[3,4,5,6] The total score based on this assessment provides a single index score reflective of quality-adjusted life years (QALY). The 36-item short-form health survey (SF-36) is another general health measure that is often used to compare across disease states.[24]

ACSD can be associated with neural compression, radiculopathy, and myelopathy. Importantly, these findings have a negative correlation with work status, EQ-5D scores, and psychological health effects such as anxiety, depression, and worsening overall quality of life based on patient's self-assessment.[20,25,28,29,30] These associations have an overall negative effect on patient's quality of life with a significant functional decline over time.[32]

As cervical deformity worsens, horizontal gaze may become altered due to changes in chin–brow vertical angle (CBVA), and subsequently require a greater degree of neck extension in an attempt to maintain a normal horizontal gaze.[25] Patients with pathologic CBVA self-report worse functional capability and

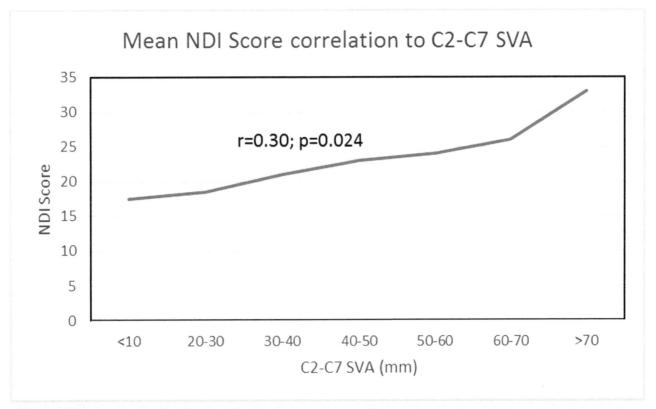

Fig. 1.2 Correlation observed between C2 and C7 sagittal vertical axis (C2–C7 SVA) and Neck Disability Index (NDI) scores showing mean NDI score per mm of SVA measurement. There is a significant positive correlation ($r = 0.30$, $p = 0.024$) with higher C2–C7 SVA and worsening NDI score, and a C2–C7 SVA of + 40 mm was demonstrated to be the threshold for moderate disability.[25]

reduced performance in activities of daily living compared to those with normal CBVA.[35] ▶ Fig. 1.3 is an example of a 70-year-old woman with prior extensive spinal procedures extending from the cervical spine to the sacrum. She presented with severe fixed chin-on-chest cervical kyphosis and pullout of her proximal-most instrumentation leading to an overall poor quality of life.

Multiple studies have demonstrated a correlation between increased cervical deformity and worse HRQOL based on SF-36, NDI, and ODI scores.[20,25,33] In a study by Smith et al, the overall

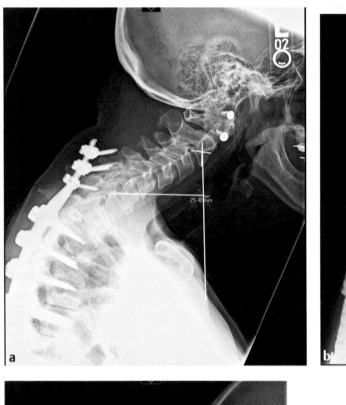
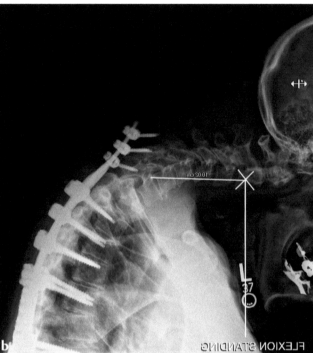
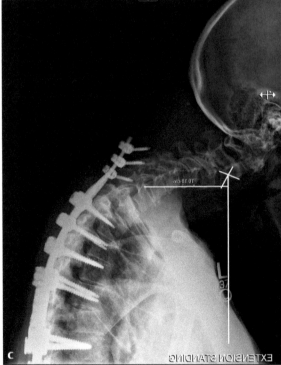
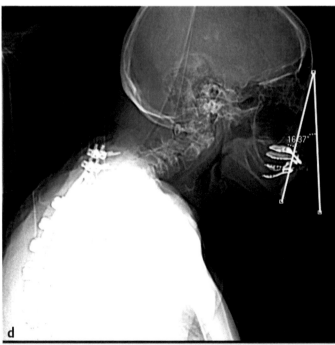

Fig. 1.3 Cervical deformity case example. This is a 70-year-old woman with prior extensive cervical thoracolumbosacral spinal instrumentation with severe chin-on-chest cervical kyphosis and pullout of her proximal-most instrumentation leading to severely affected quality of life. Preoperative cervical spine X-rays showing lateral standing (a), flexion (b), and extension (c) with respective C2–C7 sagittal vertical axis (C2–C7 SVA). (d) Image shows measurement of the chin–brow vertical angle (CBVA) to be 16 degrees and

(Continued)

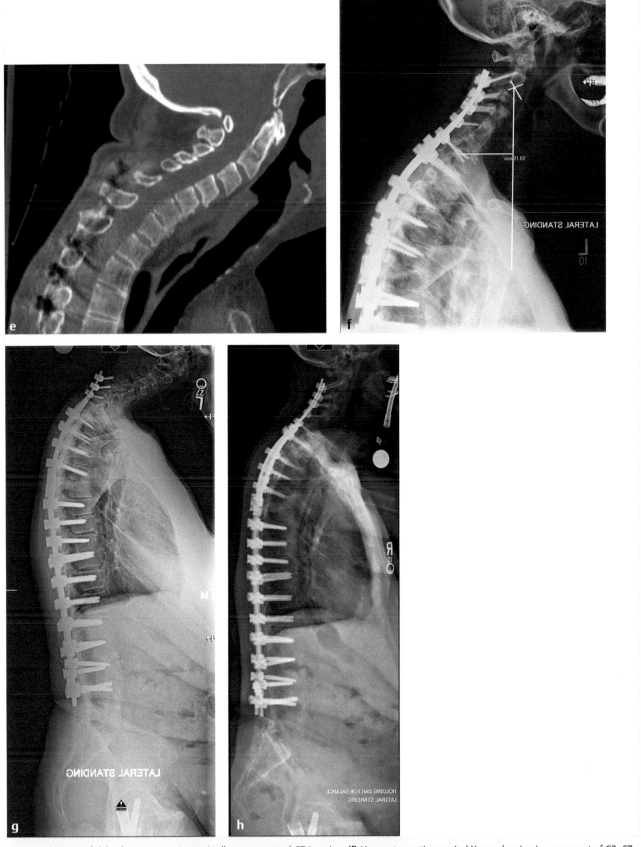

Fig. 1.3 (*Continued*) **(e)** is her preoperative sagittally reconstructed CT imaging. **(f)** Her postoperative cervical X-rays showing improvement of C2–C7 SVA and decrease in CBVA to 4 degrees. **(g,h)** Images represent preoperative and postoperative standing long-cassette sagittal radiographs.

mean EQ-5D index scores of patients with ACSD were 34% below the bottom 25th percentile for age- and gender-matched normative populations.[36] When ACSD patients were stratified by age group and compared to U.S. normative age- and gender-matched controls, patients from age 35 to 74 showed significantly worse EQ-5D index scores, and demonstrated substantial health impact that was appreciated across all five dimensions of the EQ-5D (▶ Fig. 1.4).[36]

Patients with ACSD presenting for surgical treatment were found to have average EQ-5D index health states that were comparable to patients functioning at the bottom 25th percentile for other chronic disease states including heart failure, stroke, renal failure, emphysema, and blindness/low vision (▶ Fig. 1.5). ACSD patients had a mean EQ-5D index that was significantly worse than that of patients functioning at the bottom 25th percentile for chronic ischemic heart disease, malignant breast cancer, and malignant prostate cancer (▶ Fig. 1.5).[36] The markedly negative health impact of ACSD has been demonstrated across all domains of the EQ-5D and was not significantly different based on deformity type. These disease manifestations can significantly affect the functional capabilities of ACSD patients and negatively impact overall quality of life, comparable to or worse than many other well-recognized chronic disease states based on the EQ-5D scale and the mJOA score.[4,5,6,7]

Not only can cervical deformity result in a significant decline in functional state comparable to other severe chronic diseases, but patients with cervical deformity tend to be relatively frail and have substantial comorbidities. Smith et al assessed 120 patients treated surgically for ACSD as part of a multicenter prospective study.[37] They found that the mean number of major comorbidities per patient was 1.8 and that 80% of patients had at least one major comorbidity. The most common comorbidities included current or past smoking history (38.1%), depression (31.7%), hypertension (16.7%), osteopenia or osteoporosis (16.7%), diabetes (14.2%), history of solid tumor (10.8%), chronic pulmonary disease (7.5%), and rheumatoid arthritis (6.7%). The all-cause mortality rate at a mean of 1.2 years following surgery was 9.1% in their series. The causes of death varied considerably and many were not likely directly related to the surgery, but instead may be more reflective of the overall health status of the patient population.[37]

Of patients requiring cervical spine arthrodesis, an evaluation of 87,042 patients with the Agency for Healthcare Research and Quality Elixhauser comorbidity index found that the most common comorbidities accompanying cervical deformity include hypertension (31.6%), chronic pulmonary disease (12.5%), and diabetes (10.8%).[38] Generally, patients of older age and increased comorbidities tend to have poorer outcomes. For atlantoaxial fusion, the most common patient comorbidities as defined by the Nationwide Inpatient Sample and Elixhauser comorbidity index were found to be hypertension (43.2%), electrolyte disorder (17.3%), and diabetes mellitus (11.1%).[39] For cervical fusion procedures, anterior approaches are more common for single-level pathology in relatively young, healthy patients, while posterior approaches are more typically performed on older patients with multilevel disease and more

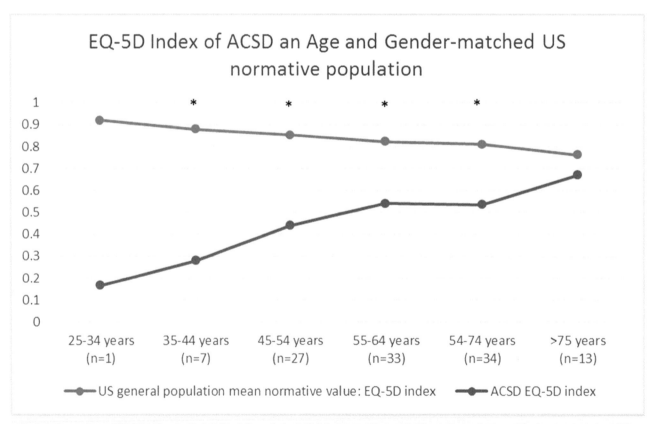

Fig. 1.4 Comparison of EQ-5D index results in 115 adult cervical spinal deformity patients with US gender- and age-matched normative values.[4] The p-values for age comparison groups of 45 to 54, 55 to 64, and 65 to 74 reached statistical significance ($p \leq 0.002$). The > 75 age-group's mean index was lower than the normative value but did not reach statistical significance ($p = 0.055$).[36]

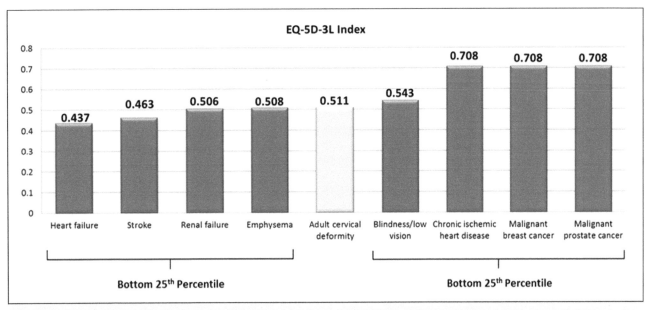

Fig. 1.5 Comparison of the mean EQ-5D index for the overall adult cervical spine deformity population index (0.511) to patients with other chronic disease states functioning at the bottom 25th percentile.[36] Values shown for disease states other than adult cervical deformity are the EQ-5D index values for the bottom 25th percentile for each disease state. (Reproduced with permission from Oxford University Press.)

comorbidities.[40] In a study of 2,742 patients undergoing posterior cervical fusion, a prolonged length of stay was most commonly associated with the comorbid conditions of alcohol abuse, congestive heart failure, obesity, and iron-deficiency anemia.[41] For patients undergoing elective anterior and posterior cervical spine procedures, unanticipated critical care management and prolonged hospitalizations were linked to patient comorbidities of pulmonary disease, hypertension, cardiovascular disease, and diabetes mellitus.[42]

1.4 Conclusion

ACSD can have a significant impact on patient's health and result in pain, myelopathy and disability, changes in head position and horizontal gaze, dysphagia, and respiratory compromise.[3] Increasing attention is being given to ACSD with regard to regional and overall spinal alignment, functional disability, HRQOL, and optimization of treatment strategies. Despite the negative effects of cervical deformity on quality of life and the associated surgical risks related to the increased comorbid status, surgery does offer an opportunity to improve quality of life.[34]

The major categories of patient-reported outcomes for ACSD have been described in relation to quality of life, pain, disability, and general health. Disease-specific measures can provide objective measure of the impact of cervical pathology, while general health measures provide the ability to compare disease impact with normative populations and across other disease states. Despite the availability of multiple PROMs that can be applied to ACSD, the disease-specific measures that are currently available for ACSD were designed primarily for cervical degenerative disease. Future efforts are needed to determine the factors most critical to the clinical outcome for ACSD patients in order to develop a truly ACSD disease-specific PROM.

References

[1] Smith JS, Shaffrey CI, Bess S, et al. Recent and emerging advances in spinal deformity. Neurosurgery. 2017; 80 3S:S70–S85

[2] Scheer JK, Tang JA, Smith JS, et al. International Spine Study Group. Cervical spine alignment, sagittal deformity, and clinical implications: a review. J Neurosurg Spine. 2013; 19(2):141–159

[3] Gusi N, Olivares PR, Rajendram R. The EQ-5D Health-Related Quality of Life Questionnaire. Handbook of Disease Burdens and Quality of Life Measures. 2010:87–99

[4] Szende AJB, Cabases J, eds. Self-Reported Population Health: An International Perspective Based on EQ-5D. New York, NY: Springer; 2014

[5] Sullivan PW, Ghushchyan V. Preference-based EQ-5D index scores for chronic conditions in the United States. Med Decis Making. 2006; 26(4):410–420

[6] Champain S, Benchikh K, Nogier A, Mazel C, Guise JD, Skalli W. Validation of new clinical quantitative analysis software applicable in spine orthopaedic studies. Eur Spine J. 2006; 15(6):982–991

[7] Bess S, Line B, Fu KM, et al. International Spine Study Group. The health impact of symptomatic adult spinal deformity: comparison of deformity types to United States population norms and chronic diseases. Spine. 2016; 41 (3):224–233

[8] Ames CP, Smith JS, Eastlack R, et al. International Spine Study Group. Reliability assessment of a novel cervical spine deformity classification system. J Neurosurg Spine. 2015; 23(6):673–683

[9] Glassman SD, Bridwell K, Dimar JR, Horton W, Berven S, Schwab F. The impact of positive sagittal balance in adult spinal deformity. Spine. 2005; 30 (18):2024–2029

[10] Briggs AM, Wrigley TV, Tully EA, Adams PE, Greig AM, Bennell KL. Radiographic measures of thoracic kyphosis in osteoporosis: Cobb and vertebral centroid angles. Skeletal Radiol. 2007; 36(8):761–767

[11] Jackson RP, McManus AC. Radiographic analysis of sagittal plane alignment and balance in standing volunteers and patients with low back pain matched for age, sex, and size. A prospective controlled clinical study. Spine. 1994; 19 (14):1611–1618

[12] Schwab F, Lafage V, Boyce R, Skalli W, Farcy JP. Gravity line analysis in adult volunteers: age-related correlation with spinal parameters, pelvic parameters, and foot position. Spine. 2006; 31(25):E959–E967

[13] Van Royen BJ, Toussaint HM, Kingma I, et al. Accuracy of the sagittal vertical axis in a standing lateral radiograph as a measurement of balance in spinal deformities. Eur Spine J. 1998; 7(5):408–412

[14] Bridwell KH. Decision making regarding Smith-Petersen vs. pedicle subtraction osteotomy vs. vertebral column resection for spinal deformity. Spine. 2006; 31(19) Suppl:S171–S178

[15] Neal CJ, McClendon J, Halpin R, Acosta FL, Koski T, Ondra SL. Predicting ideal spinopelvic balance in adult spinal deformity. J Neurosurg Spine. 2011; 15 (1):82–91

[16] El Fegoun AB, Schwab F, Gamez L, Champain N, Skalli W, Farcy JP. Center of gravity and radiographic posture analysis: a preliminary review of adult volunteers and adult patients affected by scoliosis. Spine. 2005; 30(13):1535–1540

[17] Uchida K, Nakajima H, Sato R, et al. Cervical spondylotic myelopathy associated with kyphosis or sagittal sigmoid alignment: outcome after anterior or posterior decompression. J Neurosurg Spine. 2009; 11(5):521–528

[18] Smith JS, Shaffrey CI, Lafage V, et al. International Spine Study Group. Spontaneous improvement of cervical alignment after correction of global sagittal balance following pedicle subtraction osteotomy. J Neurosurg Spine. 2012; 17 (4):300–307

[19] Ha Y, Schwab F, Lafage V, et al. Reciprocal changes in cervical spine alignment after corrective thoracolumbar deformity surgery. Eur Spine J. 2014; 23 (3):552–559

[20] Protopsaltis TS, Scheer JK, Terran JS, et al. International Spine Study Group. How the neck affects the back: changes in regional cervical sagittal alignment correlate to HRQOL improvement in adult thoracolumbar deformity patients at 2-year follow-up. J Neurosurg Spine. 2015; 23(2):153–158

[21] Protopsaltis T, Bronsard N, Soroceanu A, et al. International Spine Study Group. Cervical sagittal deformity develops after PJK in adult thoracolumbar deformity correction: radiographic analysis utilizing a novel global sagittal angular parameter, the CTPA. Eur Spine J. 2017; 26(4):1111–1120

[22] Day LM, Ramchandran S, Jalai CM, et al. Thoracolumbar realignment surgery results in simultaneous reciprocal changes in lower extremities and cervical spine. Spine. 2017; 42(11):799–807

[23] Ames CP, Blondel B, Scheer JK, et al. Cervical radiographical alignment: comprehensive assessment techniques and potential importance in cervical myelopathy. Spine. 2013; 38(22) Suppl 1:S149–S160

[24] Oh T, Scheer JK, Smith JS, et al. International Spine Study Group. Potential of predictive computer models for preoperative patient selection to enhance overall quality-adjusted life years gained at 2-year follow-up: a simulation in 234 patients with adult spinal deformity. Neurosurg Focus. 2017; 43(6):E2

[25] Tang JA, Scheer JK, Smith JS, et al. ISSG. The impact of standing regional cervical sagittal alignment on outcomes in posterior cervical fusion surgery. Neurosurgery. 2012; 71(3):662–669, discussion 669

[26] Hardacker JW, Shuford RF, Capicotto PN, Pryor PW. Radiographic standing cervical segmental alignment in adult volunteers without neck symptoms. Spine. 1997; 22(13):1472–1480, discussion 1480

[27] Benzel EC, Lancon J, Kesterson L, Hadden T. Cervical laminectomy and dentate ligament section for cervical spondylotic myelopathy. J Spinal Disord. 1991; 4 (3):286–295

[28] Tan LA, Riew KD, Traynelis VC. Cervical spine deformity-Part 1: Biomechanics, radiographic parameters, and classification. Neurosurgery. 2017; 81 (2):197–203

[29] Engquist M, Löfgren H, Öberg B, et al. Factors affecting the outcome of surgical versus nonsurgical treatment of cervical radiculopathy: a randomized, controlled study. Spine. 2015; 40(20):1553–1563

[30] Ng E, Johnston V, Wibault J, et al. Factors associated with work ability in patients undergoing surgery for cervical radiculopathy. Spine. 2015; 40 (16):1270–1276

[31] Sundseth J, Kolstad F, Johnsen LG, et al. The Neck Disability Index (NDI) and its correlation with quality of life and mental health measures among patients with single-level cervical disc disease scheduled for surgery. Acta Neurochir (Wien). 2015; 157(10):1807–1812

[32] Bakhsheshian J, Mehta VA, Liu JC. Current diagnosis and management of cervical spondylotic myelopathy. Global Spine J. 2017; 7(6):572–586

[33] Tang JA, Scheer JK, Smith JS, et al. ISSG. The impact of standing regional cervical sagittal alignment on outcomes in posterior cervical fusion surgery. Neurosurgery. 2015; 76 Suppl 1:S14–S21, discussion S21

[34] Ailon TSJ, Shaffrey C, Kim HJ, et al. ISSG. Outcomes of operative treatment for adult cervical deformity: a prospective multicenter assessment with 1-year follow-up. Neurosurgery. 2018; 83(5):1031–1039

[35] Song K, Su X, Zhang Y, et al. Optimal chin-brow vertical angle for sagittal visual fields in ankylosing spondylitis kyphosis. Eur Spine J. 2016; 25(8):2596–2604

[36] Smith JS, Line B, Bess S, et al. The health impact of adult cervical deformity in patients presenting for surgical treatment: comparison to United States population norms and chronic disease states based on the EuroQuol-5 Dimensions Questionnaire. Neurosurgery. 2017; 80(5):716–725

[37] Smith JS, Kim HJ, Passias P, et al. ISSG. Prospective multicenter assessment of all-cause mortality following surgery for adult cervical deformity. Neurosurgery. 2018; 83(6):1277–1285

[38] Derman PB, Lampe LP, Hughes AP, et al. Demographic, clinical, and operative factors affecting long-term revision rates after cervical spine arthrodesis. J Bone Joint Surg Am. 2016; 98(18):1533–1540

[39] Tanenbaum JE, Lubelski D, Rosenbaum BP, Thompson NR, Benzel EC, Mroz TE. Predictors of outcomes and hospital charges following atlantoaxial fusion. Spine J. 2016; 16(5):608–618

[40] Shamji MF, Cook C, Pietrobon R, Tackett S, Brown C, Isaacs RE. Impact of surgical approach on complications and resource utilization of cervical spine fusion: a nationwide perspective to the surgical treatment of diffuse cervical spondylosis. Spine J. 2009; 9(1):31–38

[41] De la Garza-Ramos R, Goodwin CR, Abu-Bonsrah N, et al. Prolonged length of stay after posterior surgery for cervical spondylotic myelopathy in patients over 65years of age. J Clin Neurosci. 2016; 31:137–141

[42] Harris OA, Runnels JB, Matz PG. Clinical factors associated with unexpected critical care management and prolonged hospitalization after elective cervical spine surgery. Crit Care Med. 2001; 29(10):1898–1902

2 Global Sagittal Alignment

Tejbir S. Pannu, Frank J. Schwab, and Virginie Lafage

Abstract

Sagittal alignment is one of the key elements of spinal surgery. Many publications demonstrated the relationship between the sagittal alignment and quality of life. With the analysis becoming more and more specific to particular regions of the spine, an overview of the sagittal alignment, the most important parameters and their interpretation, can be important before going deeper into any specific regional aspect. This chapter intends to describe briefly the most relevant sagittal parameters from head to toe, to show their clinical relevance, and, finally, to link them to the cervical spine.

Keywords: pelvic parameters, pelvic incidence, regional alignment, lumbar lordosis, global alignment, compensation

2.1 Slope to Slope: From Pelvis to Cervical

2.1.1 Sacral Slope: Pelvic Parameter

It is defined as the angle between the sacral endplate and the horizontal line. This parameter quantifies the sagittal inclination of the sacrum in space.

Average value: The average value of sacral slope (SS) in an asymptomatic adult is 41 degrees ± 8 degrees.[1]

SS forms the base of the spine and determines its shape. On an asymptomatic population, SS is strongly correlated to lumbar lordosis (LL; $R = 0.76$).[1]

Positional parameter: SS is affected by patient's position, as it decreases during pelvic retroversion. In addition, it cannot be used to determine the adequate lordosis in adult spinal deformity (ASD) population due to the retroversion of pelvis.

Morphological parameters, instead of the positional ones, should be used to ascertain the LL needed to stay in an aligned position.

2.1.2 Pelvic Incidence

Pelvic incidence (PI) was first described in 1992 by Duval-Beaupère.[2] It is defined as the angle between the line passing through the center of the femoral head and the center of the sacral endplate, and a line perpendicular to the sacral endplate.[3] PI quantifies the orientation of the sacrum within the ilium.

The mean value of PI in asymptomatic adults is 52 degrees ± 10 degrees (range: 35–85 degrees).[1] However, for less than 10 years old, the mean value has been shown to be 45 degrees and for more than 10 years old, the mean PI is 49 degrees.[4]

Morphological parameter: PI is not affected by patient's position.

Pelvic Incidence and Age

Increases in children: The pelvis changes shape from the fetal to the neonatal stage, and changes again in the transition to adulthood before stabilizing.[5]

Constant in adults: There is limited motion of the sacroiliac joints, thus, not affected by the orientation of the pelvis.[6] The PI can be modified in the setting of prolonged, large anterior malalignment.[3,7]

Clinical Application

Low PI: In subjects with low PI, the femoral heads are situated inferior to the sacral plate (i.e., vertical pelvis) which in turn results in low SS and, eventually, a limited ability in pelvic retroversion.[8]

High PI: In subjects with high PI, the femoral heads lie anterior to the sacral plate, resulting in large SS, and greater ability to retrovert the pelvis.

Relationship with Sacral Slope

As described earlier, these three parameters are linked via a geometrical equation[3] (▶ Fig. 2.1):

PI = pelvic tilt (PT) + SS.

Vialle et al developed predictive formulas for estimation of the theoretical PT and SS based on PI. These equations (see below) showed that with an increase in PI, both PT and SS increase. However, there is greater variation in SS as compared to PT[1] (▶ Fig. 2.2).

SS = 0.63 × PI + 7.3; SS represents around 65% of PI.

PT = 0.37 × PI - 7; PT represents around 35% of PI.

2.2 From Pelvis to Lumbar

Pelvic incidence dictates the orientation of the sacral endplate, as follows[1,3]:

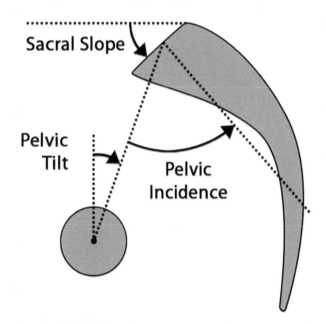

Fig. 2.1 Pelvic parameters.

Low PI: If the PI is low, S1 endplate tends to be more horizontal. In response to that, the LL flattens out to maintain a neutral sagittal alignment.

High PI: If the PI is large, S1 endplate becomes steeper. Thus, LL needs to be more prominent, in order to maintain a neutral sagittal alignment.

For characterization of the interplay between PI and LL, a simple rule was framed. It stated that the LL should match PI within 10 degrees. In other words, the mismatch between the PI and LL (PI–LL) should not exceed 10 degrees.[9] The practical application of this rule led to marked success in the treatment of ASD.

This simple rule provided acceptable clinical results[10] and decreased the risk of adjacent segment degeneration after surgery.[11]

However, in reality, this is not as simple as it seems because of the following reasons:

1. *Variation of the lordosis across LL spectrum*: LL is not uniformly distributed among different vertebrae (▶ Fig. 2.3). Most of the lordosis comes from the distal part (L4 to S1; around 65%).[12]
2. *Real lordosis is not always between L1 and S1*: This is based on a geometrical construct of LL by Roussouly et al, where LL is formed by two tangent arcs of a circle (constant superior arc [20 degrees], and variable inferior arc). SS is equal to the angle of inferior arc and determines the LL. Thus, with larger PI, larger SS is strongly associated with larger LL, chiefly in the distal segments (L4–L5, L5–S1).[13]
3. *Nonconstant value of PI–LL across PI spectrum*: On one hand, with larger PI, LL can be smaller than PI. On the other hand, with small PI, LL can be greater than PI.[14]
4. *Effect of thoracic kyphosis (TK)*: PI–LL increases with fixed large TK.[14]
5. *Impact of subject's age*: PI–LL increases with age.[15]

2.3 Lumbar to Thoracic

Going upward along the spine, the curvature of lumbar spine forms the seat of the thoracic curve, described as the TK. It is commonly measured as the angle between the upper endplate of T4 vertebra or T2 vertebra and the lower endplate of the T12 vertebra.

The mean T4–T12 TK in an asymptomatic adult varies from 34 to 44 degrees and ranges from 0 to 76 degrees. The thoracic curve is the stiffer section of the spine due to articulation of rib cage with the vertebrae.

TK and LL: The value of TK affects the LL. On one hand, large fixed hyperkyphosis results in increased LL. On the other hand, small fixed hypokyphosis results in decreased LL (▶ Fig. 2.4).

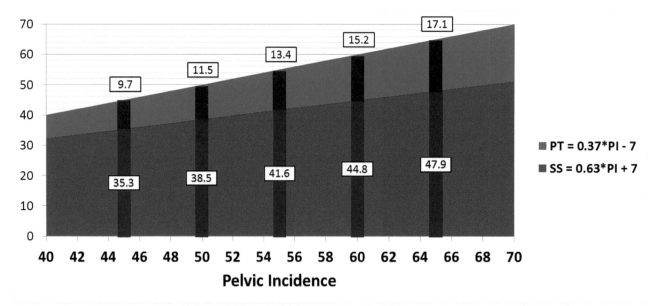

Fig. 2.2 Estimation of PT and SS based on PI. (Graph derived from formulas published in Vialle et al.[5])

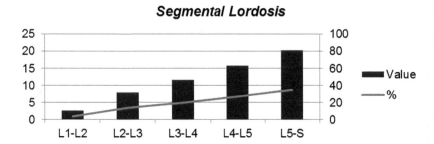

Fig. 2.3 Spectrum of the lumbar lordosis.

Patients with ASD can voluntarily decrease their TK as a compensatory mechanism for loss of LL.[16] Patients, especially young adults, recruit their extensor muscles to hyperextend the spine.[17]

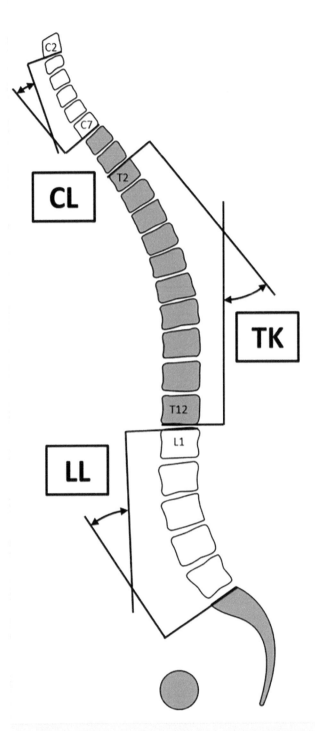

Fig. 2.4 Sagittal alignment: a chain of correlation from the pelvis to the cervical spine.

2.4 Cervical Curvature

The cervical curvature is commonly measured by an angle between the inferior endplate of C2 and the inferior endplate of C7.[18]

The cervical curvature can be lordotic, straight, or kyphotic in an asymptomatic population.[19] Up to 20% of the normal population present with a kyphotic cervical curvature.[19]

Cervical and thoracolumbar (TL) alignment: The cervical curvature is an answer to the TL alignment. As the LL is dictated by S1 slope (SS), the cervical curvature is dictated by the T1 slope.[20,21,22] Large T1 slope is associated with a lordotic cervical curvature. On the other side, horizontal T1 slope is associated with a kyphotic cervical curvature. According to Protopsaltis et al, T1–CL should be less than 17 degrees, which resonates another study from Le Huec et al, in which mean C7 slope was 19.7 degrees and for CL of 4.9 degrees.[22,23]

2.5 Global Alignment

2.5.1 Sagittal Vertical Axis

It is the most commonly used parameter to assess the global alignment. This parameter was first described in 1994 by Roger Jackson and McManus.[24] It is defined as the horizontal offset between the posterosuperior corner of S1 and a plumb line dropped from the center of C7 vertebral body.

2.5.2 Interpretation

Sagittal vertical axis (SVA) is used to assess if the patient is in neutral, positive, or negative sagittal alignment.
- If the plumb line falls in front of the sacrum, then SVA is positive and the spine is in anterior malalignment.
- If the plumb line falls behind the sacrum, then SVA is negative and the spine is in posterior malalignment.

Average value: The mean value of SVA reported by Jackson and McManus was -0.05 cm ± 2.5 cm. As of now, a threshold of + 5.0 cm is considered normal.[24]

SVA represents the end result of the TL alignment and the pelvic compensation. Loss of LL and increase in TK result in increase in SVA. Increase in pelvic retroversion results in decrease in SVA. In other words although SVA is very sensitive to change in spine curvature, it can be masked by the pelvic compensation. Thus, in addition to LL and TK, pelvic retroversion must be considered in the assessment of the SVA. It is paramount to keep in mind that the SVA is dependent on both patient position and the rotation of the pelvis.

SVA value has been proven to change a lot with age. During childhood, there is posterior progression of SVA, leading to the maximum posterior value in this population.[25] During adulthood, increasing age is correlated to a more forward SVA with loss of distal LL.[26]

2.6 From Global Alignment to Cervical Alignment

2.6.1 Objectives of the Cervical Spine

1. Maintenance of horizontal gaze independently of TL alignment.
2. 3D mobility for orientation in space.

Horizontal gaze is assessed by the following[27] (▶ Fig. 2.5):
1. *Chin–brow vertical angle (CBVA)*: An angle measured between lines from the brow and the chin and the vertical.
2. *McGregor slope (McGS)*: An angle between the line from the posterosuperior aspect of the hard palate and the caudal aspect of the opisthion and the horizontal.
3. *Slope of line of sight (SLS)*: An angle between Frankfurt line and the horizontal.

Although CBVA is measured on clinical photographs, McGS and SLS are measured on lateral radiographs.

Ranges for normal horizontal gaze: CBVA (-5 and 17 degrees), McGS (-6 and 14 degrees), or slope of light of sight (SLS; -5.1 and 18.5 degrees).[27]

Cervical curvature is affected by the TL alignment[27] (▶ Fig. 2.6):
- An increase in anterior malalignment (i.e., positive SVA) demands an increase in cervical curvature to maintain the horizontal gaze.
- Increase in TK makes T1 steeper (i.e., an increase in T1 slope). This eventually results in an increase in the cervical curvature as a compensatory mechanism to regulate the horizontal gaze.

Of note, when the compensatory mechanisms for the maintenance of gaze get saturated, patients are unable to look straight ahead, represented by an increase in CBVA. Further evidence on the relationship between the cervical and TL alignment demonstrated spontaneous correction of cervical alignment following the correction of global sagittal balance with pedicle subtraction osteotomy in lumbar region.[28]

2.7 Chain of Compensation

As the spine malaligns in a sagittal plane, several compensatory mechanisms are recruited to bring it back to harmony, termed as the "chain of compensation."

The compensatory cascade occurs in response to change in the regional alignment. The change in regional alignment can be as follows:
1. *Symptomatic change*: This group encompasses the disorders which are associated both with pain and change in sagittal balance. It includes spinal deformity (especially, ASD) and degenerative spine disease (degenerative disc disease, spinal stenosis, spondylolisthesis).[29,30]
2. *Asymptomatic change*: Aging brings tremendous changes in sagittal alignment over time. As age increases, global alignment (SVA) gets more and more anterior. In addition, TK also increases with increase in age.[31,32]

There are numerous mechanisms of compensation to sagittal malalignment.[28] The origin of these mechanisms ranges from the adjacent segment to pelvis or lower limbs. All these compensatory mechanisms have one objective, that is, to maintain a free-standing posture using minimum amount of energy (i.e., to stay within the conus of economy).

2.7.1 Curvature Compensation[33]

Lumbar curve: Hyperextension of the disc above the degenerated level.

Thoracic curve: Hyperextension. It requires back muscle and strength (usually present on young subject).

Cervical curve: Hyperlordosis to maintain horizontal gaze (proximal and distal cervical spine recruited).

2.7.2 Pelvic Compensation

Pelvic Tilt

PT quantifies the pelvic rotation around the femoral heads. It is defined as the angle between the line joining the bicoxofemoral head and the center of the sacral endplate with the vertical.

Average value: The average PT in asymptomatic subjects is 13 degrees ± 6 degrees. Similar to the PI, PT increases over the course of childhood.[4]

PT has proven to be one of the most powerful compensatory mechanisms in response to the sagittal malalignment.[16] In patients with a sagittal imbalance, loss of LL is the most common driver of the deformity. To bring the spine back in a well-aligned position, the body recruits the pelvis, in the form of increased PT, which in turn increases LL and the rest of the curves follow it.

Interpretation

Increase in PT (i.e., retroversion) is defined as the posterior rotation of the pelvis around the femoral heads. As described earlier, increase in PT is associated with anterior sagittal malalignment.

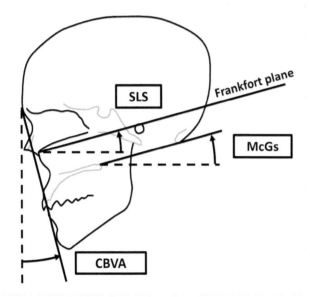

Fig. 2.5 Assessment of horizontal gaze; McGregor slope (McGS), slope of line of sight (SLS), and chin–brow vertical angle (CBVA).

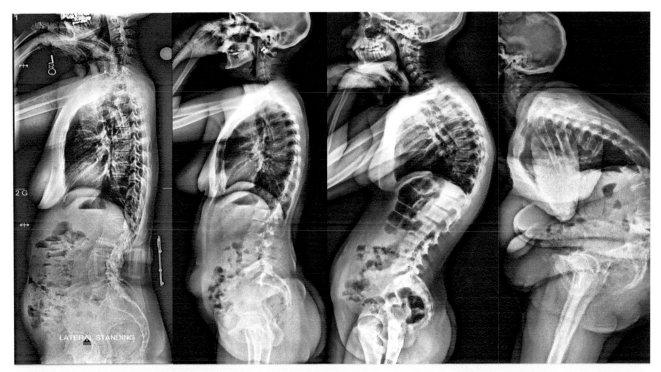

Fig. 2.6 Thoracolumbar alignment: a determinant of the cervical curvature.

Retroversion brings the spine back from the anterior malaligned position to a more posterior aligned position.

Decrease in PT (i.e., anteversion) is defined as the anterior rotation of the pelvis around the femoral heads. Opposite to the retroversion, it is associated with posterior sagittal malalignment. Anteversion functions to bring the spine back anteriorly.

2.7.3 Lower Limb Compensation

Pelvic Translation

Pelvic translation is quantified by pelvic shift (sagittal offset between the posterosuperior corner of the sacrum and anterior cortex of the distal tibia). Pelvic translation is the result of PTs, knee flexion, and ankle dorsiflexion, altogether. It is the most powerful compensation to regulate the normal gravity line position, which is in close relation to the feet. In response to the anterior malalignment, there is posterior translation of the pelvis in relation to the gravity line (▶ Fig. 2.7).[34]

Understanding of the aforementioned compensatory cascade is imperative. To maintain normal sagittal alignment and, in turn, horizontal gaze, recruited mechanisms are not limited to the spine (lumbar, thoracic, or cervical), but also involve the pelvis and lower limbs.

2.8 Clinical Relevance of Global Alignment

2.8.1 Relationship with Patient-Reported Outcomes

Numerous studies have revealed that the increase in anterior malalignment is associated with increase in pain and disability.

1. Regional malalignment (loss of LL): Schwab et al conducted the first study which developed a correlation between the loss of LL, the main driver of sagittal malalignment, and the patient-reported outcomes, visual analog scale (VAS).[35] This was soon followed by study from the same team which proved the correlation with SRS-22 and and Oswestry Disability Index (ODI).[36] Soon after this study, Glassman et al reported poor tolerance of lumbar kyphosis by patients.[29] Soon after, Schwab et al demonstrated that the lack of harmony between PI and LL represented by PI–LL is significantly correlated with pain and disability.[36]
2. Increase in compensation (PT): Lafage et al reported a significant correlation between PT and HRQOL outcome scores.[37] Steering further, Schwab et al introduced a new threshold of 20 degrees for PT to get optimal outcomes after deformity surgery and correlated increased PT with impairment in walking endurance and quality of life.[38]
3. Global spinal malalignment (SVA): Emphasizing on the global alignment, Glassman et al reported that the disability increases linearly with progressive global sagittal malalignment.[29] This was followed by revelation of high correlations between SVA and HRQOL scores by Lafage et al.[37] Progressing further, this group also showed that the SVA has the most correlation with the ODI ($r = 0.469$).[9]

2.8.2 Correction Associated with Improvement in Disability

Fakurnejad et al exhibited that substantial or complete correction of the SVA significantly improves the likelihood of reaching minimum clinically important difference for the ODI and PCS scores.[39]

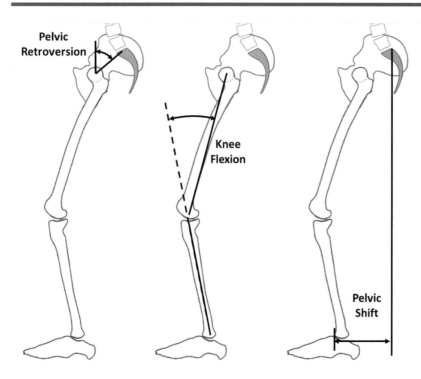

Fig. 2.7 Compensatory mechanisms in sagittal alignment: pelvis and lower limbs.

Radiographic Outcome

Undercorrection of the spinopelvic parameters (i.e., PI–LL mismatch after deformity surgery) has been observed to be associated with the following:

1. Increased risk of adjacent segment disease (proximal junctional kyphosis [PJK]).[11]
2. 10-fold higher risk for revision surgery than the controls.[11]
3. Suboptimal postoperative HRQOL outcome scores.[40]

In contrast, overcorrection of the spinopelvic parameters increases the risk of mechanical failure.[41]

An Epoch of Patient Specificity

Historically, one large "normal" value was defined for each of the sagittal alignment parameters. However, after application of new ideas, the spine community began to perceive that "one size does not fit all." This notion raised a need for some guiding principles or considerations for realignment surgery in order to make it more patient specific.

Looking back, the SRS–Schwab classification based on the spinopelvic parameters marked the beginning for an era of the patient-specific spine care.

Based on the strong bond between the sagittal malalignment and ASD, Schwab et al developed a new ASD classification (▶ Fig. 2.8).[38] This classification determined the cut-off values from the multicentric data for the most clinically relevant sagittal parameters, namely, SVA, PI–LL, and PT. In addition to the sagittal parameters, the classification has descriptive coronal curve types. The three threshold values that must be achieved after surgery for satisfactory outcomes were (1) SVA < 50 mm, (2) PT < 20 degrees, and (3) PI–LL = ±10 degrees.[38] This classification has outstanding clinical correlation with the HRQOL measurements and an excellent intra- and interobserver

reliability.[10,42] There was formation of a common language across spine specialists.

This classification was validated on several studies, both within and outside the United States.

Within the United States

Terran et al demonstrated that the SRS–Schwab classification provides a validated language to describe and categorize ASD. It reflects severity of disease state and significantly correlates with the decision whether to pursue operative or nonoperative treatment.[10]

Using the classification, Smith et al concluded that PI–LL modifier alone can act as primary indication for surgery. Patients who were operated indicated by only PI–LL despite normal SVA showed similar radiographic and HRQOL improvements versus the patients who were operated indicated by both modifiers.[43]

Outside the United States

Liu et al conducted a study on Chinese ASD subjects which revealed that the classification has good-to-excellent intra- and interobserver reliability.[44]

A year later, Nielson et al used a Danish cohort with spinal deformity. The study showed significant variation of ODI across the SVA modifiers. All modifiers were able to classify patients according to SF36 PCS in a consecutive non-U.S. cohort of ASD patients.[42]

Recently, Kyrölä et al tested the classification on a Finnish cohort with degenerative spinal disorders.[45] They showed that their range of values of the sagittal modifiers matched the values in the SRS–Schwab classification, indicating that the classification is valid even on their cohort. The study found this classification to be a practical tool to detect deformity in a cohort with no recognized ASD.

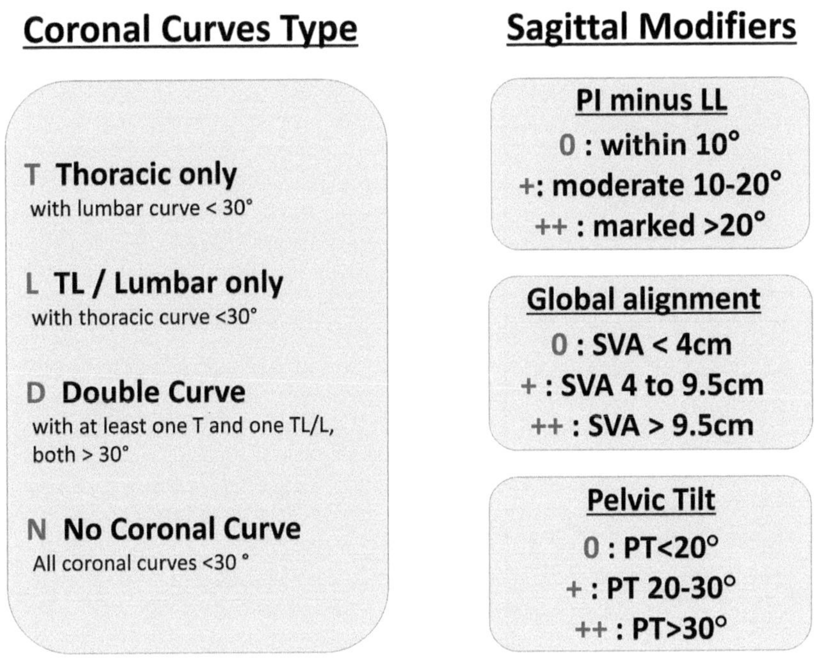

Coronal Curves Type

T Thoracic only
with lumbar curve < 30°

L TL / Lumbar only
with thoracic curve <30°

D Double Curve
with at least one T and one TL/L,
both > 30°

N No Coronal Curve
All coronal curves <30 °

Sagittal Modifiers

PI minus LL
0 : within 10°
+: moderate 10-20°
++ : marked >20°

Global alignment
0 : SVA < 4cm
+ : SVA 4 to 9.5cm
++ : SVA > 9.5cm

Pelvic Tilt
0 : PT<20°
+ : PT 20-30°
++ : PT>30°

Fig. 2.8 SRS–Schwab adult spinal deformity classification.

Table 2.1 Age-adjusted alignment thresholds of sagittal parameters

Age group	PT	PI–LL	SVA
< 35	11.0	-10.5	-30.5
35–44	15.4	-4.6	-5.5
45–54	18.8	0.5	15.1
55–64	22.0	5.8	35.8
65–74	25.1	10.5	54.5
≥ 74	28.8	17.0	79.3

Abbreviations: LL, lumbar lordosis; PI, pelvic incidence; PT, pelvic tilt; SVA, sagittal vertical axis.

Age-Specific Parameters

Treading further in the direction of patient specificity, Lafage et al concluded that the alignment targets of the sagittal modifiers proposed in the SRS–Schwab classification should be adjusted based on the age of the patient, as shown in ▶ Table 2.1.[15]

Realignment thresholds for younger ASD patients should be more rigorous than the older counterparts. Ambitious overcorrection of the older subjects can potentially lead to adjacent segment disease such as proximal junctional failure (PJF) or PJK with no added benefit in clinical improvement. The age-adjusted thresholds for the spinopelvic parameters demonstrated a positive impact on the rate of PJK and patient-reported outcome measures.[46]

2.9 Conclusion

Global spine alignment has enriched our understanding of the normal virgin spine versus the deformed spine. Sagittal balance flows from the pelvis, all the way up to the cervical spine to maintain the horizontal gaze. The evaluation of ASD should run from global to regional alignment, ultimately to the compensation. Several geometrical parameters like SVA are out there for assessment of the global sagittal balance. These parameters serve as steering principles for planning surgery and reaching a preset alignment objective. The introduction of SRS–Schwab classification, and its continuing refinement, is promising for the road to patient specificity in spine deformity care.

References

[1] Vialle R, Levassor N, Rillardon L, Templier A, Skalli W, Guigui P. Radiographic analysis of the sagittal alignment and balance of the spine in asymptomatic subjects. J Bone Joint Surg Am. 2005; 87(2):260–267

[2] Duval-Beaupère G, Schmidt C, Cosson P. A Barycentremetric study of the sagittal shape of spine and pelvis: the conditions required for an economic standing position. Ann Biomed Eng. 1992; 20(4):451–462

[3] Legaye J, Duval-Beaupère G, Hecquet J, Marty C. Pelvic incidence: a fundamental pelvic parameter for three-dimensional regulation of spinal sagittal curves. Eur Spine J. 1998; 7(2):99–103

[4] Mac-Thiong JM, Berthonnaud E, Dimar JR, II, Betz RR, Labelle H. Sagittal alignment of the spine and pelvis during growth. Spine. 2004; 29(15):1642–1647

[5] Berge C. Heterochronic processes in human evolution: an ontogenetic analysis of the hominid pelvis. Am J Phys Anthropol. 1998; 105(4):441–459

[6] Mangione P, Gomez D, Senegas J. Study of the course of the incidence angle during growth. Eur Spine J. 1997; 6(3):163–167

[7] Bao H, Liabaud B, Varghese J, et al. Lumbosacral stress and age may contribute to increased pelvic incidence: an analysis of 1625 adults. Eur Spine J. 2018; 27(2):482–488

[8] Le Huec J-CC, Aunoble S, Philippe L, Nicolas P. Pelvic parameters: origin and significance. Eur Spine J. 2011; 20 Suppl 5:564–571

[9] Schwab FJ, Blondel B, Bess S, et al. International Spine Study Group (ISSG). Radiographical spinopelvic parameters and disability in the setting of adult spinal deformity: a prospective multicenter analysis. Spine. 2013; 38(13):E803–E812

[10] Terran J, Schwab F, Shaffrey CI, et al. International Spine Study Group. The SRS-Schwab adult spinal deformity classification: assessment and clinical correlations based on a prospective operative and nonoperative cohort. Neurosurgery. 2013; 73(4):559–568

[11] Rothenfluh DA, Mueller DA, Rothenfluh E, Min K. Pelvic incidence-lumbar lordosis mismatch predisposes to adjacent segment disease after lumbar spinal fusion. Eur Spine J. 2015; 24(6):1251–1258

[12] Been E, Barash A, Marom A, et al. Vertebral bodies or discs: which contributes more to human-like lumbar lordosis? Clin Orthop Relat Res. 2010; 468 (7):1822–1829

[13] Roussouly P, Gollogly S, Berthonnaud E, et al. Classification of the normal variation in the sagittal alignment of the human lumbar spine and pelvis in the standing position. Spine (Phila Pa 1976). 2005; 30(3):346–53

[14] Schwab FJ, Diebo BG, Smith JS, et al. Fine-tuned surgical planning in adult spinal deformity: determining the lumbar lordosis necessary by accounting for both thoracic kyphosis and pelvic incidence. Spine J. San Francisco, California: Elsevier Inc; 2014 Nov [cited 2015 May 6];14(11):S73. Available at: http://linkinghub.elsevier.com/retrieve/pii/S1529943014010572. Accessed February 7, 2019

[15] Lafage R, Schwab F, Challier V, et al. International Spine Study Group. Defining spino-pelvic alignment thresholds: should operative goals in adult spinal deformity surgery account for age? Spine. 2016; 41(1):62–68

[16] Liabaud B, Liu S, Vital J, et al. Recruitment of compensatory mechanisms. 2015; 40(9):642–649

[17] Barrey C, Roussouly P, Le Huec JC, D'Acunzi G, Perrin G. Compensatory mechanisms contributing to keep the sagittal balance of the spine. Eur Spine J. 2013; 22 Suppl 6:S834–S841

[18] Ames CP, Blondel B, Scheer JK, et al. Cervical radiographical alignment: comprehensive assessment techniques and potential importance in cervical myelopathy. Spine. 2013; 38(22) Suppl 1:S149–S160

[19] Grob D, Frauenfelder H, Mannion AF. The association between cervical spine curvature and neck pain. Eur Spine J. 2007; 16(5):669–678

[20] Marnay T. Equilibre du rachis et du bassin. Cah d'enseignement la SOFCOT Masson ed. 1988:281–313

[21] Berthonnaud E, Dimnet J, Roussouly P, Labelle H. Analysis of the sagittal balance of the spine and pelvis using shape and orientation parameters. J Spinal Disord Tech. 2005; 18(1):40–47

[22] Protopsaltis T, Schwab F, Bronsard N, et al. International Spine Study Group. The T1 pelvic angle, a novel radiographic measure of global sagittal deformity, accounts for both spinal inclination and pelvic tilt and correlates with health-related quality of life. J Bone Joint Surg Am. 2014; 96(19):1631–1640

[23] Le Huec J-C, Demezon H, Aunoble S. L' équilibre sagittal du rachis cervical sur une population asymptomatique : Nouveaux paramètres et valeurs standards. (Sagittal parameters of cervical global balance. Normative values from a prospective cohort of asymptomatic volunteers). e-mémoires l'Académie Natl Chir. 2013; 12(2):18–24

[24] Jackson RP, McManus AC. Radiographic analysis of sagittal plane alignment and balance in standing volunteers and patients with low back pain matched for age, sex, and size. A prospective controlled clinical study. Spine (Phila Pa 1976). 1994; 19(14):1611–1618

[25] Cil A, Yazici M, Uzumcugil A, et al. The evolution of sagittal segmental alignment of the spine during childhood. Spine. 2005; 30(1):93–100

[26] Gelb DE, Lenke LG, Bridwell KH, Blanke K, McEnery KW. An analysis of sagittal spinal alignment in 100 asymptomatic middle and older aged volunteers. Spine. 1995; 20(12):1351–1358

[27] Diebo BG, Challier V, Henry JK, et al. Predicting cervical alignment required to maintain horizontal gaze based on global spinal alignment. Spine. 2016; 41 (23):1795–1800

[28] Smith JS, Shaffrey CI, Lafage V, et al. Spontaneous improvement of cervical alignment after correction of global sagittal balance following pedicle subtraction osteotomy. J Neurosurg Spine. 2012; 17(4):300–307

[29] Glassman SD, Bridwell KM, Dimar JR, et al. The impact of positive sagittal balance in adult spinal deformity. Spine (Phila Pa 1976). 2005; 30(18):2024–2029

[30] Barrey C, Roussouly P, Perrin G, Le Huec JC. Sagittal balance disorders in severe degenerative spine. Can we identify the compensatory mechanisms? Eur Spine J. 2011; 20 Suppl 5:626–633

[31] Mendoza-Lattes S, Ries Z, Gao Y, Weinstein SL. Natural history of spinopelvic alignment differs from symptomatic deformity of the spine. Spine. 2010; 35 (16):E792–E798

[32] Hasegawa K, Okamoto M, Hatsushikano S, Shimoda H, Ono M, Watanabe K. Normative values of spino-pelvic sagittal alignment, balance, age, and health-related quality of life in a cohort of healthy adult subjects. Eur Spine J. 2016; 25(11):3675–3686

[33] Diebo BG, Ferrero E, Lafage R, et al. Recruitment of compensatory mechanisms in sagittal spinal malalignment is age and regional deformity dependent: a full-standing axis analysis of key radiographical parameters. Spine. 2015; 40(9):642–649

[34] Ferrero E, Liabaud B, Challier V, et al. Role of pelvic translation and lower-extremity compensation to maintain gravity line position in spinal deformity. J Neurosurg Spine. 2016; 24(3):436–446

[35] Schwab FJ, Smith VA, Biserni M, Gamez L, Farcy JP, Pagala M. Adult scoliosis: a quantitative radiographic and clinical analysis. Spine. 2002; 27(4):387–392

[36] Schwab FJ, Lafage V, Farcy JP, Bridwell KH, Glassman S, Shainline MR. Predicting outcome and complications in the surgical treatment of adult scoliosis. Spine. 2008; 33(20):2243–2247

[37] Lafage V, Schwab F, Patel A, Hawkinson N, Farcy JP. Pelvic tilt and truncal inclination: two key radiographic parameters in the setting of adults with spinal deformity. Spine. 2009; 34(17):E599–E606

[38] Schwab F, Patel A, Ungar B, Farcy JP, Lafage V. Adult spinal deformity-postoperative standing imbalance: how much can you tolerate? An overview of key parameters in assessing alignment and planning corrective surgery. Spine. 2010; 35(25):2224–2231

[39] Fakurnejad S, Scheer JK, Lafage V, et al. International Spine Study Group. The likelihood of reaching minimum clinically important difference and substantial clinical benefit at 2 years following a 3-column osteotomy: analysis of 140 patients. J Neurosurg Spine. 2015; 23(3):340–348

[40] Scheer JK, Lafage R, Schwab FJ, et al. Under-correction of sagittal deformities based on age-adjusted alignment thresholds leads to worse health-related quality of life whereas over correction provides no additional benefit. Spine (Phila Pa 1976). 2018; 43(6):388–393

[41] Lafage R, Bess S, Glassman S, et al. International Spine Study Group. Virtual modeling of postoperative alignment after adult spinal deformity surgery helps predict associations between compensatory spinopelvic alignment changes, overcorrection, and proximal junctional kyphosis. Spine. 2017; 42 (19):E1119–E1125

[42] Nielsen D, Hansen L, Dragsted C, et al. Clinical correlation of SRS-Schwab Classification with HRQOL Measures in a Prospective Non-US Cohort of ASD Patients. International Meeting on Advanced Spine Techniques (IMAST); July 16–19, 2014; Valencia, Spain

[43] Smith JS, Singh M, Klineberg E, et al. International Spine Study Group. Surgical treatment of pathological loss of lumbar lordosis (flatback) in patients with normal sagittal vertical axis achieves similar clinical improvement as surgical treatment of elevated sagittal vertical axis: clinical article. J Neurosurg Spine. 2014; 21(2):160–170

[44] Liu Y, Liu Z, Zhu F, et al. Validation and reliability analysis of the new SRS-Schwab classification for adult spinal deformity. Spine. 2013; 38(11):902–908

[45] Kyrölä K, Repo J, Mecklin JP, Ylinen J, Kautiainen H, Häkkinen A. Spinopelvic changes based on the simplified SRS-Schwab adult spinal deformity classification: relationships with disability and health-related quality of life in adult patients with prolonged degenerative spinal disorders. Spine (Phila Pa 1976). 2018; 43(7):497–502

[46] Lafage R, Schwab F, Glassman S, et al. International Spine Study Group. Age-adjusted alignment goals have the potential to reduce PJK. Spine. 2017; 42 (17):1275–1282

3 Cervical Spine Alignment

Lee A. Tan, K. Daniel Riew, Vincent C. Traynelis, and Christopher P. Ames

Abstract

Cervical spine alignment plays an increasingly important role in the preoperative evaluation, surgical planning, and treatment for various cervical spine pathologies in recent years. There has been a growing body of evidence suggesting that malalignment of cervical spine is associated with poor clinical outcome and decreased quality of life. Careful preoperative assessment of cervical spine alignment can help spine surgeons in clarifying surgical goals, determining the proper surgical approach, and achieving a biomechanically sound spinal construct that ultimately optimizes clinical outcome. In this chapter, we provide a thorough review of the various cervical spine alignment parameters along with a discussion of pertinent literature. It is important for spine surgeons to be familiar with these cervical parameters during evaluation and treatment of cervical spine pathologies.

Keywords: cervical spine alignment, cervical kyphosis, cervical lordosis, SVA, T1 slope, chin–brow vertical angle, K-line, chin-on-chest

3.1 Introduction

The fundamental functions of the cervical spine include supporting the weight of the cranium, allowing normal movement of the head and neck, maintaining horizontal gaze, and protecting important neurovascular structures such as spinal cord and vertebral arteries. In recent years, cervical spine alignment has been playing an increasingly important role in the evaluation and surgical treatment of various cervical spine pathologies. There is a growing body of evidence suggesting that cervical spine malalignment is associated with poor clinical outcome and decreased quality of life.[1,2,3,4,5,6,7,8] To understand the importance of cervical alignment, it is important to be familiar with some basic concepts in cervical spine anatomy and biomechanics.

The cervical spine is a highly mobile mechanical structure with six degrees of freedom in movement. The principle motions of the cervical spine include axial rotation, flexion and extension, lateral bending, as well as a small amount of anterior-posterior translation. The cervical spine is the most mobile segment of the spinal column owing to several unique anatomical features. The atlantooccipital joint is formed by the convex-shaped occipital condyle and the concave-shaped superior articular process of the C1 facet, which allows a large degree of flexion/extension, with very little movement in lateral bending or axial rotation.[9] It accounts for about 50% of the flexion/extension motion in the cervical spine. In contrast, the atlantoaxial joint allows for a large degree of axial rotation (~ 50% of axial rotation in the normal cervical spine and can be responsible for up to 90% of axial rotation in elderly patients with more stiff subaxial spine), but with more limited flexion/extension and lateral bending.[10,11]

The total physiological range of motion (ROM) of the cervical spine allows about 90 degrees of rotation to each side, 90 degrees of flexion, 70 degrees of extension, and up to 45 degrees of lateral bending.[12] Panjabi et al[13] found that the atlantooccipital joint had an average ROM of 7.2, 3.5, 21.0, and 5.5 degrees for axial rotation, flexion, extension, and lateral bending, respectively. In contrast, the atlantoaxial joint had an average ROM of 38.9, 11.5, 10.9, and 6.7 degrees for those same parameters, respectively. The subaxial cervical spine (C3–C7) is responsible for the remainder of ROM in the cervical spine.

The center of mass (COM) of the cranium is located approximately 1 cm anterior to the supratragic notch just above the head of the mandible. The weight of the cranium is first transferred from occipital condyles to the C1 lateral masses, then to the C1–C2 facet joints, C2 lateral masses, and subsequently distributed to the subaxial spine via the intervertebral discs and facet joints. The facet joints in the subaxial cervical spine bear about two-thirds of the axial load, while the remaining one-third of the axial load is transmitted via the intervertebral discs.

In a normally aligned lordotic cervical spine, the paraspinal muscles and posterior ligamentous tension band counterbalance the forward bending movement created by the weight of the head, thus maintaining the natural, lordotic cervical alignment. When cervical kyphosis is present, the COM of the cranium moves anteriorly and the moment arm increases, creating a larger bending moment. The resultant larger bending moment requires greater energy expenditure from the paraspinal muscles to keep the head erect, which then can cause muscle fatigue and pain. Furthermore, cervical kyphosis can lead to increased tension and impaired microcirculation of the spinal cord from ventral compression and stretching, eventually leading to myelopathy over time. In addition, as cervical kyphosis shifts the axial load anteriorly, it can accelerate disc degeneration, causing decreased disc height, which in turn causes more cervical kyphosis, thus creating the notion "kyphosis begets kyphosis."

Coronal malalignment of the cervical spine is much less common compared to sagittal malalignment. However, many disease processes including cervical hemivertebra, trauma, infection, tumor, and iatrogenic causes can lead to coronal deformity, which can produce pain and disability. Recent research has also demonstrated that coronal alignment may be important in minimizing adjacent level degeneration and optimizing long-term clinical outcome in the setting of cervical arthroplasty.[7]

In this chapter, we provide an overview of the various cervical spine alignment parameters along with a discussion of pertinent literature. It is important to keep in mind that each patient may have his or her own "optimal" cervical parameters depending on patient-specific factors such age spinopelvic morphology and amount of thoracic kyphosis. The overall goal should aim to achieve a well-balanced cervical spine that has a "harmonious" and biomechanically sound relationship with the rest of spinal column rather than to achieving a specific parameter value.

3.2 Radiographic Parameters

Several radiographic parameters are frequently used to assess cervical spine alignment. Common global sagittal parameters include cervical lordosis (CL), C2–C7 sagittal vertical axis (C2–C7 SVA), T1 slope (T1S), thoracic inlet angle (TIA), neck tilt, as well as the chin–brow vertical angle (CBVA). It is important to note that segmental alignment at each level is also important, as an isolated kyphotic segment may predispose to the other levels of adjacent segment degeneration even in the setting of normal global parameter. The "K-line" is utilized by many spine surgeons to predict the likelihood of successful surgical outcome following cervical laminoplasty for the treatment of cervical stenosis. The coronal alignment of the cervical spine is typically assessed by using the well-known Cobb angle method. Although there is no universally accepted "normal values" for these parameters, current available evidence suggests that T1S–C2–C7 lordosis less than 15 degrees, C2–C7 SVA less than 40 mm, CBVA between -10 and +20 degrees are generally acceptable ranges.[3,14,15,16] Of course, each patient is unique, and the optimal amount of surgical correction should be determined on individual basis. Each of the cervical alignment parameters is discussed in detail in the following sections.

3.2.1 Cervical Lordosis

Cervical lordosis is the natural curvature present in the cervical spine. Research has suggested that CL begins to form while in utero,[17] and becomes more evident after birth as the infant learns to support the weight of the cranium, and further

increases with standing and walking. The CL also increases with aging, as a compensatory mechanism in response to decreasing lumbar lordosis and increasing thoracic kyphosis in order to maintain horizontal gaze.[2,6,15,18] Body position and posture can also affect CL. Hey et al[19] demonstrated that CL increased an average of 3.45 degrees going from standing to sitting. Of note, a lordotic alignment is usually reported as a negative angle by convention, whereas a kyphotic alignment is generally reported as a positive value.

The four most common methods for measuring CL include the modified Cobb method (mCM), Jackson physiological stress (JPS) lines, Harrison posterior tangent (HPT) method, and the Ishihara index (▶ Fig. 3.1).[2,4,20] To use the mCM, two lines are drawn along C2 and C7 inferior endplates first, then additional lines perpendicular to the first two lines are drawn respectively, and the angle subtended by the perpendicular lines equals CL. The JPS can be obtained by drawing lines along posterior vertebral walls of C2 and C7, and the angle between these two lines will give an estimate of CL. The HPT method measures CL by drawing lines along each posterior vertebral wall from C2 to C7; the segmental angles are summed to obtain the overall cervical curvature angle. The Ishihara index is obtained by first drawing a line connecting the posterior-inferior edges of C2 and C7 vertebrae, then four additional horizontal lines from the posterior-inferior edges of the C3–C6 vertebrae are drawn perpendicular to the line connecting C2 and C7. The Ishihara index is the ratio of the total length of the four horizontal segments divided by the length of the line connecting C2 and C7. A higher ratio correlates with increased lordosis, whereas a lower number correlates with decreased lordosis (Ishihara index = 0 if the spine is perfectly straight). In clinical practice, the mCM is by far the most widely used method given its simplicity and the fact that it is highly referenced in the literature. Most modern digital imaging software has built-in Cobb angle measurement capability where lordosis is obtained by simply drawing lines tangent to the endplates of the vertebrae of interest.[21]

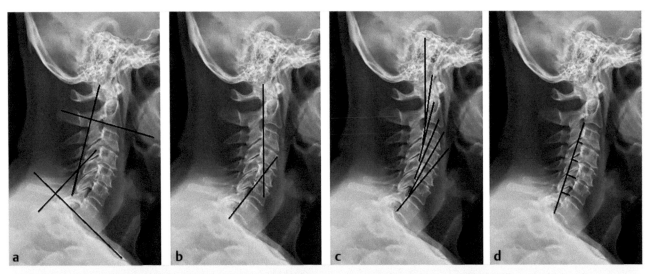

Fig. 3.1 Lateral cervical X-rays showing the four common methods for measuring cervical lordosis: the modified Cobb method **(a)**, Jackson physiological stress lines **(b)**, Harrison's posterior tangent method **(c)**, and the Ishihara index **(d)**.

Hardacker et al[22] evaluated 100 asymptomatic volunteers and found the majority of CL (77%) occurred at the C1–C2 level, while the subaxial cervical spine accounted for the remaining 23% of CL. The average C1–C7 lordosis in their study was -39.4 degrees with a standard deviation of 9.5 degrees. Iyer et al[15] studied 120 asymptomatic adults and found an average C2–C7 lordosis to be -12.2 degrees (measured with HPT method). This result is similar to the mean C2–C7 lordosis of -9.9 degrees reported by Lee et al.[23]

3.2.2 C2–C7 Sagittal Vertical Axis

C2–C7 SVA is used to measure regional sagittal alignment of the cervical spine, and it has been shown to weakly correlate with health-related quality of life.[1] The C2–C7 SVA is obtained by measuring the distance between the C2 plumb line and the posterior superior endplate of C7 (▶ Fig. 3.2). Tang et al[1] retrospectively reviewed 113 patients receiving multilevel posterior cervical fusions, and found that a C2–C7 SVA greater than 40 mm was correlated with increased disability. Interestingly, another recent study by Lee et al[24] investigated 50 patients undergoing laminoplasty for ossification of posterior longitudinal ligament (OPLL), and they did not find such correlation between increased C2–C7 SVA and worse clinical outcome. Iyer et al[15] reported a mean C2–C7 SVA of 21.3 mm in 120 asymptomatic patients from upright radiographs obtained from EOS imaging system.

Nonetheless, from the biomechanical standpoint, increased C2–C7 SVA increases the flexion bending moment of the cervical spine, and in turn increases the muscle energy expenditure required to keep the head erect; thus, it may lead to muscle fatigue, pain, and disability over time. However, level I evidence that definitively proves the correlation between increased C2–C7 SVA and increased disability is still lacking and further study on this topic is needed.

3.2.3 Thoracic Inlet Angle, T1 slope, and Neck Tilt

The concept of TIA was first introduced in 2012 by Lee et al,[23] modeled after the concept of pelvic incidence from the spino-pelvic parameters. The authors defined TIA as the angle formed by the line connecting the sternum to the midpoint of T1 upper endplate, and the line perpendicular to the T1 upper endplate (▶ Fig. 3.3). Although the TIA was originally measured on lateral X-rays, other authors[25,26] had suggested that using CT or MRI provided better visualization of reference anatomical structures and improved reliability. Lee et al[23] introduced the TIA as a fixed parameter since the thoracic inlet is relatively immobile due to articulations between the sternum, T1 ribs, and the T1 vertebral body. However, other authors have demonstrated that the TIA may change depending on neck position (neutral, flexion vs. extension),[27] standing versus sitting, as well as when the patient slept on pillows of varying heights.[28] Thus, measuring T1S on a supine CT may yield a measurement that is different from that on standing X-rays. Therefore, the TIA appears to

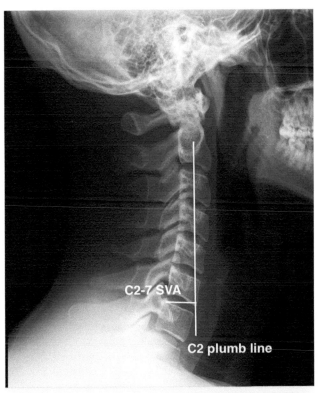

Fig. 3.2 A lateral cervical X-ray showing C2–C7 sagittal vertical axis.

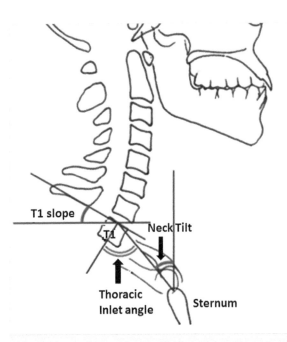

Fig. 3.3 A drawing demonstrating thoracic inlet angle, T1 slope, and neck tilt.

change with various factors and its role in clinical application is yet to be demonstrated.

The T1S is defined as the angle formed by the T1 upper endplate and the horizontal plane, analogous to the sacral slope. The neck tilt is defined as the angle formed between the line connecting the sternum to the midpoint of T1 upper endplate and the vertical axis, similar to the pelvic tilt. Oe et al[29] studied 656 volunteers aged 50 to 89 years. They found that the mean T1Ss for patients in each decade were 32, 31, 33, and 36 degrees for men, and 28, 29, 32, and 37 degrees for women, respectively. They also found that C2–C7 SVA greater than 40 mm or more, T1S greater than 40 degrees, and T1S-CL greater than 20 degrees were associated with worse EQ-5D health status scores.

3.2.4 Chin–Brow Vertical Angle

The CBVA is defined as the angle subtended by the line connecting the patient's chin (anterior mandible) to the eyebrow (superior orbital rim), and the vertical line drawn from the eyebrow. It is often used in cervical kyphotic deformity cases to help spine surgeons to determine how much correction to restore horizontal gaze and optimize daily function. The CBVA can be measured either from clinical photographs or full-body EOS X-rays (▶ Fig. 3.4). The patient must be standing with hips and knee extended and the cervical spine in the neutral position. When the head is tilted down, the CBVA is reported as a positive angle; when the head is tilted up, the CBVA is reported as a negative value. Perfect horizontal gaze would produce a CBVA of zero.

Iyer et al[15] reported a mean CBVA of -1.7 degrees after analyzing 120 asymptomatic adults. Lafage et al[30] found that a CBVA between -4.7 and + 17.7 degrees correlated with the lowest Oswestry Disability Index (ODI) after studying a series of 303 patients. Suk et al[16] conducted a prospective study including 34 patients with ankylosing spondylitis (AS) patients who had undergone pedicle subtraction osteotomy for correction of kyphotic deformity and recommended a CBVA range of -10 to + 10 degrees for optimized horizontal gaze. Interestingly, a more recent study by Song et al[3] suggested that AS patients with a postoperative CBVA between + 10 and + 20 degrees (i.e., slight flexion) had best overall results with both indoor and outdoor activities. In our experience, overcorrection of cervical kyphosis can be extremely detrimental to patients' daily activities such as cooking, walking, and toileting which require downward vision. A neutral or slight downward head tilt that balances appearance and function will most likely to achieve the optimal clinical outcome.

3.2.5 The "K-Line" and the "Modified K-Line"

Laminoplasty is a common procedure performed to treat multilevel cervical stenosis, especially in the setting of OPLL where the anterior procedure is more challenging with higher complication rates. Laminoplasty is most effective in achieving spinal cord decompression in a lordotic cervical spine, where the lordotic curve allows the spinal cord to drift dorsally to eliminate

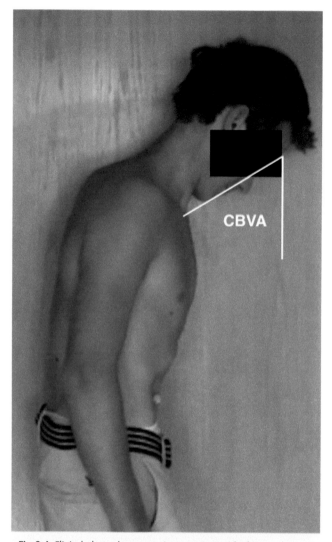

Fig. 3.4 Clinical photo demonstrating a patient with chin-on-chest deformity with chin–brow vertical angle measurement.

or reduce ventral compression indirectly. However, if there is cervical kyphosis or significant ventral compression, laminoplasty may not adequately decompress the spinal cord and lead to suboptimal clinical outcome. Suda et al reviewed a series of 114 patients, and found that when local cervical kyphosis is greater than 13 degrees, patients had worse clinical outcome after laminoplasty.[31] Posterior cervical laminectomy and fusion is another surgical technique commonly used to treat OPLL and it may offer some kyphosis correction in addition to spinal cord decompression, which essentially "shifts" the K-line more dorsally, and may yield improved outcome in some patients.

Fujiyosh et al[32] used the "K-line," which is a line drawn by connecting the midpoint of the spinal canal at C2 and C7 on standing lateral cervical X-rays, to predict clinical outcome after laminoplasty in patients with OPLL (▶ Fig. 3.5). They found that neurological recovery rate was much lower in patients with anterior compression exceeding the "K-line." Taniyama et al[33]

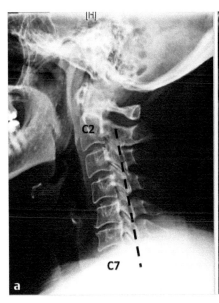
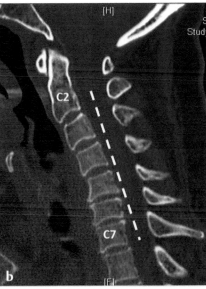

Fig. 3.5 The "K-line" (**a**) and the "modified K-line" (**b**) demonstrated on lateral cervical X-ray and CT cervical spine, respectively.

demonstrated that patients with less than 4 mm space between the anterior compression factor and the modified "K-line" (K-line drawn on sagittal MRI instead of on upright lateral X-rays) had much higher risk for persistent anterior spinal cord compression after laminoplasty. Therefore, "K-line" and "modified K-line" can help spine surgeons to predict if adequate spinal cord decompression can be achieved with laminoplasty.

3.2.6 Cervical Coronal Deformity

Coronal deformity in the cervical spine (cervical or cervicothoracic scoliosis) occurs much less commonly compared to sagittal deformity. It usually arises from a structural curve in the cervical or cervicothoracic region, causing abnormal posture of the head and neck in the coronal plane. Cervical coronal deformity typically results from bony anomalies such as a hemivertebra and/or a block vertebra, and are commonly associated with various congenital syndromes[34] including Klippel-Feil syndrome, Larsen syndrome, Goldenhar syndrome, Jarcho-Levin syndrome, congenital neuromuscular torticollis, and NF-1.

Patients with cervical coronal deformity can present with head malposition, pain, and neurological deficits. The optimal treatment strategy depends on the location and magnitude of deformity, as well as local bony and neurovascular anatomy, along with the patient's fitness for surgery. The overall goals for surgery should include prevention curve progression and restoration of spinal alignment, while decompressing neural elements and preserving neurological function.

When coronal deformity in the cervical spine is present, the magnitude of the coronal deformity can be measured and quantified by the coronal Cobb angle similar to thoracolumbar scoliosis. Two lines are drawn at the top and bottom endplates of the scoliotic curve, and then two perpendicular lines can be drawn relative to the endplate lines, respectively, and the angle subtended by the perpendicular lines is the coronal Cobb angle. In most modern imaging softwares, the angle is usually measured automatically and displaced after the lines on the endplates are drawn (▶ Fig. 3.6). The coronal Cobb angle can help spine surgeons determine the amount of cervical coronal deformity correction required, and plan for specific surgical

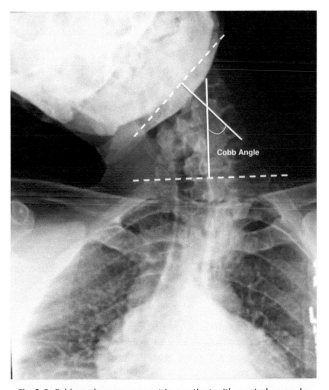

Fig. 3.6 Cobb angle measurement in a patient with cervical coronal deformity.

techniques such as asymmetric cervical corpectomy or pedicle subtraction osteotomy (PSO). With careful planning and meticulous surgical techniques, significant deformity correction can be obtained with preservation of neurological function and improvement of quality of life for patients with cervicothoracic scoliosis (▶ Fig. 3.7).

3.3 Conclusion

It is important for spine surgeons to be familiar with common cervical alignment parameters during evaluation and treatment

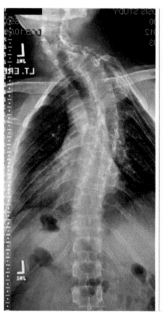
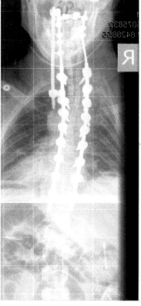
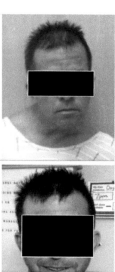

Fig. 3.7 Pre- and postoperative cervical X-rays and clinical photos demonstrating surgical correction of a patient with cervicothoracic scoliosis.

of cervical spine pathologies. Careful preoperative assessment of cervical spine alignment can help spine surgeons clarify surgical goals, determine the proper surgical approach, and achieve a biomechanically sound spinal construct that ultimately leads to improved clinical outcome.

References

[1] Tang JA, Scheer JK, Smith JS, et al. ISSG. The impact of standing regional cervical sagittal alignment on outcomes in posterior cervical fusion surgery. Neurosurgery. 2012; 71(3):662–669, discussion 669

[2] Scheer JK, Tang JA, Smith JS, et al. International Spine Study Group. Cervical spine alignment, sagittal deformity, and clinical implications: a review. J Neurosurg Spine. 2013; 19(2):141–159

[3] Song K, Su X, Zhang Y, et al. Optimal chin-brow vertical angle for sagittal visual fields in ankylosing spondylitis kyphosis. Eur Spine J. 2016; 25(8):2596–2604

[4] Ames CP, Blondel B, Scheer JK, et al. Cervical radiographical alignment: comprehensive assessment techniques and potential importance in cervical myelopathy. Spine. 2013; 38(22) Suppl 1:S149–S160

[5] Tan LA, Riew KD, Traynelis VC. Cervical spine deformity - Part 1: Biomechanics, radiographic parameters, and classification. Neurosurgery. 2017; 81(2):197–203

[6] Yuan W, Zhu Y, Zhu H, Cui C, Pei L, Huang Z. Preoperative cervical sagittal alignment parameters and their impacts on myelopathy in patients with cervical spondylotic myelopathy: a retrospective study. PeerJ. 2017; 5:e4027

[7] Kim SW, Paik SH, Oh JK, Kwak YH, Lee HW, You KH. The impact of coronal alignment of device on radiographic degeneration in the case of total disc replacement. Spine J. 2016; 16(4):470–479

[8] Oe S, Togawa D, Yoshida G, et al. Difference in spinal sagittal alignment and health-related quality of life between males and females with cervical deformity. Asian Spine J. 2017; 11(6):959–967

[9] Bogduk N, Mercer S. Biomechanics of the cervical spine. I: Normal kinematics. Clin Biomech (Bristol, Avon). 2000; 15(9):633–648

[10] Koebke J, Brade H. Morphological and functional studies on the lateral joints of the first and second cervical vertebrae in man. Anat Embryol (Berl). 1982; 164(2):265–275

[11] Mercer S, Bogduk N. Intra-articular inclusions of the cervical synovial joints. Br J Rheumatol. 1993; 32(8):705–710

[12] Swartz EE, Floyd RT, Cendoma M. Cervical spine functional anatomy and the biomechanics of injury due to compressive loading. J Athl Train. 2005; 40(3):155–161

[13] Panjabi M, Dvorak J, Duranceau J, et al. Three-dimensional movements of the upper cervical spine. Spine. 1988; 13(7):726–730

[14] Ames CP, Smith JS, Eastlack R, et al. International Spine Study Group. Reliability assessment of a novel cervical spine deformity classification system. J Neurosurg Spine. 2015; 23(6):673–683

[15] Iyer S, Lenke LG, Nemani VM, et al. Variations in occipitocervical and cervicothoracic alignment parameters based on age: a prospective study of asymptomatic volunteers using full-body radiographs. Spine. 2016; 41(23):1837–1844

[16] Suk K-S, Kim K-T, Lee S-H, Kim J-M. Significance of chin-brow vertical angle in correction of kyphotic deformity of ankylosing spondylitis patients. Spine. 2003; 28(17):2001–2005

[17] Bagnall KM, Harris PF, Jones PR. A radiographic study of the human fetal spine. 1. The development of the secondary cervical curvature. J Anat. 1977; 123(Pt 3):777–782

[18] Endo K, Suzuki H, Sawaji Y, et al. Relationship among cervical, thoracic, and lumbopelvic sagittal alignment in healthy adults. J Orthop Surg (Hong Kong). 2016; 24(1):92–96

[19] Hey HWD, Teo AQA, Tan K-A, et al. How the spine differs in standing and in sitting-important considerations for correction of spinal deformity. Spine J. 2017; 17(6):799–806

[20] Tan LA, Straus DC, Traynelis VC. Cervical interfacet spacers and maintenance of cervical lordosis. J Neurosurg Spine. 2015; 22(5):466–469

[21] Drexler L. Röntgen Anatomische Untersuchungen Über Krumming Der Halswirbelsäule in Der Verschiedenen Lebensaltern. Stuttgart: Hippokrates; 1962

[22] Hardacker JW, Shuford RF, Capicotto PN, Pryor PW. Radiographic standing cervical segmental alignment in adult volunteers without neck symptoms. Spine. 1997; 22(13):1472–1480, discussion 1480

[23] Lee SH, Kim KT, Seo EM, Suk KS, Kwack YH, Son ES. The influence of thoracic inlet alignment on the craniocervical sagittal balance in asymptomatic adults. J Spinal Disord Tech. 2012; 25(2):E41–E47

[24] Lee CK, Shin DA, Yi S, et al. Correlation between cervical spine sagittal alignment and clinical outcome after cervical laminoplasty for ossification of the posterior longitudinal ligament. J Neurosurg Spine. 2016; 24(1):100–107

[25] Qiao J, Zhu F, Liu Z, et al. Measurement of thoracic inlet alignment on MRI: reliability and the influence of body position. Clin Spine Surg. 2017; 30(4):E377–E380

[26] Jun HS, Chang IB, Song JH, et al. Is it possible to evaluate the parameters of cervical sagittal alignment on cervical computed tomographic scans? Spine. 2014; 39(10):E630–E636

[27] Janusz P, Tyrakowski M, Yu H, Siemionow K. Reliability of cervical lordosis measurement techniques on long-cassette radiographs. Eur Spine J. 2016; 25(11):3596–3601

[28] Kim HC, Jun HS, Kim JH, et al. The effect of different pillow heights on the parameters of cervicothoracic spine segments. Korean J Spine. 2015; 12(3):135–138

[29] Oe S, Togawa D, Nakai K, et al. The influence of age and sex on cervical spinal alignment among volunteers aged over 50. Spine. 2015; 40(19):1487–1494

[30] Lafage R, Challier V, Liabaud B, et al. Natural head posture in the setting of sagittal spinal deformity: validation of chin-brow vertical angle, slope of line of sight, and McGregor's slope with health-related quality of life. Neurosurgery. 2016; 79(1):108–115

[31] Suda K, Abumi K, Ito M, Shono Y, Kaneda K, Fujiya M. Local kyphosis reduces surgical outcomes of expansive open-door laminoplasty for cervical spondylotic myelopathy. Spine. 2003; 28(12):1258–1262

[32] Fujiyoshi T, Yamazaki M, Kawabe J, et al. A new concept for making decisions regarding the surgical approach for cervical ossification of the posterior longitudinal ligament: the K-line. Spine. 2008; 33(26):E990–E993

[33] Taniyama T, Hirai T, Yamada T, et al. Modified K-line in magnetic resonance imaging predicts insufficient decompression of cervical laminoplasty. Spine. 2013; 38(6):496–501

[34] Smith MD. Congenital scoliosis of the cervical or cervicothoracic spine. Orthop Clin North Am. 1994; 25(2):301–310

4 Radiographic Measurement

Nicholas D. Stekas and Themistocles S. Protopsaltis

Abstract

Sagittal malalignment of the thoracolumbar spine has long been appreciated to be a contributor to significant disability and morbidity. Recent literature has aimed to describe how sagittal malalignment of the cervical spine relates to outcomes and impairment in quality of life. However, the relationship between cervical malalignment and patient-reported outcomes has remained somewhat controversial and does not appear to be as clear as the relationship that exists in the thoracolumbar spine. While our understanding of how to best measure clinically relevant malalignment of the cervical spine has improved substantially over the last decade, more research is needed to further elucidate how to best describe cervical alignment and predict postoperative outcomes in patients with cervical deformity.

Keywords: cervical deformity, cervical lordosis, cervical sagittal vertical axis, T1 slope minus cervical lordosis, compensatory deformity, horizontal gaze, regional alignment, global alignment

4.1 Anatomy of the Cervical Spine

The cervical spine is typically composed of seven vertebrae and is anatomically complex. The articulation of the cervical vertebrae allows for mobility at the neck joint and the maintenance of horizontal gaze.[1,2] Much of the mobility of the neck comes from the articulation between the most cranial joints of the cervical spine.[3] The atlantooccipital joint, the articulation between the occiput and first cervical vertebra, accounts for approximately one-third of flexion and extension and one-half of lateral bending of the neck.[3] The articulation of the first and second cervical vertebrae accounts for approximately 50% of rotational motion of the neck.[3]

Cadaveric studies have suggested that the center of gravity of the head is located 1.8 cm anterior and 6.0 cm superior to the occipital condyle.[4] The natural curve of the cervical spine is lordosis, which begins to become significant in infancy due to the physiologic need to support the weight of the head while upright.[1] This lordotic curvature of the cervical spine is caused by wedge-shaped vertebrae in the cervical region that work to compensate for thoracic kyphosis[5] and is partly due to variance between anterior and posterior intervertebral disc height.[1,6]

Traditionally, the cervical spine has been divided into one anterior column, including the vertebral bodies and intervertebral discs, and two posterior columns, consisting of the facet joints.[7,8] It has been estimated that the anterior column is responsible for up to 82% of the weight of the head, while the posterior column is responsible for up to 33%.[8] When cervical malalignment occurs, forces can change the center of gravity of the head, leading to increased muscular energy expenditure and the potential for disability.[2]

4.2 Normal Cervical Alignment

The extreme mobility of the cervical spine makes defining normative angular measurements in the cervical region difficult. While normal ranges have been described for total and segmental angular values in the standing cervical spine,[9,10,11] alignment values that are classified as abnormal or pathologic remain contentious. Kuntz et al conducted a systematic review to suggest that normative angular alignment of total cervical lordosis was -29 degrees from the C1–C2 level and -17 degrees from the C2–C7 level.[9]

4.3 Cervical Deformity

Cervical deformity is difficult to define and to date there is no universally accepted definition. While the link between sagittal deformity of the thoracolumbar spine and clinical outcomes has been well established in the literature,[12,13,14,15] the relationship between sagittal malalignment in the cervical spine and outcome measures remains less clear. Recent research has aimed to quantify the amount of disability associated with cervical malalignment and describe the best way to classify cervical deformity.

Ames et al have developed a standardized classification system to describe cervical deformity which incorporates sagittal, regional, and global spinopelvic alignment and neurologic status.[16] This validated classification system provides a standardized nomenclature for both research and clinical purposes, which has further advanced our understanding of how to employ alignment parameters of the cervical spine for surgical planning and predicting clinical outcomes.

However, to date a universally accepted definition of cervical deformity remains somewhat elusive. One complicating factor in defining cervical deformity is distinguishing primary cervical deformity from secondary compensatory changes in cervical spine alignment due to deformity in the thoracolumbar spine. It has been suggested that currently accepted definitions of cervical deformity are insufficient due to the inherent difficulty that comes with creating an all-encompassing definition of cervical deformity to describe primary and secondary malalignment of the cervical spine.

Primary cervical deformity can result from spondylotic arthropathies, idiopathic cervical paraspinal myopathies, and iatrogenic cervical kyphosis and can create severe chin-on-chest deformity which may compromise horizontal gaze, swallowing, or even breathing.[17,18,19] However, malalignment in subjacent spine segments has been shown to induce compensatory alignment changes in the cervical region to maintain global alignment while upright.[20,21] In fact, correction of thoracic deformity has been shown to result in spontaneous resolution of cervical malalignment.[22]

While numerous alignment parameters have been described in cervical spine literature to describe clinically relevant deformity, their clinical utility remains up for debate. Great strides have been made in recent years regarding how to best describe and classify cervical deformity, but more research is needed to elucidate the optimal parameters used to describe clinically relevant sagittal malalignment of the cervical spine.

4.4 Parameters of Regional Alignment

4.4.1 Cervical Lordosis

The amount of lordotic curvature of the cervical spine can be easily quantified by measuring the angle between the inferior endplate of C2 and the inferior endplate of C7 (▶ Fig. 4.1).[23] Reported values regarding the normal range of CL in asymptomatic subjects is -16 degrees ± 16 degrees in men and -15 degrees ± 10 degrees for women between the ages of 20 and 25 years.[23,24] It has been suggested that CL increases in older patients, with the normal range of CL in patients aged 60 to 65 years -22 degrees ± 13 degrees for men and -25 degrees ± 16 degrees for women.[24]

4.4.2 Cervical Sagittal Vertical Axis

The classic measure of sagittal alignment in the cervical spine is the cervical sagittal vertical axis (cSVA). cSVA is measured as the distance between a plumb line dropped from the centroid of C2 to the posterior-superior aspect of C7 (▶ Fig. 4.2).[23]

Normative values for cSVA have been defined by Hardacker et al to range between 0.5 and 2.5 cm.[11] Tang and colleagues have reported that high postoperative cSVA correlated with poor postoperative outcomes in patients undergoing cervical fusion.[25] In the same study, linear regression was utilized to determine that a cSVA greater than 4 cm corresponds to a moderate disability threshold.[25] More recently, cSVA has also been shown to correlate with outcome measures in patients with thoracolumbar deformity[20] as well as severity of myelopathy.[26]

These findings represent rare examples of cervical malalignment correlating with postoperative outcomes in cervical spine literature and have provided valuable information regarding how spine surgeons can classify and define cervical deformity. As such, a cSVA greater than 4 cm and increased cervical

kyphosis have been the most commonly published descriptors of cervical deformity in cervical spine literature. However, recent research has alluded to the fact that these definitions of cervical deformity may not be a sufficient description of clinically relevant malalignment.

For one, cervical kyphosis has been shown to exist in up to 34% of asymptomatic patients and may be a normal feature of standing alignment in young patients.[27] Additionally, malalignment of the cervical spine can be skewed by deformity in the thoracolumbar spine due to compensatory changes to maintain global alignment when standing at rest.[21] To date, cSVA remains a commonly accepted definition of cervical deformity, but it is often considered in relation to other measures of malalignment in order to address these shortcomings.

4.4.3 T1 Slope minus Cervical Lordosis

Given the limitations associated with using the cSVA and cervical kyphosis as metrics for defining cervical deformity, there has been an attempt to account for the confounding effect of thoracolumbar deformity and compensatory cervical alignment that these parameters fail to address. Recent literature has begun to focus on the importance of the relationship between T1 slope and cervical lordosis in describing cervical malalignment.[28,29]

The relationship between pelvic incidence and lumbar lordosis has been used effectively as a descriptor of lumbopelvic alignment and has been shown to be an effective tool for correction of lumbar flatback deformity.[30] Analogously, T1 slope minus cervical lordosis (TS-CL) attempts to quantify the amount of cervical

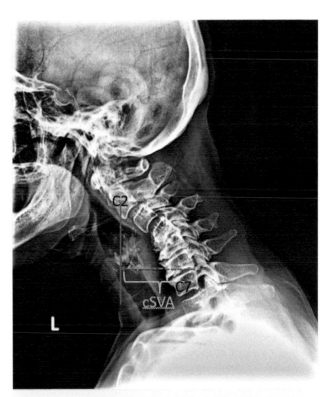

Fig. 4.2 Cervical sagittal vertical axis. The cervical sagittal vertical axis (cSVA) is measured as the distance between a plumb line from the center of C2 and a horizontal line at the level of the superior-posterior corner of the C7 endplate.

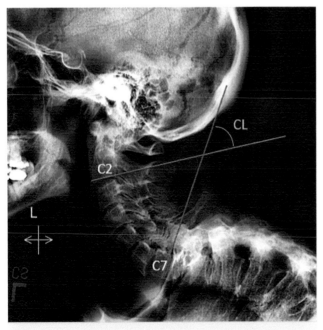

Fig. 4.1 Cervical lordosis. Cervical lordosis is measured as the angle between the lower (caudal) endplate of C2 and the lower endplate of~C7.

malalignment in the sagittal plane while accounting for underlying thoracolumbar alignment. TS-CL can be measured as the slope of the superior endplate of T1, minus the angle between the lower endplate of C2 and the lower endplate of C7 (CL) (▶ Fig. 4.3).[23]

T1 slope has been shown to correlate with cervical lordosis. It is hypothesized that as thoracic kyphosis increases, cervical lordosis increases in order to maintain compensatory alignment of the axial skeleton. However, an excessively large T1 slope may overcome the ability of the cervical spine to compensate for excessive thoracic kyphosis. As such, it is important to take into account the mismatch between T1 slope and cervical lordosis (TS-CL) when attempting to understand cervical malalignment in the setting of thoracic deformity. When a mismatch exists between T1 slope and cervical lordosis, either thoracolumbar deformity is so severe that changes in cervical spine alignment can no longer compensate or underlying cervical deformity is present.[28,29,31] However, given cervical deformity in the presence of underlying thoracic deformity, it is important to identify which values of TS-CL correspond to cervical deformity, rather than cervical compensation, and which values correspond to pathologic alignment.

Protopsaltis et al demonstrated that even in the presence of underlying thoracolumbar deformity, if the mismatch between T1 slope and cervical lordosis is greater than 17 degrees, cervical deformity is present.[28] One study of 31 patients with multilevel posterior cervical fusion showed that a TS-CL mismatch greater than 22.2 degrees corresponded to severe disability and a cSVA greater than 4.35 cm.[32]

More recently, TS-CL has also been used to determine the deficit of cervical lordosis in a given deformity for the purpose of surgical planning.[28] By subtracting normative values from the measured TS-CL, a lordosis deficit can be obtained. The lordosis deficit can be utilized by spine surgeons to plan alignment targets in patients undergoing surgery for cervical deformity.[28]

4.4.4 C2 Slope

Like TS-CL, C2 slope can be utilized to measure cervical malalignment in the setting of preexisting thoracolumbar deformity. C2 slope is a mathematical approximation of TS-CL which has recently been proposed as a simplified, singular measurement of cervical deformity.[33] Assuming that the slope of the upper endplate of T1 is similar to the slope of the upper endplate of C7, TS-CL can be simplified to C2 slope.[33] C2 slope can be measured as the angle between the slope of the lower endplate of C2 and the horizontal (▶ Fig. 4.4).[23] Recent research has suggested that C2 slope is very strongly correlated to TS-CL and may act as a useful marker of overall cervical alignment, acting as a link between the occipitocervical and cervicothoracic spine.[33] While preliminary research has been encouraging, more investigation is needed to identify the utility of C2 slope in predicting postoperative outcomes and establishing alignment targets after surgery.

4.4.5 Chin–Brown Vertical Angle

The chin–brow vertical angle (CBVA) is a commonly used parameter to assess a patient's horizontal gaze following malalignment of the cervical spine. CBVA can be measured by the angle between a line from the chin to the brow, and a line from the vertical. Kuntz et al reported a normal neutral value for CBVA to be -1 degrees.[9] However, a more recent study conducted analyzing sagittal visual fields in 25 patients with ankylosing spondylitis found that the best satisfaction occurred when CBVA fell between 10 and 20 degrees.[34] CBVA measurements of less than -10 degrees have been linked to poor outcome measures.[35]

CBVA is traditionally described using clinical photographs of a patient's line of sight and is not always readily available on

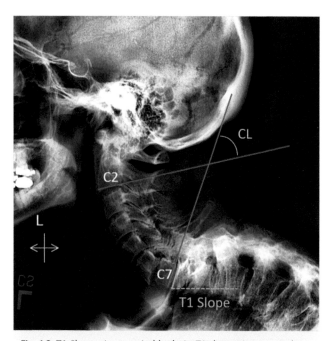

Fig. 4.3 **T1** Slope minus cervical lordosis. T1 slope minus cervical lordosis is measured as the angle between the upper endplate of T1 and the horizontal subtracted by cervical lordosis (the angle between the lower endplate of C2 and the lower endplate of C7).

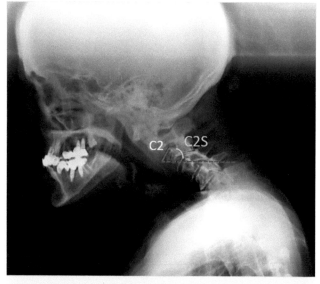

Fig. 4.4 **C2** Slope. C2 slope is calculated as the angle between the upper endplate of C2 and the horizontal.

traditional sagittal radiographs.[23] As such, surrogate markers of horizontal gaze, including McGregor's slope (McGS) and the slope of line of sight (SLS), have been proposed as descriptors of horizontal gaze that can be readily described using traditional radiography.[23] SLS is defined as the angle between a line from the anterior inferior margin of the orbit to the top of the external auditory meatus and the horizontal.[23] The McGS can be described as the angle between a line from the upper surface of the posterior edge of the hard palate and the most caudal point of the occipital curve.[23] Recent studies have shown that McGS and SLS correlate strongly with CBVA and are associated with similar disability scores.[36]

4.5 Parameters of Global Alignment

In assessing cervical deformity, it is imperative to differentiate primary cervical deformities from compensatory changes in alignment due to deformity in subjacent spinal regions. Research has shown that thoracolumbar deformity can induce compensatory changes in the cervical spine to maintain global alignment.[20,21,22]

In recent years, the importance of long cassette radiographs has been recognized in the evaluation of cervical deformity. Full spine radiography can identify concurrent thoracic and lumbar

deformities that contribute to compensatory deformity in the cervical spine. As a result, a firm understanding of global alignment and compensatory mechanisms is crucial for surgical planning of cervical malalignment.

Ramchandran et al have reported that long cassette radiography has the potential to change surgical planning in as many as 30% of cases due to the presence of thoracolumbar malalignment.[37] While the clinical scenarios that suggest the use of full spine radiographs have not been well established, Klineberg and colleagues have shown that when T1 slope exceeds 32 degrees, concomitant thoracolumbar is likely to be present with a sensitivity and specificity of 69%.[38] Knott et al have suggested utilizing long cassette radiographs when T1 tilt falls outside of the range of 13 to 25 degrees.[39]

4.5.1 C2–T1 Pelvic Angle

Global alignment of the thoracolumbar spine has been assessed using the T1 pelvic angle (TPA), which is the angle formed between a line from the femoral heads to the T1 centroid and a line from the femoral heads to the sacral endplate. Similarly, the C2–T1 pelvic angle (CTPA) has been proposed as a means of determining the relative amount of cervical deformity. The CTPA can be described by the angle between a line from the femoral heads to the C2 centroid and a line from the femoral heads to the T1 centroid (▶ Fig. 4.5).

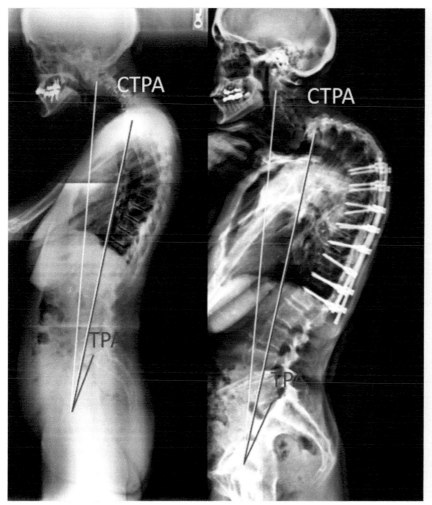

Fig. 4.5 C2–T1 pelvic angle (CTPA) and T1 pelvic angle. T1 pelvic angle is measured as the angle between a line from the femoral heads to the middle of the sacral endplate and a line from the femoral heads to the centroid of T1. Its cervical counterpart, the C2–T1 pelvic angle, is measured as the angle from the femoral heads to centroid of C2 and a line from the femoral heads to the centroid of T1.

The relationship between regional alignment parameters in the cervical region (such as C2 slope) and regional alignment parameters at the cervicothoracic junction (such as T1 slope) can be used to distinguish primary cervical deformity from compensatory malalignment due to thoracolumbar deformity. In situations where C2 slope is low and T1 slope is high, thoracolumbar deformity may be present and full-length spine films should be obtained to evaluate CTPA and global alignment (▶ Fig. 4.6).

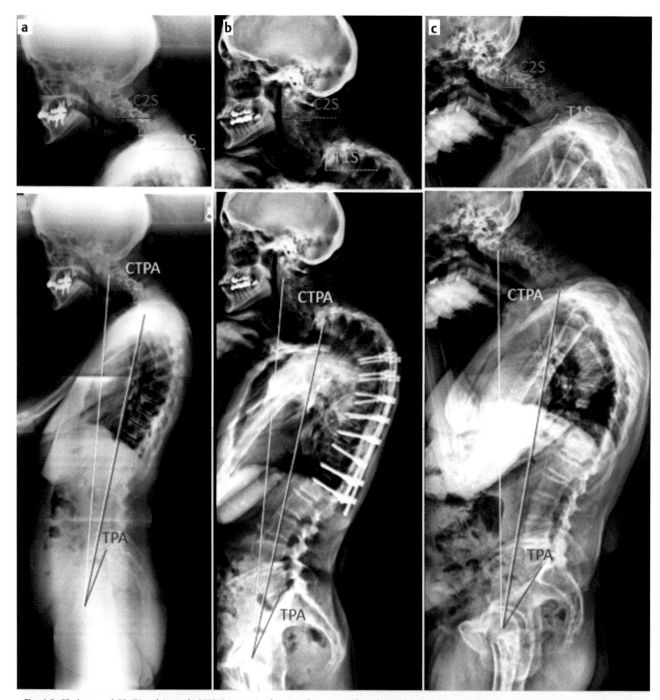

Fig. 4.6 C2 slope and C2–T1 pelvic angle (CTPA) in cervicothoracic alignment. The relationship between C2 slope and T1 slope can help differentiate cervical malalignment resulting underlying thoracolumbar deformity versus primary cervical deformity. When T1 slope is high and C2 slope is low, deformity in the thoracolumbar spine is likely and full-body imaging of the axial skeleton is indicated. However, when C2 slope is high and T1 slope is low, primary cervical deformity is more likely. (**a**) A patient with high C2 slope and low T1 slope implies primary cervical deformity. In this case, full-body imaging may not be necessary. (**b**) A patient with low C2 slope and high T1 slope implies thoracolumbar deformity with appropriate cervical compensation. Full-body imaging is necessary to evaluate thoracolumbar deformity. (**c**) A patient with high C2 tilt and high T1 slope implies deformity is in both the cervical and thoracolumbar spine without cervical compensation. Full-length spine films are necessary to evaluate thoracolumbar deformity. T1 pelvic angle (TPA) assesses thoracolumbar alignment and CTPA assesses cervical alignment.

4.6 The Future of Cervical Alignment Research

While several useful alignment parameters have been identified to describe sagittal deformity of the cervical spine, their clinical utility remains controversial. To date few studies have been able to show a distinct link between various alignment parameters and clinical outcomes. As such, surgical planning for cervical deformity is difficult and is not made on the basis of alignment alone but instead taken in context of the clinical picture associated with each case.

The wide range of etiologies and clinical impacts of various cervical spine pathologies does not lend itself to a one-size-fits-all definition of cervical deformity. However, many recent advancements in cervical spine literature have played an important role in furthering our understanding of cervical deformity and improving surgical outcomes. Technologic improvements including the wide spread use of full-spine imaging and measurement software to quantify malalignment has made studying cervical deformity much more feasible. However, more research is needed to identify which alignment parameters will prove most valuable in surgical planning and predicting outcomes.

References

[1] Nguyen NM, Baluch DA, Patel AA. Cervical sagittal balance: a review. Contemporary Spine Surgery. 2014; 15(1):1–8

[2] Scheer JK, Tang JA, Smith JS, et al. International Spine Study Group. Cervical spine alignment, sagittal deformity, and clinical implications: a review. J Neurosurg Spine. 2013; 19(2):141–159

[3] Monahan JJ, Waite RJ. Orthopaedics in primary care. In: Steinberg GG, Akins CM, eds. Orthopaedics in Primary Care. Baltimore, MD: Lippincott Williams & Wilkins; 1999

[4] Beier G, Schuck M, Schuller E, Spann W. Determination of Physical Data of the Head. I. Center of Gravity and Moments of Inertia of Human Heads. 1979. Available at: http://oai.dtic.mil/oai/oai?verb=getRecord&metadataPrefix=html&identifier=ADA080333. Accessed April 19, 2014

[5] Gay RE. The curve of the cervical spine: variations and significance. J Manipulative Physiol Ther. 1993; 16(9):591–594

[6] Broberg KB. On the mechanical behaviour of intervertebral discs. Spine. 1983; 8(2):151–165

[7] Louis R. Spinal stability as defined by the three-column spine concept. Anat Clin. 1985; 7(1):33–42

[8] Pal GP, Sherk HH. The vertical stability of the cervical spine. Spine. 1988; 13 (5):447–449

[9] Kuntz C, IV, Levin LS, Ondra SL, Shaffrey CI, Morgan CJ. Neutral upright sagittal spinal alignment from the occiput to the pelvis in asymptomatic adults: a review and resynthesis of the literature. J Neurosurg Spine. 2007; 6(2):104–112

[10] Gore DR, Sepic SB, Gardner GM. Roentgenographic findings of the cervical spine in asymptomatic people. Spine. 1986; 11(6):521–524

[11] Hardacker JW, Shuford RF, Capicotto PN, Pryor PW. Radiographic standing cervical segmental alignment in adult volunteers without neck symptoms. Spine. 1997; 22(13):1472–1480, discussion 1480

[12] Glassman SD, Bridwell K, Dimar JR, Horton W, Berven S, Schwab F. The impact of positive sagittal balance in adult spinal deformity. Spine. 2005; 30(18):2024–2029

[13] Lafage V, Schwab F, Patel A, Hawkinson N, Farcy JP. Pelvic tilt and truncal inclination: two key radiographic parameters in the setting of adults with spinal deformity. Spine. 2009; 34(17):E599–E606

[14] Protopsaltis TS, Schwab FJ, Smith JS, et al. The T1 pelvic angle (TPA), a novel radiographic parameter of sagittal deformity, correlates strongly with clinical measures of disability. Spine J. 2013; 13(9):S61

[15] Schwab FJ, Lafage V, Farcy JP, Bridwell KH, Glassman S, Shainline MR. Predicting outcome and complications in the surgical treatment of adult scoliosis. Spine. 2008; 33(20):2243–2247

[16] Ames CP, Smith JS, Eastlack R, et al. International Spine Study Group. Reliability assessment of a novel cervical spine deformity classification system. J Neurosurg Spine. 2015; 23(6):673–683

[17] Moore RE, Dormans JP, Drummond DS, Shore EM, Kaplan FS, Auerbach JD. Chin-on-chest deformity in patients with fibrodysplasia ossificans progressiva. A case series. J Bone Joint Surg Am. 2009; 91(6):1497–1502

[18] Lee JS, Youn MS, Shin JK, Goh TS, Kang SS. Relationship between cervical sagittal alignment and quality of life in ankylosing spondylitis. Eur Spine J. 2015; 24(6):1199–1203

[19] Gerling MC, Bohlman HH. Dropped head deformity due to cervical myopathy: surgical treatment outcomes and complications spanning twenty years. Spine. 2008; 33(20):E739–E745

[20] Protopsaltis TS, Scheer JK, Terran JS, et al. International Spine Study Group. How the neck affects the back: changes in regional cervical sagittal alignment correlate to HRQOL improvement in adult thoracolumbar deformity patients at 2-year follow-up. J Neurosurg Spine. 2015; 23(2):153–158

[21] Oh T, Scheer JK, Eastlack R, et al. International Spine Study Group. Cervical compensatory alignment changes following correction of adult thoracic deformity: a multicenter experience in 57 patients with a 2-year follow-up. J Neurosurg Spine. 2015; 22(6):658–665

[22] Smith JS, Shaffrey CI, Lafage V, et al. International Spine Study Group. Spontaneous improvement of cervical alignment after correction of global sagittal balance following pedicle subtraction osteotomy. J Neurosurg Spine. 2012; 17(4):300–307

[23] Lafage V, Diebo BSF. Sagittal Spino-Pelvic Alignment: From Theory to Clinical Application. (Quintanilla, ed.). Madrid, Spain: Editorial Medica Panamericana; 2015

[24] Gore DR. Roentgenographic findings in the cervical spine in asymptomatic persons: a ten-year follow-up. Spine. 2001; 26(22):2463–2466

[25] Tang JA, Scheer JK, Smith JS, et al. ISSG. The impact of standing regional cervical sagittal alignment on outcomes in posterior cervical fusion surgery. Neurosurgery. 2015; 76 Suppl 1:S14–S21, discussion S21

[26] Smith JS, Lafage V, Ryan DJ, et al. Association of myelopathy scores with cervical sagittal balance and normalized spinal cord volume: analysis of 56 preoperative cases from the AOSpine North America Myelopathy study. Spine. 2013; 38(22) Suppl 1:S161–S170

[27] Le Huec JC, Demezon H, Aunoble S. Sagittal parameters of global cervical balance using EOS imaging: normative values from a prospective cohort of asymptomatic volunteers. Eur Spine J. 2015; 24(1):63–71

[28] Protopsaltis TS, Terran J, Bronsard N, et al. T1 slope minus cervical lordosis (TS-CL), the cervical answer to PI-LL, defines cervical sagittal deformity in patients undergoing thoracolumbar osteotomy. In: Cervical Spine Research Society (CSRS) Annual Meeting; December 5–7, 2013

[29] Kim T-H, Lee SY, Kim YC, Park MS, Kim SW. T1 slope as a predictor of kyphotic alignment change after laminoplasty in patients with cervical myelopathy. Spine. 2013; 38(16):E992–E997

[30] Legaye J, Duval-Beaupère G, Hecquet J, Marty C. Pelvic incidence: a fundamental pelvic parameter for three-dimensional regulation of spinal sagittal curves. Eur Spine J. 1998; 7(2):99–103

[31] Blondel BSF, Ames CP, LeHuec JC, et al. The crucial role of cervical alignment in regulating sagittal spino-pelvic alignment in human standing posture. In: Podium Presented at 19th International Meeting on Advanced Spine Techniques. Istanbul, Turkey; 2012

[32] Hyun SJ, Kim KJ, Jahng TA, Kim HJ. Clinical impact of T1 slope minus cervical lordosis after multilevel posterior cervical fusion surgery: a minimum 2-year follow up data. Spine. 2017; 42(24):1859–1864

[33] Protopsaltis TS, Ramchandran S, Lafage R, et al. The importance of C2-Slope as a singular marker of cervical deformity and the link between upper- cervical and cervico-thoracic alignment among cervical deformity patients. Cervical Spine Research Society Annual Meeting (CSRS). Toronto, Canada; 2016

[34] Song K, Su X, Zhang Y, et al. Optimal chin-brow vertical angle for sagittal visual fields in ankylosing spondylitis kyphosis. Eur Spine J. 2016; 25(8):2596–2604

[35] Suk KS, Kim KT, Lee S-HS, Kim JM. Significance of chin-brow vertical angle in correction of kyphotic deformity of ankylosing spondylitis patients. Spine. 2003; 28(17):2001–2005

[36] Lafage R, Challier V, Liabaud B, et al. Natural head posture in the setting of sagittal spinal deformity: validation of chin-brow vertical angle, slope of line of sight, and McGregor's slope with health-related quality of life. Neurosurgery. 2016; 79(1):108–115

[37] Ramchandran S, Smith JS, Ailon T, et al. AOSpine North America, International Spine Study Group. Assessment of impact of long-cassette standing X-rays on surgical planning for cervical pathology: an International Survey of Spine Surgeons. Neurosurgery. 2016; 78(5):717–724

[38] Klineberg Eric O, Carlson Brandon B, Protopsaltis Themistocles S, et al; International Spine Study Group. Can Measurements on Cervical Radiographs Predict Concurrent Thoracolumbar Deformity and Provide a Threshold for Acquiring Full-Length Spine Radiographs? Chicago; 2015

[39] Knott PT, Mardjetko SM, Techy F. The use of the T1 sagittal angle in predicting overall sagittal balance of the spine. Spine J. 2010; 10(11):994–998

5 Cervical Disability Assessment

Nicholas D. Stekas and Themistocles S. Protopsaltis

Abstract

As the American healthcare climate continues to shift toward a model that emphasizes quality of care relative to cost, patient-reported outcome measures have become increasingly important as a way to quantify outcomes and assess baseline disability. Capturing disability in patients with cervical deformity has proven to be challenging. While patients with cervical deformity have been shown to be significantly disabled, few studies have shown a distinct relationship between sagittal malalignment and disability. As our understanding of patient-reported outcome measures and cervical deformity continues to evolve, further investigation will be required to develop outcome metrics that capture clinical symptoms that are important to patients with cervical deformity.

Keywords: cervical deformity, patient-reported outcome measures, health-related quality-of-life measures, Numeric Rating Scale, Visual Analog Scale, Neck Disability Index, Oswestry Disability Index, modified Japanese Orthopaedic Association Scale

5.1 Introduction

While the effects of thoracolumbar deformity on disability have been well studied,[1,2,3] recent research has aimed to describe the effect of cervical deformity on health status.[4,5] The analysis of outcomes and disability in cervical deformity patients have been less conclusive than those described in thoracolumbar literature, patients who undergo cervical deformity correction have been shown to have significant improvement.[6] However, the best methods to describe the morbidity associated with malalignment of the cervical spine have yet to be been fully elucidated. Given the recent importance placed on the assessments of both outcomes and disability in the American healthcare system, it is of paramount importance to identify the optimal methods to capture the disability inherent and specific to cervical deformity and quantify the benefits of correction.

In recent decades, the American healthcare climate has shifted from a volume based focus to a value-based model that emphasizes quality of care over quantity.[7] In the current healthcare landscape, the value of care is determined by the outcome obtained following intervention relative to cost.[8] In years past, outcome metrics were measured in the form of mortality rates but, more recently, health-related outcome questionnaires have gained popularity as a way to quantify patient outcomes.[8] Health-related outcome questionnaires ask relevant questions about a patient's general health and how a patient's life has been limited by his or her pathological symptoms.

A number of instruments have since been developed to measure pain, disability, and improvement following treatment in spine surgery, as well as other medical specialties, that have been used in both the clinical and research setting.[9] The goal of outcome assessment is to establish baseline disability, evaluate the effectiveness of various treatment options, and educate patients about their anticipated recovery following surgical or medical intervention.[9,10]

In the spine surgery literature, many outcome metrics have been assessed for their ability to capture disability and postoperative improvement with varying success. In both cervical and thoracolumbar literature, outcome measures have been shown to improve following spine surgery.[11,12,13,14] However, the disability inherent in patients with thoracolumbar deformity and cervical deformity is polyfactorial resulting from general frailty, neurologic compromise, as well as spinal malalignment; thus, an optimal outcome metric for sagittal malalignment has not been established.

In thoracolumbar spine literature, various health-related quality-of-life (HRQOL) measures have been shown to correlate with disability resulting from sagittal malalignment of the spine. Radiographic parameters to describe thoracolumbar malalignment have been shown to correlate with various HRQOL scores, with published correlation coefficients ranging from 0.3 to 0.5.[2,3,15,16,17] While several outcome metrics have shown significant correlation with sagittal malalignment of the thoracolumbar spine, studies that have managed to correlate sagittal malalignment with disability in the cervical spine have been much rarer and show more modest correlations.[18,19,20]

In a study of 113 patients undergoing posterior cervical fusion, Tang et al demonstrated that positive cervical sagittal alignment greater than 40 mm was associated with greater disability by the NDI and SF-36.[18] Additionally, in a cohort of 122 patients undergoing anterior cervical decompression and fusion (ACDF), Villavicencio et al demonstrated that improved or maintained cervical sagittal alignment was associated with superior outcomes in SF-36 and NDI.[19] Still, the association between outcome metrics and sagittal malalignment of the cervical spine remains elusive and an all-encompassing outcome metric to describe cervical deformity is yet to be found in the literature.

5.2 Challenges to Capturing Disability from Cervical Deformity

Surgical correction of cervical deformity is associated with increased potential for morbidity and neurologic injury. As such, the need for functional outcome assessment in patients with cervical deformity is great.[21] One contributing factor complicating the ability to capture disability from cervical deformity is the nature of neck pain itself. While neck pain is one of the most common complaints nationwide and one of the largest socioeconomic burdens on our current healthcare system,[22] several factors make assessing neck pain difficult. Neck pain is often a multifactorial condition and may be influenced by many factors outside of the cervical neck itself.[23,24] Indeed, most causes of common neck pain are unknown.[9,25] It has also been suggested that many complaints of primary neck pain have nonorganic causes, which may be associated with psychosocial factors.[26]

While neck pain can be difficult to capture with modern disability metrics, capturing disability from cervical deformity has proven to be even more difficult. Primary cervical deformity can result from a myriad of causes, including degenerative causes, congenital causes, or iatrogenic causes.[21] Additionally, cervical deformity can lead to a huge range of symptoms such as myelopathy, dysphagia, dyspnea, or severe chin-on-chest deformity which compromises horizontal gaze.[4,27,28] It is possible that the complex symptom profile of cervical deformity has contributed to the difficulty in developing an all-encompassing outcome metric to describe disability associated with this debilitating condition.

Finally, the applicability of currently utilized disability assessment measures in cervical spine literature has not been sufficiently investigated in cervical deformity populations. While many outcome assessment tools have been investigated for their correlation to various cervical pathologies and cervical malalignment, existing outcome questionnaires were not designed to capture cervical deformity specifically. Existing questionnaires are limited in that they do not currently address disabilities that are unique and debilitating to cervical deformity patients specifically, including symptoms like gaze limitation or swallowing.

It has been suggested that, eventually, a cervical deformity-specific outcome questionnaire may be necessary to assess baseline disability and the success of corrective surgery. Studies reporting on outcomes following cervical spine problems utilize several different outcome metrics in an attempt to best capture the patient's pain and disability. In general, outcome metrics for patients undergoing cervical deformity correction should capture neck pain, arm pain, and compensatory back pain in addition to limitations in quality of life until more specific outcome metrics to capture the disability inherent in cervical deformity are developed.

5.3 Important Terminology in Describing Outcome Metrics

The utility and applicability of outcome metrics are often assessed based on validity, reliability, and ability to detect change in health.[29] Validity refers to the agreeability of an outcome metric with previously reported outcome metrics.[30] Assessment tools that correlate very strongly with other published measures (associated with Pearson correlations > 0.8) are considered to have strong validity.[30]

Reliability is a term used to describe the reproducibility of an outcome metric in capturing a given pathology within the same study subject.[31] Outcome metrics with good reliability are associated with a great degree of consistency between questionnaire scores at two different time points in the same subject or when measured by two different observers.[31] Traditionally, a Pearson coefficient of 0.75 indicates acceptable reliability.[32]

The ability of an outcome metric to detect change in health status is measured using the minimum clinically important different (MCID). In the technical sense, the MCID was defined by Jaeschke et al in 1989 as "The smallest difference in score in the domain of interest which patients perceive as beneficial...."[33,34] While there are several methods of calculating the MCID for an outcome metric, calculations attempt to use the metric in question to measure a patient's internal values and predict changes in medical management.[33]

5.4 Currently Utilized Outcome Metrics of Cervical Deformity

5.4.1 Pain Outcome Metrics

Numeric Rating Scale and Visual Analog Scale

The numeric rating scale (NRS) is one of the most commonly used outcome metrics to capture pain in the clinical setting.[35] Using the NRS Neck, patients are asked to grade their neck pain on a scale of 0 to 10 with 0 being no pain and 10 being the worst pain possibly imaginable.[9] The visual analog scale (VAS) is similar to the NRS Neck, but instead pain is graded using visual cues rather than a numeric scale. Most commonly, patients are asked to mark their pain on a continuous 10-cm line, which the evaluator will then measure to obtain a VAS score ranging from 1 to 100 mm.[36]

The NRS and VAS are the most common pain metrics used clinically today due to ease of use and success in capturing pain.[9] The VAS Neck pain scale has been shown to have strong test–retest reliability, estimated to be 0.95.[37] However, more recent studies have suggested that the reliability of VAS Neck and VAS Arm pain is closer to 0.874 and 0.810, respectively.[36] In general, the VAS Neck pain is believed to be both valid and reliable in regard to assessing pain intensity in the neck and is often used as the gold standard when comparing new rating methods.[9,38] However, it is associated with several limitations.

It is well known that symptoms resulting from cervical neck pathologies, like cervical radiculopathy or myelopathy, may manifest as symptoms in the arms or subjacent spine structures. As such, when investigating pathologies of the cervical neck, it is important to capture pain in the neck, the back, and the limbs separately whenever possible. Despite ease of use, strong reliability, and good validity, the NRS and VAS pain scales are limited by the fact that they do not capture disability or symptoms other than pain. For a more comprehensive disability assessment, it is important to assess for motor pathologies, sensory pathologies, autonomic insufficiency, as well as how symptoms are affecting daily life.

5.4.2 Disability Outcome Metrics

Neck Disability Index

The Neck Disability Index (NDI) was developed in 1991 and is the oldest questionnaire developed to measure disability from neck pathologies.[39,40,41,42] As of 2008, the NDI had been translated into 22 languages and had been cited in over 300 publications.[43] Unlike the NRS Neck and VAS Neck pain assessment metrics, the NDI has the advantage of measuring cumulative disability rather than simply intensity of pain. The NDI was modeled after the Oswestry Disability Index (ODI), which is a validated and reliable outcome metric widely considered to be the gold standard in capturing disability from back pain.[39,40,41] Since its development, the NDI has become the most widely used scale in describing neck disability and is widely considered to be one of the most reliable neck disability metrics.[39,42,43]

Originally, the NDI was designed with six items from the ODI scale including pain intensity, lifting, sleeping, driving, personal care, and sex life.[44] Later, four more items were added: headache, concentration, reading, and working resulting in a complete 10-item questionnaire.[39,44] The NDI questionnaire was then finalized after being specifically tailored to patients who had undergone whiplash injury to the cervical neck.[39,42] Each of the 10 questions in the NDI is evaluated on a scale of 0 to 5, with 0 being no disability and 5 being maximal disability. The total score, which ranges from 0 to 50, may then be doubled to calculate a disability percentage, which has been used to help account for missing questions that have not been answered.[45,46] An NDI score of 0 to 4 indicates no disability, a score of 5 to 24 indicates mild disability, a score of 15 to 25 is considered moderate disability, a score of 25 to 34 is considered severe disability, and a score greater than 35 is considered complete disability.[42,43]

Despite being much more tailored to capturing total disability than the VAS and NRS Neck pain scores, the NDI has been shown to have a relatively small burden in terms of the difficulty in completing the questionnaire. Current literature has suggested that the time needed to complete the questionnaire is less than 10 minutes and the time needed to analyze the questionnaire is about five minutes.[39,47]

In addition to being accessible and easy to complete, the NDI has also been shown to have strong validity. A systematic review conducted by Macdermid et al found that the NDI correlated strongly with VAS acute pain scores and moderately with the Short-Form 36 questionnaire as well as VAS chronic pain scores.[39] However, measurements of the retest reliability of the NDI have been slightly more ambiguous. While several studies report reliability coefficients greater than 0.9,[46,48,49] more recent high-powered studies have shown lower reliability.[45,50] It has been postulated that the utility of the NDI is pathology specific and may be more reliable for chronic pain than acute pain.[39,46,49]

Given that disability assessment with the NDI has shown variability based on different pathological states, more research is needed to analyze how well the NDI captures disability in cases of cervical deformity. The NDI was validated in patients presenting to a chiropractic practice and has since been classically used to describe disability from whiplash injuries.[42] Unfortunately, the NDI does not account for several crucial pathologic symptoms relevant to cervical deformity, including arm pain, weakness, sensory pain, horizontal gaze, or difficulty swallowing. However, in recent years, an attempt has been made to apply the NDI to cervical deformity literature with mixed results.

While HRQOL outcomes generally fail to correlate substantially with malalignment of the cervical spine, NDI scores have been shown to be decreased at baseline in patients with substantial deformity. Increased cervical sagittal vertical axis in particular has been implicated in poor NDI scores. Tang et al used the NDI to define a threshold of disability of a cSVA greater than 4 cm.[18] Iyer et al reported that increasing T1S cervical lordosis mismatch (TS-CL) and increased cSVA were both independent risk factors for decreased NDI at baseline.[51] Another recent study found that the most important alignment parameters of the cervical neck in impacting outcome metrics, including NDI scores, were the cSVA, C0–C2 angle, and the C2–C7 angle.[52]

While current cervical deformity literature is not conclusive regarding direct correlations between cervical alignment parameters and outcome metrics, there has been considerable progress made in understanding how cervical malalignment and corrective surgery for cervical deformity affects quality of life. While the NDI remains a key measure of disability from cervical deformity, it does have limitations to its use to describe how sagittal imbalance of the cervical spine influences health outcomes.

Modified Japanese Orthopaedic Association Scale

The Japanese Orthopaedic Association (JOA) score was developed in 1975 to measure disability associated specifically with cervical myelopathy and has since been modified to be more applicable to western cultures.[53,54,55] The Modified Japanese Orthopaedic Association (mJOA) assesses both motor and sensory neurologic impairment in the limbs, the trunk, and autonomic function in an attempt to grade severity associated with cervical myelopathy.[53] The scale is scored from a minimum of 0 (indicating maximum disability) to 18 (normal function). mJOA scores greater than or equal to 15 are considered mild myelopathy, scores from 12 to 14 are considered moderate myelopathy, and scores below 12 are considered severe myelopathy.[56]

While the mJOA is somewhat limited as a disability tool due to the fact that it is specifically designed to capture symptoms of myelopathy, it has been shown to be associated with similar scores for other reported outcome measures of the cervical spine. In a study of 757 patients with cervical myelopathy, mJOA scores lower than 11 were associated with significantly worse quality of life as measured by the NDI and SF-36.[57] In cervical deformity literature, a study conducted by Liu et al showed that mJOA scores correlated with spondylolisthesis, maximum kyphotic segment angulation, and segmental cones of kinesis in cervical myelopathy paitents.[58] However, as outcome assessment in cervical deformity continues to improve, it is becoming increasingly important to discover how cervical deformity affects one's overall health and how to best predict postoperative outcomes.

5.4.3 Quality-of-Life Outcome Metrics
Short-Form 36 Survey

The Short-Form 36 Survey (SF-36) was developed as part of the Rand Health Insurance Study, in an attempt to quantify the effects of different insurance plans on health outcomes.[59] Since then, the SF-36 survey has been utilized to quantify health status in many different disease states, including various cervical and thoracolumbar spine pathologies.[60] Unlike traditional disability assessment metrics like the NDI and mJOA, the SF-36 survey was designed to measure total health status that is standardized across all disease states, rather than specific to certain pathologies.[60] To date, the SF-36 has been cited by thousands of journal articles.

The survey measures general disability as it relates to eight major categories: vitality, physical functioning, bodily pain, general health perceptions, physical role functioning, emotional role functioning, social role functioning, and mental health.[60,61]

Unlike the ODI and NDI, the SF-36 questionnaire is scored with a summary score rather than a raw score, which functions as a direct comparison to the standard deviation of answers obtained from the general population.[62]

The SF-36 is one of the most commonly used outcome metrics used in modern medicine and has been used successfully as an outcome metric in both cervical and thoracolumbar literature.[63,64] It has been shown that the SF-36 is comparable in its ability to capture disability from cervical pathologies similarly to the NDI[64] and mJOA.[64,65] However, the SF-36 questionnaire is unique to these outcome metrics in its generalizability to compare neck pathologies to other disease states as well as its ability to account for both physical and mental morbidities associated with spinal disease.[60,66]

Like the NDI, the SF-36 has shown limited utility in capturing disability from cervical deformity. The SF-36 has also been shown to correlate with increased cSVA at baseline.[18] In a recent study of 757 patients with undergoing cervical fusion, cervical deformity postoperatively was associated with significantly lower SF-36 scores.[67] One of the most important contributions to cervical deformity literature using the SF-36 questionnaire has been the defining of age-adjusted alignment parameters. Lafage et al used normative values of the SF-36 to define age-adjusted alignment thresholds in thoracolumbar deformity patients to conclude that elderly patients benefit from less rigorous deformity corrections.[68]

EuroQuol-5 Dimension

The EuroQuol-5 Dimension (EQ-5D) survey was first developed by the Euro-QOL group in 1990 in an attempt to capture generic health status in a concise and easily accessible questionnaire.[69] Like the SF-36, the EQ-5D attempts to quantify overall health status independent of particular pathologies.[70] As such, both questionnaires can be used to compare overall health across different disease states. With the current healthcare climate's emphasis on cost-effective treatment, the questionnaire has become an important outcome metric to assess quality-of-life years, a standard metric used to define cost-effectiveness care by the U.S. Panel on Cost-Effectiveness in Health and Medicine.[71,72] The EQ-5D assesses five dimensions of overall health status, including mobility, self-care, usual activities, pain/discomfort, and anxiety/depression.[73]

In addition to capturing overall health status, the EQ-5D has several other advantages as well, including its wide applicability and ease of completion.[70] To date, the EQ-5D has been translated into 171 languages[73] and is a simple questionnaire consisting of only five questions with three response categories, taking only a few minutes to complete.[71,73]

While the EQ-5D has gained popularity across many specialties, its validation and utility in cervical spine pathologies requires further investigation. One high-power study of 3,732 patients with degenerative cervical spine disorders found only a modest regression model predicting the EQ-5D using NDI scores, neck pain scores, and arm pain scores.[74] Another study found that the EQ-5D was inferior to the SF-6D score (a shortened version of the SF-36) when capturing quality of life in patients undergoing elective cervical spine surgery.[75]

While the EQ-5D has generally not shown excellent correlations with previously described outcome metrics in cervical literature, it has been utilized effectively to describe overall health status of cervical deformity compared to other disease states. A recent study by Smith et al has shown that EQ-5D patients are significantly disabled at baseline, with health scores similar to pathologies such as blindness, emphysema, renal failure, and stroke.[76]

5.4.4 Patient-Reported Outcomes Measurement Information System

Patient-Reported Outcomes Measurement Information System (PROMIS) was developed in 2004 by the National Institutes of Health to address the shortcomings of previously established outcome metrics and establish a more reliable, valid, and generalizable measures of clinical outcomes.[77] The PROMIS survey has gained recent popularity in part due to computer adaptive testing (CAT). Using CAT, response theory is utilized to customize the questionnaire based on the patient's previous responses.[30]

The PROMIS CAT questionnaire measures general health status in three main domains: physical health, mental health, and social health.[78] The scores from the questionnaire are then reported as a T-score, which is normalized to the general population with the mean set to 50 and a standard deviation set to 10.[78] The PROMIS CAT algorithm has several advantages for both questionnaire administrators and patients alike, including ease of questionnaire completion, greater precision for patients, and an intuitive scoring scale.[78]

Given the relative novelty of the PROMIS questionnaire, more research is needed to elucidate its utility in cervical spine pathology. One study of 148 patients undergoing cervical spine surgery found moderate to strong correlations between PROMIS scores and the NDI and SF-12v2 (a modified version of the SF-36 survey).[79] Another recent study of 59 patients with degenerative cervical spine disorders found that PROMIS demonstrated strong validity and comparable responsiveness to previously described outcome metrics including the NDI and the SF-12.[80] While conclusive data regarding how well PROMIS captures cervical deformity has yet to be published, future investigations will likely be aimed at investigating how PROMIS scores correlate with sagittal imbalance of the cervical spine.

5.5 The Future of Disability Assessment in Adult Cervical Deformity

While cervical deformity has been shown to be associated with severe morbidity and poor health status, quantifying outcome measures have been challenging. Several outcome measures of disability, including the NRS Neck, VAS Neck, NDI, mJOA, SF-36, EQ-5D, and PROMIS, have all been used in cervical deformity literature with some success. However, none of these metrics are without their limitations. In comparison to thoracolumbar literature, outcome and disability assessment has proven a great challenge for cervical deformity. To date, few studies have managed to correlate outcome metrics with sagittal imbalance of the cervical spine or predict surgical outcomes using currently available outcome metrics.

Current outcome metrics used in cervical deformity literature fail to capture certain crucial symptoms that cervical deformity patients commonly find disabling, including gaze restriction and dysphagia. As a result, it is important to use multiple disability assessment metrics to assess pain, disability, and health status in patients afflicted with cervical deformity to gain maximum understanding of health status. However, as the literature evolves, the development of a cervical deformity–specific outcome metric will likely, one day, play a large role in establishing a full understanding of this complex pathology.

References

[1] Protopsaltis TS, Schwab FJ, Smith JS, et al. The T1 pelvic angle (TPA), a novel radiographic parameter of sagittal deformity, correlates strongly with clinical measures of disability. Spine J. 2013; 13:S61

[2] Lafage V, Schwab F, Patel A, Hawkinson N, Farcy JP. Pelvic tilt and truncal inclination: two key radiographic parameters in the setting of adults with spinal deformity. Spine. 2009; 34(17):E599–E606

[3] Glassman SD, Bridwell K, Dimar JR, Horton W, Berven S, Schwab F. The impact of positive sagittal balance in adult spinal deformity. Spine. 2005; 30 (18):2024–2029

[4] Lee JS, Youn MS, Shin JK, Goh TS, Kang SS. Relationship between cervical sagittal alignment and quality of life in ankylosing spondylitis. Eur Spine J. 2015; 24(6):1199–1203

[5] Scheer JK, Tang JA, Smith JS, et al. International Spine Study Group. Cervical spine alignment, sagittal deformity, and clinical implications: a review. J Neurosurg Spine. 2013; 19(2):141–159

[6] Smith JS, Shaffrey CI, Kim HJ, et al. Outcomes of operative treatment for adult cervical deformity: a prospective multicenter assessment with one-year follow-up. Spine J. 2016; 16:S351–S352

[7] Porter ME. What is value in health care? N Engl J Med. 2010; 363(26):2477–2481

[8] Porter ME, Larsson S, Lee TH. Standardizing patient outcomes measurement. N Engl J Med. 2016; 374(6):504–506

[9] Misailidou V, Malliou P, Beneka A, Karagiannidis A, Godolias G. Assessment of patients with neck pain: a review of definitions, selection criteria, and measurement tools. J Chiropr Med. 2010; 9(2):49–59

[10] Liebenson C, Yeomans S. Outcomes assessment in musculoskeletal medicine. Man Ther. 1997; 2(2):67–74

[11] Mokhtar SA, McCombe PF, Williamson OD, Morgan MK, White GJ, Sears WR. Health-related quality of life: a comparison of outcomes after lumbar fusion for degenerative spondylolisthesis with large joint replacement surgery and population norms. Spine J. 2010; 10(4):306–312

[12] Bohtz C, Meyer-Heim A, Min K. Changes in health-related quality of life after spinal fusion and scoliosis correction in patients with cerebral palsy. J Pediatr Orthop. 2011; 31(6):668–673

[13] Schroeder GD, Boody BS, Kepler CK, et al. Comparing health-related quality of life outcomes in patients undergoing either primary or revision anterior cervical discectomy and fusion. Spine. 2018; 43(13):E752–E757

[14] Poorman GW, Passias PG, Horn SR, et al. International Spine Study Group. Despite worse baseline status depressed patients achieved outcomes similar to those in nondepressed patients after surgery for cervical deformity. Neurosurg Focus. 2017; 43(6):E10

[15] Protopsaltis T, Schwab F, Bronsard N, et al. International Spine Study Group. The T1 pelvic angle, a novel radiographic measure of global sagittal deformity, accounts for both spinal inclination and pelvic tilt and correlates with health-related quality of life. J Bone Joint Surg Am. 2014; 96(19):1631–1640

[16] Legaye J, Duval-Beaupère G, Hecquet J, Marty C. Pelvic incidence: a fundamental pelvic parameter for three-dimensional regulation of spinal sagittal curves. Eur Spine J. 1998; 7(2):99–103

[17] Terran J, Schwab F, Shaffrey CI, et al. International Spine Study Group. The SRS-Schwab adult spinal deformity classification: assessment and clinical correlations based on a prospective operative and nonoperative cohort. Neurosurgery. 2013; 73(4):559–568

[18] Tang JA, Scheer JK, Smith JS, et al. ISSG. The impact of standing regional cervical sagittal alignment on outcomes in posterior cervical fusion surgery. Neurosurgery. 2015; 76 Suppl 1:S14–S21, discussion S21

[19] Villavicencio AT, Babuska JM, Ashton A, et al. Prospective, randomized, double-blind clinical study evaluating the correlation of clinical outcomes and cervical sagittal alignment. Neurosurgery. 2011; 68(5):1309–1316, discussion 1316

[20] Protopsaltis TS, Terran J, Bronsard N, et al. T1 slope minus cervical lordosis (TS-CL), the cervical answer to PI-LL, defines cervical sagittal deformity in patients undergoing thoracolumbar osteotomy. In: Cervical Spine Research Society (CSRS) Annual Meeting; December 5–7, 2013

[21] Etame AB, Wang AC, Than KD, La Marca F, Park P. Outcomes after surgery for cervical spine deformity: review of the literature. Neurosurg Focus. 2010; 28 (3):E14

[22] Hoy D, March L, Woolf A, et al. The global burden of neck pain: estimates from the global burden of disease 2010 study. Ann Rheum Dis. 2014; 73 (7):1309–1315

[23] MacDermid JC, Walton DM, Bobos P, Lomotan M, Carlesso L. A qualitative description of chronic neck pain has implications for outcome assessment and classification. Open Orthop J. 2016; 10:746–756

[24] Guzman J, Hurwitz EL, Carroll LJ, et al. Bone and Joint Decade 2000–2010 Task Force on Neck Pain and Its Associated Disorders. A new conceptual model of neck pain: linking onset, course, and care: the Bone and Joint Decade 2000–2010 Task Force on neck pain and its associated disorders. Spine. 2008; 33(4) Suppl:S14–S23

[25] Bogduk NMB. Management of acute and chronic neck pain: an evidence based approach. 2006

[26] Ariëns GA, van Mechelen W, Bongers PM, Bouter LM, van der Wal G. Psychosocial risk factors for neck pain: a systematic review. Am J Ind Med. 2001; 39 (2):180–193

[27] Moore RE, Dormans JP, Drummond DS, Shore EM, Kaplan FS, Auerbach JD. Chin-on-chest deformity in patients with fibrodysplasia ossificans progressiva. A case series. J Bone Joint Surg Am. 2009; 91(6):1497–1502

[28] Gerling MC, Bohlman HH. Dropped head deformity due to cervical myopathy: surgical treatment outcomes and complications spanning twenty years. Spine. 2008; 33(20):E739–E745

[29] Hawkins RJ. Recommendations for evaluating and selecting appropriately valued outcome measures. Instr Course Lect. 2016; 65:587–591

[30] Fidai MS, Saltzman BM, Meta F, et al. Patient-reported outcomes measurement information system and legacy patient-reported outcome measures in the field of orthopaedics: a systematic review. Arthroscopy. 2018; 34(2):605–614

[31] Alrubaiy L, Hutchings HA, Williams JG. Assessing patient reported outcome measures: A practical guide for gastroenterologists. United European Gastroenterol J. 2014; 2(6):463–470

[32] Health measurement scales: a practical guide to their development and use (5th edition). Aust N Z J Public Health. 2016; 40(3):294–295

[33] Cook CE. Clinimetrics Corner: the Minimal Clinically Important Change Score (MCID): a necessary pretense. J Manual Manip Ther. 2008; 16(4):E82–E83

[34] Jaeschke R, Singer J, Guyatt GH. Measurement of health status. Ascertaining the minimal clinically important difference. Control Clin Trials. 1989; 10 (4):407–415

[35] Teles AR, Khoshhal KI, Falavigna A. Why and how should we measure outcomes in spine surgery? J Taibah Univ Med Sci. 2016; 11(2):91–97

[36] MacDowall A, Skeppholm M, Robinson Y, et al. Validation of the visual analog scale in the cervical spine. J Neurosurg Spine. 2018; 28(3):227–235

[37] McDowell INC. Measuring Health. A Guide to Rating Scales and Questionnaires. New York, NY: Oxford University Press; 1996

[38] Nordin M, Carragee EJ, Hogg-Johnson S, et al. Assessment of neck pain and its associated disorders: results of the Bone and Joint Decade 2000–2010 Task Force on neck pain and its associated disorders. J Manipulative Physiol Ther. 2009; 32(2) Suppl:S117–S140

[39] MacDermid JC, Walton DM, Avery S, et al. Measurement properties of the neck disability index: a systematic review. J Orthop Sports Phys Ther. 2009; 39(5):400–417

[40] Fairbank JC, Pynsent PB. The Oswestry Disability Index. Spine. 2000; 25 (22):2940–2952, discussion 2952

[41] Maughan EF, Lewis JS. Outcome measures in chronic low back pain. Eur Spine J. 2010; 19(9):1484–1494

[42] Vernon H, Mior S. The Neck Disability Index: a study of reliability and validity. J Manipulative Physiol Ther. 1991; 14(7):409–415

[43] Vernon H. The Neck Disability Index: state-of-the-art, 1991–2008. J Manipulative Physiol Ther. 2008; 31(7):491–502

[44] Howell ER. The association between neck pain, the Neck Disability Index and cervical ranges of motion: a narrative review. J Can Chiropr Assoc. 2011; 55 (3):211–221

[45] Cleland JA, Fritz JM, Whitman JM, Palmer JA. The reliability and construct validity of the Neck Disability Index and patient specific functional scale in patients with cervical radiculopathy. Spine. 2006; 31(5):598–602

[46] Ackelman BH, Lindgren U. Validity and reliability of a modified version of the neck disability index. J Rehabil Med. 2002; 34(6):284–287

[47] Jorritsma W, de Vries GE, Geertzen JHB, Dijkstra PU, Reneman MF. Neck Pain and Disability Scale and the Neck Disability Index: reproducibility of the Dutch language versions. Eur Spine J. 2010; 19(10):1695–1701

[48] Wlodyka-Demaille S, Poiraudeau S, Catanzariti J-F, Rannou F, Fermanian J, Revel M. French translation and validation of 3 functional disability scales for neck pain. Arch Phys Med Rehabil. 2002; 83(3):376–382

[49] Cook C, Richardson JK, Braga L, et al. Cross-cultural adaptation and validation of the Brazilian Portuguese version of the Neck Disability Index and Neck Pain and Disability Scale. Spine. 2006; 31(14):1621–1627

[50] Cleland JA, Childs JD, Whitman JM. Psychometric properties of the Neck Disability Index and Numeric Pain Rating Scale in patients with mechanical neck pain. Arch Phys Med Rehabil. 2008; 89(1):69–74

[51] Iyer S, Nemani VM, Nguyen J, et al. Impact of cervical sagittal alignment parameters on neck disability. Spine. 2016; 41(5):371–377

[52] Bao H, Varghese J, Lafage R, et al. Principal radiographic characteristics for cervical spinal deformity: a health-related quality of life analysis. Spine. 2017; 42(18):1375–1382

[53] Kato S, Oshima Y, Oka H, et al. Comparison of the Japanese Orthopaedic Association (JOA) score and modified JOA (mJOA) score for the assessment of cervical myelopathy: a multicenter observational study. PLoS One. 2015; 10(4): e0123022

[54] Japanese Orthopaedic Association. Scoring system for cervical myelopathy. J Jpn. 1994:490–503

[55] Boos N, Aebi ME. Degenerative Disorders of the Cervical Spine. New York, NY: Springer-Verlag Berlin Heidelberg; 2008

[56] Fehlings MG, Wilson JR, Kopjar B, et al. Efficacy and safety of surgical decompression in patients with cervical spondylotic myelopathy: results of the AOSpine North America prospective multi-center study. J Bone Joint Surg Am. 2013; 95(18):1651–1658

[57] Tetreault L, Kopjar B, Nouri A, et al. The modified Japanese Orthopaedic Association scale: establishing criteria for mild, moderate and severe impairment in patients with degenerative cervical myelopathy. Eur Spine J. 2017; 26 (1):78–84

[58] Liu S, Lafage R, Smith JS, et al. The Impact of Dynamic Alignment, Motion, and Center of Rotation on Myelopathy Grade and Regional Disability in Cervical Spondylotic Myelopathy. In: International Meeting on Advanced Spine Techniques (IMAST); July 16–19, 2014; Valencia, Spain

[59] Ware JE, Jr, Sherbourne CD. The MOS 36-item short-form health survey (SF-36). I. Conceptual framework and item selection. Med Care. 1992; 30(6):473–483

[60] Guilfoyle MR, Seeley H, Laing RJ. The Short Form 36 health survey in spine disease–validation against condition-specific measures. Br J Neurosurg. 2009; 23(4):401–405

[61] Ware J, Kosinski M, Dewey J, et al. SF-36 health survey: manual and interpretation guide. Boston. Available at: http://scholar.google.com/scholar? hl=en&btnG=Search&q=intitle:SF-36+Health+Survey+Manual+and+Interpretation+Guide#0. 2000. Accessed April 5, 2015

[62] Liem YS, Bosch JL, Arends LR, Heijenbrok-Kal MH, Hunink MG. Quality of life assessed with the Medical Outcomes Study Short Form 36-Item Health Survey of patients on renal replacement therapy: a systematic review and meta-analysis. Value Health. 2007; 10(5):390–397

[63] Grevitt M, Khazim R, Webb J, Mulholland R, Shepperd J. The short form-36 health survey questionnaire in spine surgery. J Bone Joint Surg Br. 1997; 79 (1):48–52

[64] McCarthy MJH, Grevitt MP, Silcocks P, Hobbs G. The reliability of the Vernon and Mior neck disability index, and its validity compared with the short form-36 health survey questionnaire. Eur Spine J. 2007; 16(12):2111–2117

[65] Singh A, Crockard HA. Comparison of seven different scales used to quantify severity of cervical spondylotic myelopathy and post-operative improvement. J Outcome Meas. 2001–2002; 5(1):798–818

[66] Stoll T, Kauer Y, Büchi S, Klaghofer R, Sensky T, Villiger PM. Prediction of depression in systemic lupus erythematosus patients using SF-36 Mental Health scores. Rheumatology (Oxford). 2001; 40(6):695–698

[67] Kato S, Nouri A, Wu D, et al. Impact of cervical spine deformity on preoperative disease severity and post-operative outcomes following fusion surgery for degenerative cervical myelopathy - sub-analysis of AOSpine North America and International Studies. Spine (Phila Pa 1976). 2018 Feb 15; 43(4):248–254

[68] Lafage R, Schwab F, Challier V, et al. International Spine Study Group. Defining spino-pelvic alignment thresholds: should operative goals in adult spinal deformity surgery account for age? Spine. 2016; 41(1):62–68

[69] EuroQol Group. EuroQol–a new facility for the measurement of health-related quality of life. Health Policy. 1990; 16(3):199–208

[70] Rabin R, de Charro F. EQ-5D: a measure of health status from the EuroQol Group. Ann Med. 2001; 33(5):337–343

[71] Payakachat N, Ali MM, Tilford JM. Can The EQ-5D detect meaningful change? A systematic review. Pharmacoeconomics. 2015; 33(11):1137–1154

[72] Weinstein MC, Siegel JE, Gold MR, Kamlet MS, Russell LB. Recommendations of the panel on cost-effectiveness in health and medicine. JAMA. 1996; 276 (15):1253–1258

[73] van Reenen M, Oppe M. EQ-5D-3 L user guide: basic information on how to use the EQ-5D-3 L instrument. Euro Qol Res Found 2015:22

[74] Carreon LY, Bratcher KR, Das N, Nienhuis JB, Glassman SD. Estimating EQ-5D values from the Neck Disability Index and numeric rating scales for neck and arm pain. J Neurosurg Spine. 2014; 21(3):394–399

[75] Chotai S, Parker SL, Sivaganesan A, Godil SS, McGirt MJ, Devin CJ. Quality of life and general health after elective surgery for cervical spine pathologies: determining a valid and responsive metric of health state utility. Neurosurgery. 2015; 77(4):553–560, discussion 560

[76] Smith JS, Line B, Bess S, et al. The health impact of adult cervical deformity in patients presenting for surgical treatment: comparison to United States population norms and chronic disease states based on the EuroQuol-5 Dimensions Questionnaire. Neurosurgery. 2017; 80(5):716–725

[77] Cella D, Yount S, Rothrock N, et al. PROMIS Cooperative Group. The Patient-Reported Outcomes Measurement Information System (PROMIS): progress of an NIH Roadmap cooperative group during its first two years. Med Care. 2007; 45(5) Suppl 1:S3–S11

[78] Brodke DJ, Saltzman CL, Brodke DS. PROMIS for orthopaedic outcomes measurement. J Am Acad Orthop Surg. 2016; 24(11):744–749

[79] Purvis TE, Andreou E, Neuman BJ, Riley LH, III, Skolasky RL. Concurrent validity and responsiveness of PROMIS health domains among patients presenting for anterior cervical spine surgery. Spine. 2017; 42(23):E1357–E1365

[80] Boody BS, Bhatt S, Mazmudar AS, Hsu WK, Rothrock NE, Patel AA. Validation of Patient-Reported Outcomes Measurement Information System (PROMIS) computerized adaptive tests in cervical spine surgery. J Neurosurg Spine. 2018; 28(3):268–279

6 Cervical Malalignment and Disability Scores

Sravisht Iyer, Han Jo Kim, and K. Daniel Riew

Abstract

As our understanding of cervical deformity has grown over the past several years, so too has our appreciation for the significant disability these deformities can cause. This chapter explores this aspect of cervical malalignment. We review the current outcome measures used to measure disability, the Neck Disability Index, and the Short-Form 36 Physical Component Score. We discuss the limitations of these measurements in the context of cervical deformity and discuss the characteristics of an ideal outcome measure. Finally, we explore three areas of cervical alignment: occipitocervical, subaxial, and cervicothoracic that have received increasing attention as drivers of disability. The importance of the line of sight parameters, C0–C2 angle, C2–C7 angle, C2–C7 sagittal vertical axis, and T1 slope minus cervical lordosis, are all discussed in the context of harmonious spinal alignment. Lastly, we discuss the substantial dysphagia experienced by adult cervical deformity patients preoperatively.

Keywords: cervical alignment, disability scores, cervical lordosis, C2–C7 SVA, TS–CL, line of sight, NDI, SF-36

6.1 Introduction

Cervical deformity and malalignment is a topic that has been receiving increased interest in the recent years. It has become apparent that a significant number of patients with thoracolumbar adult spinal deformity have concomitant cervical deformity.[1,2,3,4] As more attention has been paid to compensatory changes in spine surgery, there has been a growing understanding of reciprocal changes in cervical alignment with thoracolumbar deformity surgery.[5,6] There has been a growing appreciation of the fact that these changes in alignment can have a real correlation with patient disability.

The importance of cervical alignment is not surprising given the paramount importance of horizontal gaze in day-to-day life. Many of the compensatory mechanisms described in the adult deformity literature serve one of two purposes: (1) to enable standing within a cone of economy and (2) to maintain horizontal gaze.[1,7,8] While the thoracolumbar spine responds to the first goal, the cervical spine must often make reciprocal changes to enable the second.[8] These reciprocal changes, however, can sometimes result in neck pain, dysphagia, or other complaints that can cause significant disability. This chapter seeks to organize the existing literature on cervical malalignment and its impact on disability as quantified by health-related quality-of-life (HRQOL) scores.

6.2 The Challenge of Measuring Disability in the Cervical Spine

While there is no question that cervical deformity can cause significant disability, measuring the degree of disability can frequently be challenging. This difficulty represents a key limitation of much of the literature discussed in this chapter.

Currently, the disability caused by cervical pathology is measured using a number of disease-specific patient-reported outcome (PROs) measures or surgeon-administered tools to evaluate functional status.[9,10] None of these measures, however, have proven themselves to be a "gold standard" for cervical pathology.[11,12] Examples of widely used PROs include the Neck Disability Index (NDI), the neck and arm pain Visual Analog Scale (VAS), and the 36-Item Short-Form Health Survey (SF-36). Examples of investigator-administered tools include the modified Japanese Orthopedic Association (mJOA) and Nurick scales.

The NDI, the most commonly used PRO,[13] illustrates many of the limitations of the current generation of PROs. Because the NDI was originally developed as an instrument for patients with neck pain and whiplash-associated disorders, the majority of validation of the NDI has focused on this patient population.[13] The authors could not identify any study that has validated the psychometric properties of NDI in patients with myelopathy, although it has been used to describe outcomes in this patient population.[14,15,16] Furthermore, the literature on NDI in patients with cervical radiculopathy has yielded mixed results.[9,17,18,19,20] For instance Young et al have shown that the NDI has poor construct validity in patients with cervical radiculopathy and may suffer from limited test–retest reliability (intraclass correlation coefficient [ICC] = 0.55).[21] Other authors have suggested that the NDI may be multidimensional instrument making it difficult to calculate change of score and other parametric statistics with NDI data.[20] And although NDI has been shown to be responsive to cervical surgery, there is no clear definition of a minimum clinically important difference (MCID); values calculated in the literature vary from 3.5 to 9.5 on a 0 to 50 scale.[9,11,17,22] The difficulty in calculating MCID and larger MCIDs has been attributed to the fact that the NDI was not designed with cervical radiculopathy patients in mind.[13] The NDI may also have significant floor effects in patients with cervical spine disorders.[23]

To our knowledge, there are no studies that have validated or attempted to validate the utility of NDI in patients with cervical deformity. The NDI functions as a pain-interference (PI) scale; that is, it seeks to examine how neck pain affects functions of daily living. Therefore, it may serve to measure how cervical deformity affects neck pain. It does not, however, directly address important consequences of cervical deformity (e.g., in ability to maintain horizontal gaze and difficulty swallowing).

General outcome measures such as the SF-36 also have substantial shortcomings. In a survey of 147 patients, Baron and colleagues found that SF-36 scores in cervical patients did not follow the same patterns as the general population.[24] Additionally, in the cervical population, the two components of the SF-36 score (mental and physical) did not explain as much of the variance in SF-36 scales as required. These authors also found significant floor/ceiling effect in multiple scales of the SF-36 and concluded that reporting SF-36 summary scores in patients with neck disease was inappropriate and misleading.[24]

The alternatives to PROs have been surgeon-administered instruments such as the mJOA and Nurick scales. These have undergone only limited psychometric evaluation; validation of the mJOA is limited to a single, recently published study.[25] Although this study described the mJOA as a useful tool in assessing functional status in patients with myelopathy, the outcome measure had only moderate internal consistency (Cronbach $\alpha = 0.63$) and was multidimensional. The authors also found that this functional measure of disability was poorly correlated with patient-related outcome measures such as the NDI and SF-36. In addition, the authors were not able to evaluate inter- and intra-rater reliability of this surgeon-administered tool.[25] The JOA and mJOA, however, have been used to measure disability in the cervical spine.

Newer PROs such as the National Institutes of Health (NIH) Patient Reported Outcomes Measurement Information System (PROMIS) may have the potential to overcome the aforementioned shortcomings. The PROMIS was developed to allow practitioners to determine global and domain-specific outcome measures; additionally, it uses tools such as computer adaptive testing (CAT) to minimize floor and ceiling effects and reduce questionnaire burden. While there has been some preliminary work performed on the NIH PROMIS in cervical spine patients, there are currently no studies on cervical deformity patients.

In addition to the NIH PROMIS, it might also be useful to devise a disease-specific measure to utilize in patients with cervical deformity. An ideal measure would measure impairment due to limitations in achieving horizontal gaze, range of motion, and dysphagia. There is currently no single outcome measure to address each of these domains; all of which have special relevance to cervical deformity patients.

While the development of such disability measures might represent an interesting area of future research, there have been several recent publications that have examined the impact of cervical malalignment on disability. Cervical malalignment can be considered in one of three different regions: occipitocervical and upper cervical alignment, subaxial cervical alignment, and cervicothoracic alignment.

6.3 Occipitocervical and Upper Cervical Alignment and Measures of Horizontal Gaze

As noted earlier, horizontal gaze is an important requirement for most activities of daily living. The alignment between the occiput and the cervical spine serves as an important regulator of this function. The first occipitocervical parameter to be correlated to disability was the chin–brow vertical angle (CBVA). Suk et al described the significance of the CBVA in a series of ankylosing spondylitis patients. They showed that patients with elevated CBVA had significantly lower scores for horizontal gaze compared to patients with corrected CBVA.[26] Several authors have since commented on the importance of horizontal gaze and other similar parameters have been described that are closely correlated to the CBVA. These include the slope line of sight (SLS) and McGregor slope (McGS).[27,28,29] Although Suk et al found no correlation between CBVA and HRQOL in a modified arthritis scale,[26] other authors have used a regression analysis to suggest optimal targets for CBVA, SLS, and McGS in patients with cervical deformity. Lafage et al used regression analysis in

303 patients presenting to a deformity clinic and determined that CBVA ranging from -4.7 to 17.7 degrees, SLS ranging from -5.1 to 18.5 degrees, and McGS ranging from -5.7 to 14.3 degrees correlated to lower patient disability scores on the Oswestry Disability Index (ODI).[27] It should be noted, however, that the ODI measures lower back dysfunction and may not be broadly applicable to patients with cervical deformity.

Bao et al recently published a principal components analysis of all patients with cervical deformity.[30] Their goal was to determine which components of cervical alignment were mostly correlated to disability. They compared 171 asymptomatic and 107 symptomatic patients and attempted to determine which cervical alignment parameters were best able to discriminate between the two groups. In their analysis, SLS and McGS were different between the symptomatic and asymptomatic cohorts and SLS was an independent predictor of cervical disability. The principal component revealed three principal components: cranial orientation (SLS, McGS, CBVA), occipitocervical orientation (C0–C2), and lower cervical alignment (C2–C7 Cobb, C2–C7 SVA).

The C0–C2 angle is an additional occipitocervical parameter that has been correlated to disability in patients with cervical malalignment. As noted earlier, C0–C2 is an important component of cervical alignment in patients with neck complaints. Izeki et al showed the importance of the C0–C2 angle in setting the oropharyngeal space. In their experience, patients who are fused with a more kyphotic C0–C2 angle were more likely to have a narrowed oropharyngeal space and more likely to experience dysphagia and disability.[31]

6.4 Subaxial Cervical Alignment

Historically, "malalignment" in the subaxial cervical spine was considered to mean cervical kyphosis. This focus on cervical kyphosis stems partially from the disability experienced by patients suffering from post-laminectomy kyphosis.[32,33,34,35] More recent data, however, have shown that cervical kyphosis may not necessarily represent "abnormal" alignment. Diebo and colleagues showed that cervical kyphosis might represent a normal alignment profile in a significant number of patients, particularly those with low thoracic kyphosis (TK).[8] Studies of asymptomatic patients have also shown that a significant number (up to 35%) can have cervical kyphosis[36] and additional studies have since shown that cervical curvature has a poor correlation with measures of disability in postoperative patients.[37,38,39]

That said, it is important to consider C2–C7 curvature in patients with cervical disability. In the principal components analysis by Bao et al, the C2–C7 angle was an important component of disability when considered in conjunction with upper cervical alignment and the C2–C7 sagittal vertical axis (SVA).[30] Similarly, Iyer et al reported on a series of 90 preoperative patients who were presented to a cervical spine clinic for surgery. In this series, an increased C2–C7 lordosis was correlated to increased disability as measured by the NDI.[40] This finding has since been corroborated in a series of postoperative patients as well.[37]

The C2–C7 SVA has emerged as an important predictor of disability in patients with cervical malalignment. The C7–S1 SVA is one of the most well-described predictors of disability in patients with thoracolumbar deformity[1,41,42,43] and it appears that the C2–C7 SVA might be an analog in the cervical spine.

Tang et al were the first to describe this relationship in a series of postoperative patients undergoing posterior cervical fusion.[39] They conducted a retrospective study of patients undergoing a long-segment posterior cervical procedure and measured how various radiographic parameters (C1–C2 angle, C2–C7 angle, C2–C7 SVA, and center of gravity of the head [CGH]–C7 SVA) correlated with HRQOL at 2 months and 1 year. In their series of 113 patients, increasing C2–C7 SVA and CGH–C7 SVA was significantly correlated to increasing disability on the NDI and the SF-36 Physical Component Score (PCS). This finding first brought to light the potential impact of C2–C7 SVA. Several studies have since corroborated this finding.[30,37,38,40,44] Iyer et al reproduced the findings of Tang et al in a series of preoperative patients.[40] In their series, they examined how radiographic parameters affected patient-reported NDI scores *before* surgery. As with Tang et al, they found that increasing C2–C7 SVA was an independent predictor of increasing NDI scores (increasing disability). This finding in conjunction with the data on postoperative patients suggests that increasing C2–C7 SVA might be an important driver of disability. The importance was again emphasized by Bao et al when they found that C2–C7 SVA was an important factor of disability in their principal components analysis.[30] Hyun et al have shown that a C2–C7 SVA greater than 45 to 50 mm likely corresponds to severe disability (NDI > 25).[37,38] In general, the current literature suggests that C2–C7 SVA greater than 4 cm may be considered abnormal cervical spine parameters.[37,39,45,46,47]

6.5 Cervicothoracic Alignment

As C2–C7 SVA parallels the C7–S1 SVA, recent papers have begun focusing on the T1 slope (TS)–cervical lordosis (CL) mismatch (TS-CL) as an analog of the pelvic incidence–lumbar lordosis (PI-LL) mismatch in thoracolumbar deformity. As with the pelvis, the T1 vertebra is a relatively immobile spinal segment. The orientation of T1 is influenced by TK and the thoracic inlet (TI)—a ring comprising the sternum, the ribs, and the muscular attachments of the neck. Because the TS is set by these various factors, there is growing evidence to suggest that its orientation might be an important local regulator of cervical alignment. TS has been strongly correlated to TK, CL, and the C0–C2 angle.[29,48] Functionally, a large TS requires a large CL to provide harmonious alignment and allow for horizontal gaze. A low CL in this setting would create a high TS-CL which, in turn, would compromise horizontal gaze and have a negative impact on disability scores.

In addition to C2–C7 SVA, a number of similar studies have shown that TS–CL has an important relationship with cervical disability scores. Iyer et al were among the first to show the impact that TS–CL can have on disability scores. In their analysis of preoperative patients, they found that a higher TS–CL (in addition to C2–C7 SVA) was an independent predictor of increased disability.[40] Hyun et al found a similar relationship in postoperative patients undergoing multilevel posterior surgery.[37,38] In their analysis, a TS–CL over approximately 20 degrees corresponds to severe disability.[37,38] In general, a TS–CL over 16.5 degrees may be considered an abnormal cervical parameter.[37,39,45,46,47]

6.6 Cervical Deformity and Dysphagia

Dysphagia can be an important source of disability in patients with cervical deformity that has not yet been studied rigorously. To date, few studies have measured dysphagia in this subset of patients, however. One study by the International Spine Study Group sought to determine if surgery to correct cervical deformity would have an impact on postoperative dysphagia.[49] In this series, the investigators used the Quality of Life in Swallowing Disorders (SWAL-QoL).[50] The SWAL-QoL is a validated outcome instrument to quantify dysphagia; it utilizes 44 questions across 11 domains. This score has been validated in patients with oropharyngeal dysphagia[51,52,53] and has been previously utilized in the cervical literature.[50,54,55,56] Interestingly, while these authors did not find a change in SWAL-QoL scores at 3-month follow-up, they found that patients with cervical deformity had a significant amount of dysphagia preoperatively. The baseline SWAL-QoL of patients in this study (78) was similar to a group of patients with oropharyngeal cancer receiving chemotherapy and radiation.[57] Indeed, the level of disability experienced by cervical deformity patients *preoperatively* was the same as that of ACDF patients *postoperatively*.[55]

While it is reasonable to conclude that certain cervical deformities (e.g., chin-on-chest) have a significant impact on dysphagia, the impact of individual alignment parameters on dysphagia is incompletely understood. The most well-established relationship between alignment and dysphagia is the link between the C0–C2 angle and oropharyngeal stenosis.[31] Some recent studies in fusion patients suggest that a pharyngeal inlet angle may be able to predict dysphagia in patients with occipitocervical fusions.[58] These authors developed a swallowing line (S-line) that might be helpful in predicting dysphagia in postoperative patients. Overcorrection of CL is thought to increase the risk for postoperative dysphagia; however, the impact of *preoperative* alignment and dysphagia is still poorly understood.[58,59,60]

6.7 Conclusion

Cervical malalignment can have a significant impact on disability scores. Although the tools to measure disability resulting from cervical deformity are limited, there are several alignment measures such as C2–C7 SVA, TS–CL, SLS, and C2–C7 angle that have been shown to correlate with disability in pre- and postoperative patients. These findings serve to reinforce the clinical relevance of cervical deformity and the importance of harmonious spinous alignment.

References

[1] Scheer JK, Tang JA, Smith JS, et al. International Spine Study Group. Cervical spine alignment, sagittal deformity, and clinical implications: a review. J Neurosurg Spine. 2013; 19(2):141–159

[2] Passias PG, Jalai CM, Lafage V, et al. Primary drivers of adult cervical deformity: prevalence, variations in presentation, and effect of surgical treatment strategies on early postoperative alignment. Neurosurgery. 2018; 83(4):651–659

[3] Jalai CM, Passias PG, Lafage V, et al. International Spine Study Group (ISSG). A comparative analysis of the prevalence and characteristics of cervical malalignment in adults presenting with thoracolumbar spine deformity based on variations in treatment approach over 2 years. Eur Spine J. 2016; 25(8): 2423–2432

[4] Passias PG, Soroceanu A, Smith J, et al. International Spine Study Group. Postoperative cervical deformity in 215 thoracolumbar patients with adult spinal deformity: prevalence, risk factors, and impact on patient-reported outcome and satisfaction at 2-year follow-up. Spine. 2015; 40(5):283–291

[5] Ha Y, Schwab F, Lafage V, et al. Reciprocal changes in cervical spine alignment after corrective thoracolumbar deformity surgery. Eur Spine J. 2014; 23 (3):552–559

[6] Smith JS, Shaffrey CI, Lafage V, et al. International Spine Study Group. Spontaneous improvement of cervical alignment after correction of global sagittal balance following pedicle subtraction osteotomy. J Neurosurg Spine. 2012; 17 (4):300–307

[7] Dubousset J. Three-dimensional analysis of the scoliotic deformity. Pediatr Spine. 1994; 1994:479–496

[8] Diebo BG, Challier V, Henry JK, et al. Predicting cervical alignment required to maintain horizontal gaze based on global spinal alignment. Spine. 2016; 41 (23):1795–1800

[9] Cleland J, Gillani R, Bienen EJ, Sadosky A. Assessing dimensionality and responsiveness of outcomes measures for patients with low back pain. Pain Pract. 2011; 11(1):57–69

[10] Singh A, Tetreault L, Casey A, Laing R, Statham P, Fehlings MG. A summary of assessment tools for patients suffering from cervical spondylotic myelopathy: a systematic review on validity, reliability and responsiveness. Eur Spine J. 2015; 24 Suppl 2:209–228

[11] Schellingerhout JM, Verhagen AP, Heymans MW, Koes BW, de Vet HC, Terwee CB. Measurement properties of disease-specific questionnaires in patients with neck pain: a systematic review. Qual Life Res. 2012; 21(4):659–670

[12] Pietrobon R, Coeytaux RR, Carey TS, Richardson WJ, DeVellis RF. Standard scales for measurement of functional outcome for cervical pain or dysfunction: a systematic review. Spine. 2002; 27(5):515–522

[13] Vernon H. The Neck Disability Index: state-of-the-art, 1991–2008. J Manipulative Physiol Ther. 2008; 31(7):491–502

[14] Sasso RC, Smucker JD, Hacker RJ, Heller JG. Clinical outcomes of BRYAN cervical disc arthroplasty: a prospective, randomized, controlled, multicenter trial with 24-month follow-up. J Spinal Disord Tech. 2007; 20(7):481–491

[15] Heller JG, Sasso RC, Papadopoulos SM, et al. Comparison of BRYAN cervical disc arthroplasty with anterior cervical decompression and fusion: clinical and radiographic results of a randomized, controlled, clinical trial. Spine. 2009; 34(2):101–107

[16] Davis RJ, Nunley PD, Kim KD, et al. Two-level total disc replacement with Mobi-C cervical artificial disc versus anterior discectomy and fusion: a prospective, randomized, controlled multicenter clinical trial with 4-year follow-up results. J Neurosurg Spine. 2015; 22(1):15–25

[17] Young IA, Michener LA, Cleland JA, Aguilera AJ, Snyder AR. Manual therapy, exercise, and traction for patients with cervical radiculopathy: a randomized clinical trial. Phys Ther. 2009; 89(7):632–642

[18] Cleland JA, Childs JD, Whitman JM. Psychometric properties of the Neck Disability Index and Numeric Pain Rating Scale in patients with mechanical neck pain. Arch Phys Med Rehabil. 2008; 89(1):69–74

[19] Cleland JA, Fritz JM, Whitman JM, Palmer JA. The reliability and construct validity of the Neck Disability Index and patient specific functional scale in patients with cervical radiculopathy. Spine. 2006; 31(5):598–602

[20] van der Velde G, Beaton D, Hogg-Johnston S, Hurwitz E, Tennant A. Rasch analysis provides new insights into the measurement properties of the neck disability index. Arthritis Rheum. 2009; 61(4):544–551

[21] Young IA, Cleland JA, Michener LA, Brown C. Reliability, construct validity, and responsiveness of the neck disability index, patient-specific functional scale, and numeric pain rating scale in patients with cervical radiculopathy. Am J Phys Med Rehabil. 2010; 89(10):831–839

[22] Young BA, Walker MJ, Strunce JB, Boyles RE, Whitman JM, Childs JD. Responsiveness of the Neck Disability Index in patients with mechanical neck disorders. Spine J. 2009; 9(10):802–808

[23] Hung M, Cheng C, Hon SD, et al. Challenging the norm: further psychometric investigation of the neck disability index. Spine J. 2015; 15(11):2440–2445

[24] Baron R, Elashaal A, Germon T, Hobart J. Measuring outcomes in cervical spine surgery: think twice before using the SF-36. Spine. 2006; 31(22): 2575–2584

[25] Kopjar B, Tetreault L, Kalsi-Ryan S, Fehlings M. Psychometric properties of the modified Japanese Orthopaedic Association scale in patients with cervical spondylotic myelopathy. Spine. 2015; 40(1):E23–E28

[26] Suk K-S, Kim K-T, Lee S-H, Kim J-M. Significance of chin-brow vertical angle in correction of kyphotic deformity of ankylosing spondylitis patients. Spine. 2003; 28(17):2001–2005

[27] Lafage R, Challier V, Liabaud B, et al. Natural head posture in the setting of sagittal spinal deformity: validation of chin-brow vertical angle, slope of line of sight, and McGregor's slope with health-related quality of life. Neurosurgery. 2016; 79(1):108–115

[28] Song K, Su X, Zhang Y, et al. Optimal chin-brow vertical angle for sagittal visual fields in ankylosing spondylitis kyphosis. Eur Spine J. 2016; 25(8): 2596–2604

[29] Lee S-HH, Son E-SS, Seo E-MM, Suk K-SS, Kim K-TT. Factors determining cervical spine sagittal balance in asymptomatic adults: correlation with spinopelvic balance and thoracic inlet alignment. Spine J. 2015; 15(4):705–712

[30] Bao H, Varghese J, Lafage R, et al. Principal radiographic characteristics for cervical spinal deformity: a health-related quality-of-life analysis. Spine. 2017; 42(18):1375–1382

[31] Izeki M, Neo M, Takemoto M, et al. The O-C2 angle established at occipitocervical fusion dictates the patient's destiny in terms of postoperative dyspnea and/or dysphagia. Eur Spine J. 2014; 23(2):328–336

[32] Albert TJ, Vacarro A. Postlaminectomy kyphosis. Spine. 1998; 23(24): 2738–2745

[33] Deutsch H, Haid RW, Rodts GE, Mummaneni PV. Postlaminectomy cervical deformity. Neurosurg Focus. 2003; 15(3):E5

[34] Park DK, An HS. Problems related to cervical fusion: malalignment and nonunion. Instr Course Lect. 2009; 58:737–745

[35] Butler JC, Whiteclod TS, III. Postlaminectomy kyphosis. Causes and surgical management. Orthop Clin North Am. 1992; 23(3):505–511

[36] Iyer S, Lenke LG, Nemani VM, et al. Variations in occipitocervical and cervicothoracic alignment parameters based on age: a prospective study of asymptomatic volunteers using full-body radiographs. Spine. 2016; 41(23): 1837–1844

[37] Hyun S-J, Kim K-J, Jahng T-A, Kim HJ. Relationship between T1 slope and cervical alignment following multilevel posterior cervical fusion surgery: impact of T1 slope minus cervical lordosis. Spine. 2016; 41(7):E396–E402

[38] Hyun S-J, Kim K-J, Jahng T-A, Kim H-J. Clinical impact of T1 slope minus cervical lordosis after multilevel posterior cervical fusion surgery: a minimum 2-year follow up data. Spine. 2017; 42(24):1859–1864

[39] Tang JA, Scheer JK, Smith JS, et al. ISSG. The impact of standing regional cervical sagittal alignment on outcomes in posterior cervical fusion surgery. Neurosurgery. 2012; 71(3):662–669, discussion 669

[40] Iyer S, Nemani VM, Nguyen J, et al. Impact of cervical sagittal alignment parameters on neck disability. Spine. 2016; 41(5):371–377

[41] Glassman SD, Bridwell K, Dimar JR, Horton W, Berven S, Schwab F. The impact of positive sagittal balance in adult spinal deformity. Spine (Phila Pa 1976). 2005; 30(18):2024–2029

[42] Glassman SD, Carreon L, Dimar JR. Outcome of lumbar arthrodesis in patients sixty-five years of age or older. Surgical technique. J Bone Joint Surg Am. 2010; 92 Suppl 1, Pt 1:77–84

[43] Schwab F, Lafage V, Patel A, Farcy J-PP. Sagittal plane considerations and the pelvis in the adult patient. Spine. 2009; 34(17):1828–1833

[44] Gum JL, Glassman SD, Douglas LR, Carreon LY. Correlation between cervical spine sagittal alignment and clinical outcome after anterior cervical discectomy and fusion. Am J Orthop. 2012; 41(6):E81–E84

[45] Glassman SD, Berven S, Bridwell K, Horton W, Dimar JR. Correlation of radiographic parameters and clinical symptoms in adult scoliosis. Spine (Phila Pa 1976). 2005; 30(6):682–688

[46] Ames CP, Smith JS, Scheer JK, et al. Impact of spinopelvic alignment on decision making in deformity surgery in adults: a review. J Neurosurg Spine. 2012; 16(6):547–564

[47] Lee SH, Kim KT, Seo EM, Suk KS, Kwack Y-HH, Son E-SS. The influence of thoracic inlet alignment on the craniocervical sagittal balance in asymptomatic adults. J Spinal Disord Tech. 2012; 25(2):E41–E47

[48] Protopsaltis TS, Terran JS, Bronsard N, et al. T1 Slope Minus Cervical Lordosis (TS-CL), the Cervical Analog of PI-LL Defines Cervical Sagittal Deformity in Patients Undergoing Thoracolumbar Osteotomy. In: Cervical Spine Research Society, 41st Annual Meeting; 2013

[49] Smith MW, Annis P, Lawrence BD, Daubs MD, Brodke DS. Acute proximal junctional failure in patients with preoperative sagittal imbalance. Spine J. 2015; 15(10):S165–S166

[50] Siska PA, Ponnappan RK, Hohl JB, Lee JY, Kang JD, Donaldson WF, III. Dysphagia after anterior cervical spine surgery: a prospective study using the swallowing-quality of life questionnaire and analysis of patient comorbidities. Spine. 2011; 36(17):1387–1391

[51] McHorney CA, Bricker DE, Robbins J, Kramer AE, Rosenbek JC, Chignell KA. The SWAL-QOL outcomes tool for oropharyngeal dysphagia in adults: II. Item reduction and preliminary scaling. Dysphagia. 2000; 15(3):122–133

[52] McHorney CA, Robbins J, Lomax K, et al. The SWAL-QOL and SWAL-CARE outcomes tool for oropharyngeal dysphagia in adults: III. Documentation of reliability and validity. Dysphagia. 2002; 17(2):97–114

[53] McHorney CA, Bricker DE, Kramer AE, et al. The SWAL-QOL outcomes tool for oropharyngeal dysphagia in adults: I. Conceptual foundation and item development. Dysphagia. 2000; 15(3):115–121

[54] Lu DC, Tumialán LM, Chou D. Multilevel anterior cervical discectomy and fusion with and without rhBMP-2: a comparison of dysphagia rates and outcomes in 150 patients. J Neurosurg Spine. 2013; 18(1):43–49

[55] Fengbin Y, Xinwei W, Haisong Y, Yu C, Xiaowei L, Deyu C. Dysphagia after anterior cervical discectomy and fusion: a prospective study comparing two anterior surgical approaches. Eur Spine J. 2013; 22(5):1147–1151

[56] Kukreja S, Ahmed OI, Haydel J, Nanda A, Sin AH. Complications of anterior cervical fusion using a low-dose recombinant human bone morphogenetic protein-2. Korean J Spine. 2015; 12(2):68–74

[57] de Campos RJ, Palma PV, Leite IC. Quality of life in patients with dysphagia after radiation and chemotherapy treatment for head and neck tumors. J Clin Exp Dent. 2013; 5(3):e122–e127

[58] Kaneyama S, Sumi M, Takabatake M, et al. The prediction and prevention of dysphagia after occipitospinal fusion by use of the S-line (swallowing line). Spine. 2017; 42(10):718–725

[59] Tian W, Yu J. The role of C2-C7 and O-C2 angle in the development of dysphagia after cervical spine surgery. Dysphagia. 2013; 28(2):131–138

[60] Tian W, Yu J. The role of C2–C7 angle in the development of dysphagia after anterior and posterior cervical spine surgery. Clin Spine Surg. 2017; 30(9):E1306–E1314

7 Physical Examination of Cervical Deformity

Amanda N. Sacino, Corinna C. Zygourakis, and Christopher P. Ames

Abstract

The cervical spine provides structural support and is essential for the performance of daily tasks and maintenance of patients' quality of life. Therefore, the ability to assess cervical spine deformity both clinically and radiographically is imperative for deciding appropriate treatment. Clinical assessment begins with a physical exam to evaluate for posture, range of motion, and neurologic function. Radiologic assessment includes evaluation of different alignment parameters including those for cervical lordosis, sagittal vertical axis, chin–brow vertical angle, and T1 slope. These factors contribute to formation of the surgical plan for correction of cervical spine deformity.

Keywords: cervical deformity, cervical lordosis, sagittal vertical axis, chin–brow vertical angle, T1 slope

7.1 Introduction

The cervical spine is composed of seven vertebrae, which articulate in a manner that supports head and neck movement, axial cranial loads, and maintenance of horizontal gaze while providing structural support for the spinal cord and associated neurovascular structures.[1] As the most mobile spinal region, the cervical spine is essential for the performance of daily tasks and maintenance of patients' quality of life.[2] Therefore, patients with cervical spine deformities (▶ Fig. 7.1) can have a severely negatively impacted quality of life secondary to pain, motor or sensory deficits, inability to perform acts of daily living, and inability to maintain horizontal gaze. The ability to assess cervical spine deformity both clinically and radiographically is imperative for deciding appropriate treatment.

7.2 Neurologic/Musculoskeletal Exam

7.2.1 General Observation

Routine physical exam begins with general observation of the patient. The patient should be observed in dynamic and static situations (▶ Fig. 7.2), noting the patient's posture and quality of movement. Posture should be observed with both sitting and standing. In addition, it is extremely important to ask the patient to stand in a comfortable position, which may be significantly different from their forced upright posture (▶ Fig. 7.3). An abnormal posture that may be indicative of cervical spine deformity is upper crossed syndrome. Chronic poor posture leads to tightness of the upper trapezius, levator scapula, and pectoralis major and minor crossed with weakness of the middle and lower trapezius. Over time, this imbalance may lead to joint dysfunction, particularly at the atlantooccipital joint, C4–C5 segment, and cervicothoracic junction.[3]

The patient's horizontal gaze should also be assessed, as worsening cervical deformity alters the gaze level and decreases quality of life. Horizontal gaze is assessed by having the patient stand with the neck in a neutral or fixed position while the hips or knees are extended. In this position, parameters for horizontal gaze can be measured, such as the chin–brow vertical angle (CBVA; ▶ Fig. 7.4), described in further detail later; the slope of sight or the Frankfort line, from the anteroinferior margin of the orbit to the top of the external auditory meatus; and the McGregor slope, from the posterior margin of the hard palate to the most caudal part of the occiput.

Any movement of the upper and lower extremities should be fluid and symmetric. Asymmetry may be due to underlying

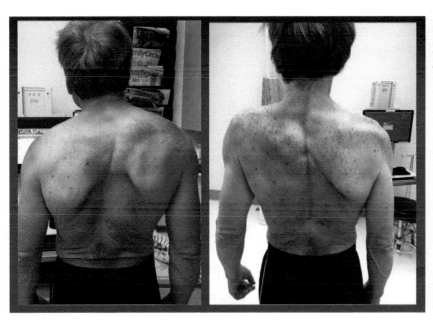

Fig. 7.1 Example of a patient with cervicothoracic deformity before and after surgical correction. This patient presented with severe neck pain and was unhappy with his appearance.

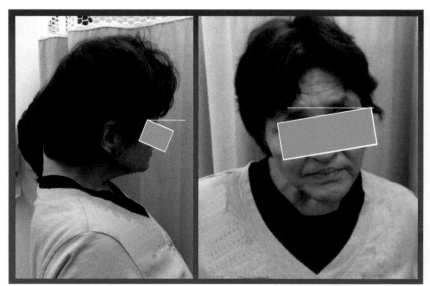

Fig. 7.2 Abnormal static posture in a patient with cervical spinal deformity. She experiences neck pain and head position fatigue that is worse at the end of the day.

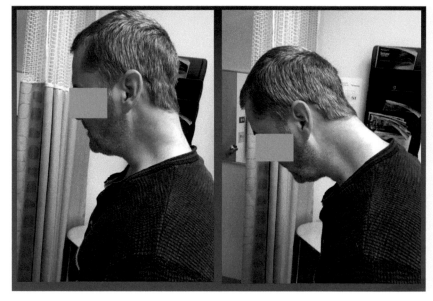

Fig. 7.3 On the left is the patient's posture when asked to stand straight; on the right, when he stands comfortably.

pain and/or weakness. While assessing posture and movement, the clinician should also observe muscle form and soft tissue surrounding the cervical spine. Muscle bulk and tone should be assessed for right and left symmetry. In response to chronic stress from deformity, muscles may shorten, weaken, or become tender to palpation. For example, trapezius muscle tenderness and increased tone are seen in patients with a dorsal kyphotic deformity (▶ Fig. 7.5). Strain from deformity can also result in swelling and tenderness of soft tissues surrounding the cervical spine.

7.2.2 Range of Motion

Neck rotation along with lateral bending, flexion, and extension are important for gauging the extent of cervical spine deformity. The clinician should assess both active and passive range of motion. While assessing the range of motion, the clinician should also note the quality of the movement, pain or resistance to movement, and muscle spasm in response to movement. Normal parameters for neck range of motion are as follows: rotation up to 90 degrees but on average 13 to

57 degrees; lateral bending up to 43 degrees but on average 9 to 21 degrees; and flexion up to 60 degrees but on average 13 to 32 degrees.[4,5] While decreases in the degree of neck range of motion can be an indicator of cervical spine pathology (▶ Fig. 7.6), it must be used in conjunction with the rest of the physical exam and imaging in order to distinguish deformity from other disorders and to decipher the exact deformity.

7.2.3 Neurologic Exam

Muscle Strength, Sensation, and Reflex

A decrease in muscle strength, particularly in the upper extremities, may be indicative of spinal cord or nerve root compression secondary to cervical spine deformity. Basic testing of strength in the physical exam is testing of movement against resistance using the following scoring scale: 5, able to fully overcome resistance; 4 (+ or -), able to overcome resistance to varying degrees, but not fully; 3, able to move antigravity, but not able to overcome resistance; 2, muscle contraction present,

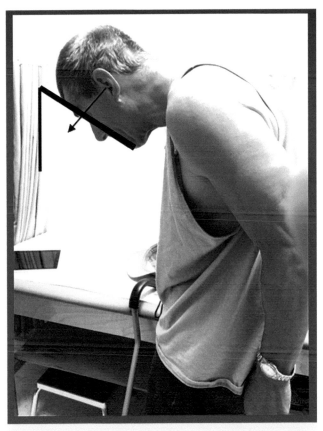

Fig. 7.4 Patient with 70 degrees CBVA and severely compromised line of site.

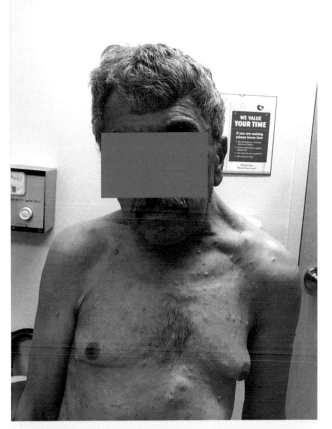

Fig. 7.5 Patient with asymmetric left trapezius activation and hypertrophy due to cervical spine deformity.

Fig. 7.6 Patient with rigid neck deformity, 2 years after motorcycle accident resulting in amputations of right arm and left leg.

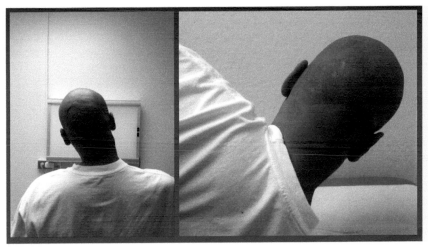

but limb cannot move against gravity; 1, muscle twitch present, but no substantial movement of the limb; and 0, no movement. Each joint of the upper extremities should be tested in isolation on both the right and left sides for shoulder abduction, elbow flexion and extension, wrist flexion and extension, and hand intrinsic strength. Lower extremity strength may also be tested in the same manner.

Similarly, reflexes should be tested for presence, grade, and symmetry. The following grading scale is used: 4, clonus; 3, hyperreflexic; 2, normoreflexic; 1, hyporeflexic; and 0, no

reflex. Reflexes in the upper extremities that should be tested include biceps, triceps, and brachioradialis. Additionally, sensation to touch should be grossly tested on the scalp, neck, and upper extremities. To further discriminate which spinal cord tracts are available, touch may be further separated into light touch, pinprick, vibration, and proprioception. Lower extremity sensation and reflexes should be tested in the same manner.

Weakness, changes in reflexes, and loss of sensation in specific muscle groups and dermatomal distributions may be indicative of the spinal level affected by cervical deformity. Damage to C1–C3 may cause no symptoms or decreased sensation over the scalp and neck. Damage to the C4 level would result in weakness in shoulder elevation, with decreased sensation over the top of the shoulders and back of the neck, and no associated change in reflex. An isolated injury to C5 would result in weakness of shoulder abduction and external rotation with decreased sensation over the lateral arm and forearm, and a decreased biceps reflex. C6 injury may cause weaker shoulder abduction along with weakened elbow flexion and wrist extension. Decreased sensation extends further down the lateral arm to the thumb. The brachioradialis reflex may be diminished in addition to the biceps reflex. Damage to nerve roots from C7–T1 would cause additional weakness in wrist flexion and in the intrinsic hand muscles. Decreased sensation would include the more medial aspect of the arm, forearm, and hand. The triceps reflex might also be decreased.

Special Provocation Maneuvers

There are additional signs present on the physical exam that can implicate spinal cord compression in cervical spine deformity. The most well-known is the Hoffman sign. The Hoffman sign is elicited by flicking the nail of the middle finger. Subsequent flexion of the ipsilateral index finger and/or thumb is considered a positive sign and suggests underlying pyramidal tract pathology secondary to cervical spine compression.[6,7] Additionally, Spurling test may be used to assess for cervical nerve root compression. The patient's neck is flexed 30 degrees to the affected side if a downward axial compressive force is applied. A positive test is pain radiating down the affected dermatome.[8]

7.3 Radiographic Parameters

7.3.1 Cervical Lordosis

Cervical lordosis (CL) is measured as a negative angle on imaging, as compared to kyphosis, which is a positive angle. There are multiple methods used for measuring CL: the modified Cobb method (mCM), the Jackson physiological stress (JPS) line, the Ishihara index, and the Harrison posterior tangent (HPT) method[2,9] as seen in ▶ Fig. 7.7. All measurements can be obtained using sagittal views on X-rays or CT scans of the cervical spine. The mCM (▶ Fig. 7.7a) is calculated by first drawing lines along the inferior endplates of C2 and C7, and then drawing vertical lines perpendicular to both. The angle formed at the intersection of the vertical lines is the CL. The JPS (▶ Fig. 7.7b) is the intersection of two lines drawn along the posterior vertebral walls of C2 and C7.[10,11] The HPT (▶ Fig. 7.7c) is calculated by drawing vertical lines parallel to the posterior surfaces of C2 to C7 vertebral bodies, and adding all the segmental angles.[12]

Finally, the Ishihara index is a ratio where a higher value corresponds to a more lordotic spine. It is calculated by drawing a vertical line from the posterior-inferior body of C2 to that of C7, followed by drawing perpendicular, horizontal lines across the posterior-inferior vertebrae from C3 to C6. The lengths of each horizontal line should be added and then divided by the length of the vertical line.[13]

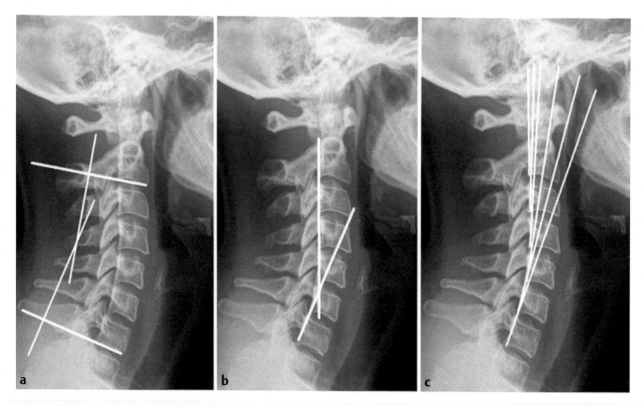

Fig. 7.7 Sagittal radiographs showing the modified Cobb method (**a**), Jackson physiological stress line (**b**), and Harrison posterior tangent (**c**) for determining cervical lordosis. (Reproduced with permission from Scheer et al.[2])

The CL changes with age to compensate for thoracic kyphosis and reduced lumbar lordosis (LL). Multiple studies have revealed a wide range for CL based on age and gender. One study reported CL values of 15 and 16 degrees in men and women, respectively, aged 20 to 25, with values increasing to 22 and 25 degrees in men and women, respectively, aged 60 to 65 years.[2] When looking at the contributions of each segment of the cervical spine to overall lordosis, C1–C2 is the most significant lordotic angle, whereas C4–C7 is the least.[14] Comparison of each method for measuring the CL suggests that HPT may be the most accurate estimate[12]; however, mCM is the most commonly used method due to feasibility and reliability.[15]

7.3.2 C2–C7 Sagittal Vertical Axis

The sagittal vertical axis (SVA), as the name suggests, focuses on the sagittal alignment of the cervical spine. The value is obtained by first drawing a vertical line from the C2 plumb line and another vertical line from the posterior superior C7 endplate. The SVA is the distance between these two lines (▶ Fig. 7.8). While several studies have been conducted to determine a normal range for the SVA, there still is no consensus. Normative values have been estimated at 1.5 cm ± 1 cm.[2,4] The measurement is easy to use; however, it is affected by concomitant thoracolumbar deformity, which must be taken into account in surgical planning.

Cervical SVA has been one of the most important cervical spinal parameters correlating with factors measuring health-related quality of life (HRQoL) such as the Neck Disability Index (NDI), SF-36 mental and physical component scores, and visual analog scale for neck pain.[2] For example, a study by Villavicencio et al reported improvement in clinical outcomes with improvement in cervical sagittal alignment.[16] Glassman et

al found that the C7 plumb line is the most reliable when correlating with HRQoL scores, and that there is a correlation between increased sagittal malalignment and severity of symptoms.[17] Additionally, studies showed that a C2–C7 SVA value of greater than 40 mm correlates with worse health status[18] and a worse NDI score.[19]

7.3.3 Chin–Brow Vertical Angle

The CBVA is based on the patient's horizontal gaze. It is measured by first drawing a diagonal line connecting the patient's chin to eyebrow followed by a vertical line from the eyebrow. The CBVA is the angle formed by the connection between the two lines (▶ Fig. 7.9). The goal of surgical correction is a neutral head position. A neutral head position corresponds to a CBVA of zero, with a positive value corresponding to the head tilted down and a negative value corresponding to the head tilted up. Although studies for determining normal ranges for CBVA values have not been completed in asymptomatic patients, normal values for postoperative patients are -10 to 10 degrees.[2,4]

Chin-on-chest deformity is a severe, rigid kyphotic deformity of the cervical spine. CBVA is typically used for preoperative planning. CBVA in these patients can range as high as 96 degrees with an average of 35.5 degrees.[20] Correction of the deformity leads to objective improvement in horizontal gaze. Of note, overcorrection of the CBVA to less than -10 degrees also had a negative impact on horizontal gaze.[20]

7.3.4 T1 Slope

The T1S is useful in characterizing cervical spinal deformity when paired with other measurements such as the SVA. It is calculated as the angle formed by the T1 upper endplate and

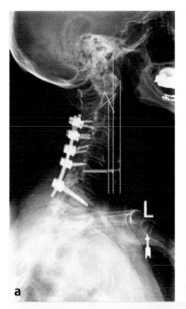 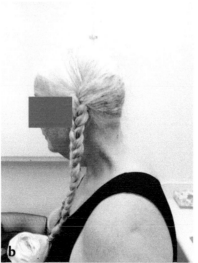 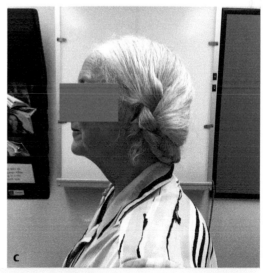

Fig. 7.8 (a) Sagittal radiograph showing cervical SVA measurement. (Reproduced with permission from Scheer et al.[2]) Clinical example of SVA in a patient with a cervical kyphotic deformity before **(b)** and after **(c)** surgery.

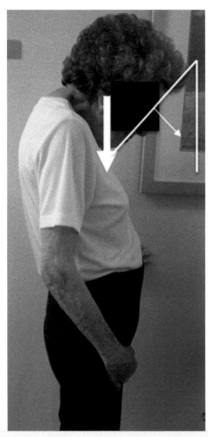

Fig. 7.9 Clinical photographic representation of CBVA measurement with the patient standing with neck in a neutral or flexed position and hips and knees extended. (Reproduced with permission from Scheer et al.[2])

the horizontal plane (▶ Fig. 7.10). The T1S directly correlates with the magnitude of CL. This relationship is similar to that of the pelvic incidence (PI), which also correlates with LL. When analyzing the magnitude of the CL in the context of the whole spine, studies have shown that the above values are largely proportional. For example, a large PI requires a large LL, which increases thoracic kyphosis, therefore causing an increase in the T1S and CL. The overall change in CL with a change in LL is not enough to maintain the position of the head over the pelvis and will cause increase in muscle tension and pain; however, it should be enough to maintain horizontal gaze.[2,4] Oe et al found that a T1S greater than 40 degrees or a T1S-CL greater than 20 degrees is associated with worse HRQoL.[18]

7.4 Conclusion

Appropriate measurement of the extent of cervical spinal deformity on imaging is imperative for preoperative planning. In this chapter, we summarized clinical and radiographic findings associated with cervical spine deformity. Important points to take from the chapter are as follows: (1) the physical exam should focus not only on the aesthetic presentation but also the sequelae of symptoms related to the deformity, such as disruption of horizontal gaze, myelopathy, and weakness; (2) the CL is most commonly measured by the mCM with normal values ranging from 15 to 25 degrees, which vary with age and gender; (3) the normal range for the cervical SVA is 1.5 cm ± 1 cm, and this measurement is most accurate for correlating with HRQoL; (4) the normal range for the CBVA, which helps determine appropriate horizontal gaze, is -10 to 10 degrees; and (5) the T1S values influence the magnitude of the CL in relation to changes in the PI and LL.

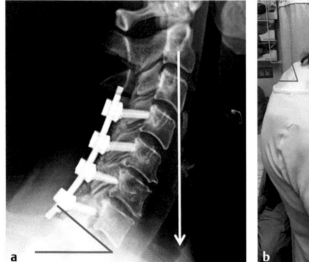
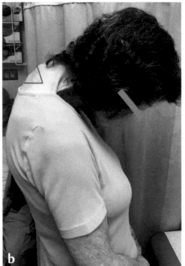
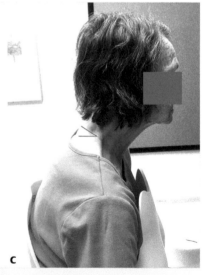

Fig. 7.10 (a) Sagittal radiograph depicting the angle of the T1 slope in relation to the cervical SVA. (Reproduced with permission from Scheer et al.[2]) Clinical example of T1 slope in a patient with severe cervicothoracic deformity before (**b**) and after (**c**) surgery.

References

[1] Haines DE. Neuroanatomy: An Atlas of Structures, Sections, and Systems. 2007

[2] Scheer JK, Tang JA, Smith JS, et al. International Spine Study Group. Cervical spine alignment, sagittal deformity, and clinical implications: a review. J Neurosurg Spine. 2013; 19(2):141–159

[3] V J. Muscles and motor control in cervicogenic headache: traumatic vs. nontraumatic onset. Cephalalgia. 1994; 21:195–215

[4] Passias P. Cervical Myelopathy. Philadelphia, PA: Jaypee Brothers Medical Publishers; 2016

[5] Bible JE, Biswas D, Miller CP, Whang PG, Grauer JN. Normal functional range of motion of the cervical spine during 15 activities of daily living. J Spinal Disord Tech. 2010; 23(1):15–21

[6] Tejus MN, Singh V, Ramesh A, Kumar VR, Maurya VP, Madhugiri VS. An evaluation of the finger flexion, Hoffman's and plantar reflexes as markers of cervical spinal cord compression - a comparative clinical study. Clin Neurol Neurosurg. 2015; 134:12–16

[7] Houten JK, Noce LA. Clinical correlations of cervical myelopathy and the Hoffmann sign. J Neurosurg Spine. 2008; 9(3):237–242

[8] Shah KC, Rajshekhar V. Reliability of diagnosis of soft cervical disc prolapse using Spurling's test. Br J Neurosurg. 2004; 18(5):480–483

[9] Tan LA, Riew KD, Traynelis VC. Cervical spine deformity-Part 1: Biomechanics, radiographic parameters, and classification. Neurosurgery. 2017; 81(2):197–203

[10] Jackson R. The Cervical Syndrome. 2nd ed. Springfield, IL: Charles C Thomas; 1958

[11] Jackson RP, McManus AC. Radiographic analysis of sagittal plane alignment and balance in standing volunteers and patients with low back pain matched for age, sex, and size. A prospective controlled clinical study. Spine. 1994; 19(14):1611–1618

[12] Harrison DE, Harrison DD, Cailliet R, Troyanovich SJ, Janik TJ, Holland B. Cobb method or Harrison posterior tangent method: which to choose for lateral cervical radiographic analysis. Spine. 2000; 25(16):2072–2078

[13] Takeshita K, Murakami M, Kobayashi A, Nakamura C. Relationship between cervical curvature index (Ishihara) and cervical spine angle (C2–7). J Orthop Sci. 2001; 6(3):223–226

[14] Hardacker JW, Shuford RF, Capicotto PN, Pryor PW. Radiographic standing cervical segmental alignment in adult volunteers without neck symptoms. Spine. 1997; 22(13):1472–1480, discussion 1480

[15] Polly DW, Jr, Kilkelly FX, McHale KA, Asplund LM, Mulligan M, Chang AS. Measurement of lumbar lordosis. Evaluation of intraobserver, interobserver, and technique variability. Spine. 1996; 21(13):1530–1535, discussion 1535–1536

[16] Villavicencio AT, Babuska JM, Ashton A, et al. Prospective, randomized, double-blind clinical study evaluating the correlation of clinical outcomes and cervical sagittal alignment. Neurosurgery. 2011; 68(5):1309–1316, discussion 1316

[17] Glassman SD, Berven S, Bridwell K, Horton W, Dimar JR. Correlation of radiographic parameters and clinical symptoms in adult scoliosis. Spine. 2005; 30(6):682–688

[18] Oe S, Togawa D, Nakai K, et al. The influence of age and sex on cervical spinal alignment among volunteers aged over 50. Spine. 2015; 40(19):1487–1494

[19] Tang JA, Scheer JK, Smith JS, et al. ISSG. The impact of standing regional cervical sagittal alignment on outcomes in posterior cervical fusion surgery. Neurosurgery. 2012; 71(3):662–669, discussion 669

[20] Suk KS, Kim KT, Lee SH, Kim JM. Significance of chin-brow vertical angle in correction of kyphotic deformity of ankylosing spondylitis patients. Spine. 2003; 28(17):2001–2005

8 Cervical Osteotomy Types

Marcus D. Mazur, Christopher I. Shaffrey, K. Daniel Riew, Christopher P. Ames, and Justin S. Smith

Abstract

A wide variety of anterior and posterior osteotomy techniques to correct cervical spine deformities have been described. The cervical osteotomy classification system is a validated grading scale, which categorizes cervical osteotomy types into seven grades according to the extent of anatomical resection and destabilization. The system is designed to be comprehensive and to encompass the wide range of anterior and posterior resections that are used to correct cervical deformities. It provides a standardized nomenclature to enable more effective communication between surgeons and to facilitate research on patients with cervical spine deformities.

Keywords: cervical osteotomy types, cervical deformity, classification system, nomenclature, spine deformities

8.1 Introduction

Cervical spine osteotomies are powerful techniques to correct deformities. Correcting cervical deformities can be technically challenging and require extensive operations. Several anterior and posterior osteotomy techniques and their variations have been described to correct a wide variety of cervical deformities.[1,2,3,4,5,6,7,8,9,10,11,12] Recently, a validated classification system has been developed to standardize the descriptions of cervical osteotomy types.[13] The cervical osteotomy classification system is similar to that developed by Schwab et al[14] to describe osteotomies to correct deformities of the thoracic and lumbar spine.

Much like the standardized classification systems developed for other spinal conditions (e.g., scoliosis, spondylolisthesis, and trauma), a comprehensive classification system for cervical spine osteotomy types provides a valuable tool to facilitate effective research and communication between physicians on the clinical and radiographic findings in patients undergoing surgical management of cervical spine deformities.

8.2 Description of Cervical Osteotomy Classification System

The cervical osteotomy classification system provides a common nomenclature to more effectively and objectively communicate the type of surgical resection(s) performed. It is not intended to provide indications for surgery or to assist in the determination of the appropriate surgical approaches. The system is a 7-point scale based on anatomical resections that are graded according to the potential for destabilization (▶ Table 8.1, ▶ Fig. 8.1). It is designed to be comprehensive as to include the wide range of surgical resections that may be performed for cervical deformity correction.

A given case may involve multiple resection types. The highest grade of osteotomy performed is designated as the major osteotomy, whereas other lower grades of osteotomies performed are designated as minor osteotomies. Additionally, modifiers are used to designate the surgical approach(es): anterior (A), posterior (P), anterior-posterior (AP), posterior-anterior (PA), anterior-posterior-anterior (APA), and posterior-anterior-posterior (PAP).

Table 8.1 Cervical osteotomy types

Osteotomy grade	Resection	Description	Surgical approach modifiers
1	Partial facet joint resection or anterior discectomy and partial uncovertebral joint resection	Anterior cervical discectomy and partial uncovertebral joint resection, or partial facet resection	A, P, AP, PA, APA, PAP
2	Complete facet joint resection	Resection of both superior and inferior facets at a given segment	P, AP, PA, APA, PAP
3	Partial or complete corpectomy	Partial or complete corpectomy including discs above and below	A, AP, PA, APA, PAP
4	Complete uncovertebral joint resection to transverse foramen	Anterior osteotomy through lateral vertebral body and uncovertebral joints into transverse foramen	A, AP, PA, APA, PAP
5	Opening wedge osteotomy	Complete posterior element resection with osteoclastic fracture and open wedge creation	P, AP, PA, APA, PAP
6	Closing wedge osteotomy	Complete posterior element resection and pedicle resection with closing wedge creation	P, AP, PA, APA, PAP
7	Vertebral column resection	Resection of one or more entire vertebral bodies and discs including complete uncovertebral joint and posterior lamina and facets	AP, PA, APA, PAP

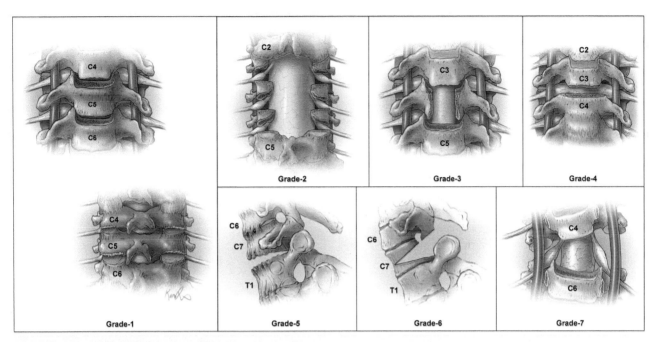

Fig. 8.1 Illustrations depicting the 7 cervical osteotomy types, which are based on anatomical resections according to progression of destabilization. Used with permission from Xavier Studio.

8.2.1 Grade 1: Partial Facet Joint Resection or Discectomy and Partial Uncovertebral Joint Resection

A Grade 1 osteotomy involves a partial joint resection. It may be performed via an anterior approach that includes a discectomy and partial uncovertebral joint resection, a posterior approach that includes partial resection of the facet joint, or through combinations of both approaches. A Grade 1 osteotomy has limited capacity for deformity correction, but it may be applied over multiple levels to cumulatively facilitate realignment. When performed posteriorly, it offers the potential to promote fusion by removing cartilage from the facet surfaces.

Grade 1 osteotomies may be performed through anterior or posterior approaches (modifiers A or P), or a combination of both approaches (AP, PA, APA, or PAP). Whether performed anteriorly or posteriorly, Grade 1 osteotomies require mobility of the opposite column (posterior or anterior, respectively) to achieve correction.

Case Example: Grade 1, Modifier A

A 51-year-old man presented with signs of cervical myelopathy and left upper extremity weakness and atrophy. Imaging demonstrated a loss of cervical lordosis with multilevel disc degeneration but no evidence of facet ankylosis (▶ Fig. 8.2). He underwent preoperative traction for 48 hours followed by a multilevel anterior cervical discectomy with partial uncovertebral joint resection and interbody fusion at C3–C4, C4–C5, C5–C6, and C6–C7.

8.2.2 Grade 2: Complete Facet Resection

A Grade 2 osteotomy involves resection of both superior and inferior facets at a given segment. Other posterior elements (i.e.,

the lamina, ligamentum flavum, and spinous process) may be performed as part of a Grade 2 osteotomy, but this grade of resection does not include any portion of the vertebral body. This type of resection is analogous to those commonly performed for deformity correction in the thoracic and lumbar spine, which have several variations and terms, including Smith-Petersen, Ponte, polysegmental, chevron, and extension osteotomies among others.[15,16,17] Grade 2 osteotomies are often performed at multiple levels to facilitate a greater magnitude of deformity correction.

A posterior approach (modifier P) is used for Grade 2 osteotomies, but anterior column mobility is necessary. Thus, Grade 2 osteotomies may be performed in combination with anterior soft-tissue release procedures (modifiers AP, PA, APA, or PAP).

Case Example: Grade 2, Modifier P

A 64-year-old man presented with neck pain and difficulty maintaining horizontal gaze. Imaging demonstrated a loss of cervical lordosis (▶ Fig. 8.3) but no evidence of ankylosis of the anterior disc spaces (not shown). The deformity was considered to be partially reducible. A single-stage operation was performed consisting of posterior instrumentation and fusion from C2 to T10 and posterior column osteotomies with complete facet joint resections from C3–C4 to C7–T1.

8.2.3 Grade 3: Partial or Complete Corpectomy

A Grade 3 osteotomy involves partial or complete resection of a vertebral body, including the adjacent discs. In addition to providing anterior release, performing a corpectomy facilitates decompression of the spinal canal and foramina. A structural graft or expandable cage is then inserted into the corpectomy

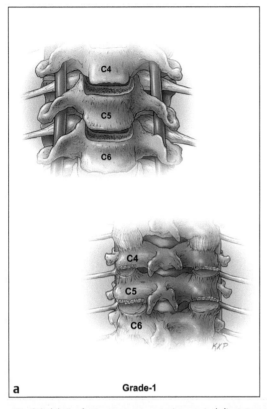
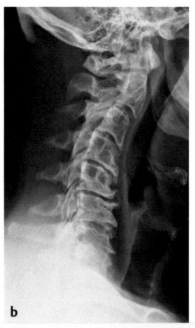
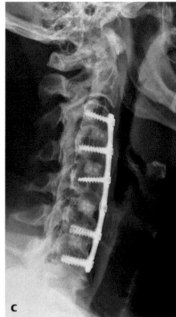

a   **Grade-1**   **b**   **c**

Fig. 8.2 **(a)** Grade 1 osteotomy, anterior cervical discectomy, partial uncovertebral joint resection, or partial facet joint resection. Pre- **(b)** and postoperative radiographs **(c)** depicting anterior cervical discectomies with partial uncovertebral joint resections at C3–C4, C4–C5, C5–C6, and C6–C7 (Grade 1, modifier A).

defect to enable restoration of cervical lordosis and provide arthrodesis. A ventral strategy provides an optimal approach for decompression of the spinal cord and enables placement of the interbody graft in a structurally favorable location for correction of the deformity.

An anterior approach (modifier A) is used for Grade 3 osteotomies, but mobility of the posterior column (i.e., facet joints) is necessary to maximize deformity correction. Thus, Grade 3 osteotomies may be performed in combination with posterior release procedures (modifiers AP, PA, APA, or PAP).

Case Example: Grade 3, Modifier A

A 72-year-old woman presented with neck pain and cervical myelopathy. Imaging demonstrated a Grade 3 spondylolisthesis of C3 in the setting of an autofusion across the disc space at C4 and C5 (▶ Fig. 8.5). A single-stage anterior procedure was performed with corpectomies at C4 and C5 (major osteotomy, Grade 3, modifier A), discectomy at C6–C7 (minor osteotomy, Grade 1, modifier A), placement of a fibular strut allograft between C3 and C6, placement of a bone allograft spacer between C5 and C6, and plating from C3 to C7.

8.2.4 Grade 4: Complete Uncovertebral Joint Resection to the Transverse Foramen

A Grade 4 osteotomy involves an anterior bony resection that is carried laterally across the uncovertebral joint and into the

transverse foramen. This provides a complete anterior release. Posteriorly, the bony resection is taken all the way to the posterior longitudinal ligament. Laterally, the osteotomy is continued through the disc space and the uncinates to the transverse foramen. This type of osteotomy may put the vertebral artery at risk for injury. Skeletonization of the vertebral arteries bilaterally is sometimes needed to decrease the risk of arterial kinking, particularly if the osteotomy is performed at the apex of the deformity in cases of severe kyphosis for which a large focal correction is performed. However, if a gradual correction is performed over several levels, vertebral artery exposure may not be necessary.[18] Anterior foraminotomies are often performed to prevent nerve root compression as lordosis is restored during the deformity correction. A Grade 4 osteotomy should be considered in patients with ankylosis at the lateral margins of the anterior column, such as in the setting of a previous anterior surgical arthrodesis, diffuse idiopathic skeletal hyperostosis, or fixed kyphosis.

An anterior approach (modifier A) is used for Grade 4 osteotomies, but these require mobility of the posterior column. Thus, they may be combined with a posterior release procedure (modifiers AP, PA, APA, or PAP).

Case Example: Grade 4, Modifier AP

A 59-year-old man presented with neck pain and the inability to maintain horizontal gaze (▶ Fig. 8.4). Imaging demonstrated a loss of cervical lordosis with evidence of diffuse idiopathic skeletal hyperostosis and extensive ankylosis across the disc

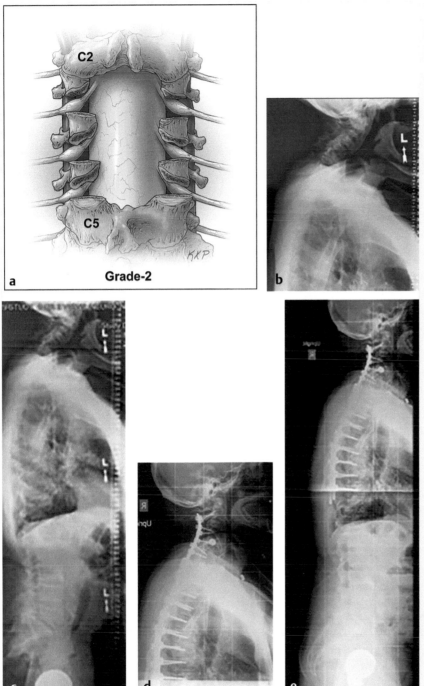

Fig. 8.3 **(a)** Grade 2 osteotomy, complete facet joint resection. Pre- **(b,c)** and postoperative radiographs **(d,e)** depicting osteotomies with complete facet joint resections at C3–C4, C4–C5, C5–C6, C6–C7, and C7–T1 and posterior instrumentation and fusion from C2 to T10 (Grade 2, modifier P).

spaces between C3 and C6. A two-staged operation was performed. First, a complete anterior release was performed laterally out to the transverse foramen bilaterally with resection of the discs and uncovertebral joints, followed by placement of interbody grafts at C3–C4, C4–C5, C5–C6. Second, posterior instrumentation and fusion was performed from C2 to T3.

8.2.5 Grade 5: Opening Wedge Osteotomy

A grade 5 osteotomy involves complete resection of the posterior elements (i.e., lamina, spinous process, and facets)

followed by a controlled osteoclastic fracture and creation of an anterior open wedge in the anterior column. Complete laminectomies and foraminotomies as well as undercutting of the pedicles are performed to permit the nerve roots sufficient space during closure of the osteotomy. The osteotomy is performed by extending the patient's head to induce the osteoclasis in a controlled fashion while monitoring the spinal cord for changes. In this fashion, the middle column acts as the fulcrum with elongation of the anterior column, opening the wedge anteriorly, and shortening of the posterior column. Care must be taken during the correction because elongation of the anterior column could potentially stretch the soft

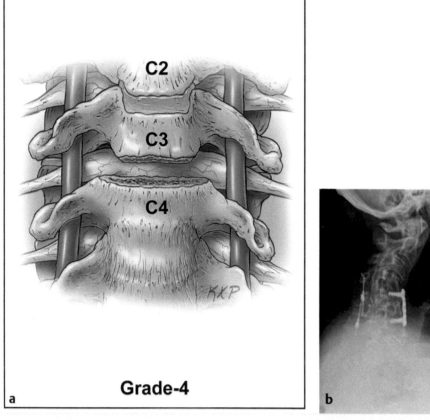

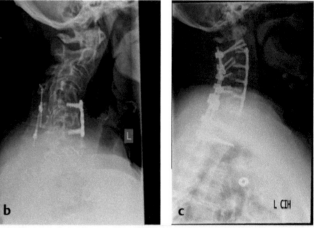

Fig. 8.4 **(a)** Grade 4 osteotomy, complete uncovertebral joint resection to transverse foramen. Pre- **(b)** and postoperative radiographs **(c)** depicting complete anterior release carried out laterally to the transverse foramen at C3–C4, C4–C5, and C5–C6, followed by posterior instrumented fusion from C2 to T3 (Grade 4, modifier AP).

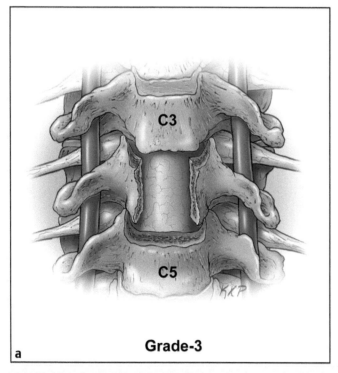

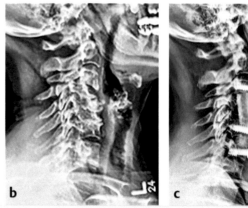

Fig. 8.5 **(a)** Grade 3 osteotomy, partial or complete corpectomy. Pre- **(b)** and postoperative radiographs **(c)** depicting complete anterior corpectomies at C4 and C5 (Grade 3, modifier A).

tissues, which may cause neurovascular complications or injury to the trachea or esophagus.

Typically, a grade 5 osteotomy is performed at C7, which is below the most common entrance of the vertebral arteries into the transverse foramen at C6. However, a vertebral artery originating at C7 has been reported in up to 5% of patients[19]; so, a preoperative vascular study is warranted for surgical planning. The C7 lamina is resected completely along with the inferior portion of the C6 lamina and the superior portion of the T1 lamina. The C7–T1 foramina are decompressed to prevent compression of the C8 nerve roots during closure of the osteotomy. Performing the osteotomy at C7 rather than T1 also avoids dissecting out the T1 rib for removal, which can be tedious.

A posterior approach (modifier P) is used for Grade 5 osteotomies, but these may be performed in combination with anterior release procedures (modifiers AP, PA, APA, or PAP).

Case Example: Grade 5, Modifier PA

A man with ankylosing spondylitis presented with a chin-on-chest deformity. Images demonstrated a fixed kyphotic deformity with fusion across multiple facet joints and disc spaces (▶ Fig. 8.6). A multistaged operation was performed using combined posterior and anterior approaches. First, a posterior approach was used to remove the posterior elements of C6, C7, and T1, including the C6–C7 and C7–T1 facet joints. The

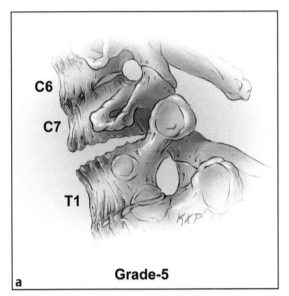

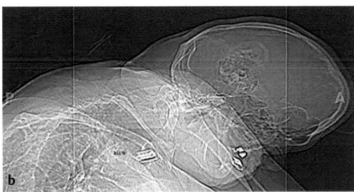

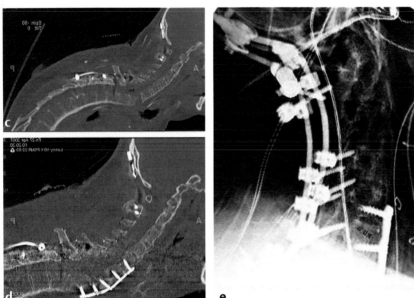

Fig. 8.6 (a) Grade 5 osteotomy, opening wedge osteotomy. Pre- **(b)** and postoperative images **(c–e)** depicting an opening wedge osteotomy at C7 in a patient with ankylosing spondylitis and chin-on-chest deformity (Grade 5, modifier PA). Posterior instrumentation and fusion from the occiput to T5 and anterior interbody fusion and plating from C5 to T2 were also performed.

vertebral closing wedge osteotomy was then performed and closed. However, the degree of correction was not sufficient; so, an opening wedge osteotomy was performed by extending the neck to create an osteoclastic fracture in a controlled fashion under neuromonitoring guidance. The result was a significant increase in cervical lordosis. Cervical alignment was secured in the desired position using posterior instrumentation from the occiput to T5. Later, an anterior approach was used for insertion of an interbody graft at C6–C7 with anterior plating from C5–T2 to provide anterior column support and to help prevent anterior displacement.

8.2.6 Grade 6: Closing Wedge Osteotomy

A Grade 6 osteotomy involves complete removal of the posterior elements (i.e., lamina, spinous process, and facets), decancellation of the pedicles and a portion of the vertebral body, followed by removal of the walls of the pedicles and vertebral body, and creation of a closing wedge. This type of osteotomy is also called a pedicle subtraction osteotomy. Decancellation of the pedicles and vertebral bodies can be performed using taps, curettes, high-speed bur, and osteotomes. As in the Grade 5 osteotomy, after obtaining a preoperative vascular study to confirm the absence of an anomalous pathway of the vertebral arteries, the osteotomy is typically performed at C7 to avoid manipulation of the vertebral arteries and to obviate tedious dissection to disarticulate the ribs. Wide foraminotomies and pedicle resection should be performed to avoid compression of the C8 nerve roots during closure of the wedge. Depending on the type of cervical deformity, a Grade 6 osteotomy may also be performed at the T2 or T3 vertebral levels to minimize the risks of compromise to upper extremity innervation.

In theory, a Grade 6 osteotomy may be safer than a Grade 5 osteotomy because a closing wedge should not stretch the anterior structures to the same extent as an opening wedge osteotomy. The closure may proceed in a more controlled fashion because no osteoclastic fracture is necessary. Moreover, a closing wedge may provide better biomechanical stability than an opening wedge, considering that the former is less likely to cause an anterior gap that compromises the integrity of the anterior longitudinal ligament and it provides a wider surface area for bone-on-bone load bearing interface.[2,20]

A posterior approach (modifier P) is used for Grade 6 osteotomies, but these may be performed in combination with anterior release procedures (modifiers AP, PA, APA, or PAP).

Case Example: Grade 6, Modifier P

A woman with a previous T4–ilium fusion suffered a C7 compression fracture with resultant loss of cervical lordosis, cord compression, and myelopathy (▶ Fig. 8.7). The posterior bone

resection included the C6, C7 and T1 posterior elements, the C6–C7 and C7–T1 facet joints, the C7 pedicles, and a wedge-shaped section of the C7 vertebral body that included the fractured portion. The closing wedge osteotomy was performed by extending the neck to hinge on the anterior cortex of the vertebral body to correct the deformity by increasing lordosis. The new cervical alignment was secured in position by extending the fusion to C2.

8.2.7 Grade 7: Complete Vertebral Column Resection

A Grade 7 osteotomy includes complete resection of one or more vertebral bodies, including adjacent discs, uncovertebral joints, facets, and lamina. A combination of anterior and posterior approaches is used for ventral and dorsal release, removal of any potential compression on the spinal cord, and reconstruction of the affected segment by lengthening the anterior column and shortening the posterior column. Anterior column support is provided using a custom-cut fibular allograft or cage. Vertebral column resection operations are technically challenging to perform safely and have relatively few indications. Consequently, there is limited information in the literature.

Combined approaches are required for Grade 7 osteotomies (modifiers AP, PA, APA, or PAP).

Case Example: Grade 7, Modifier PAP

A woman in her 60 s presented with erosive arthritis and cervical kyphosis with fusion across multiple disc spaces and facet joints (▶ Fig. 8.8). A multistaged operation was performed. First, posterior fixation was performed at C2, C3, C6, and C7. The posterior elements of C3, C4, C5, and C6 were removed as well as the C4–C5 facet joints and the C4 and C5 pedicles. Temporary stabilizing rods were inserted. Next, an anterior approach was used to complete the C4 and C5 vertebrectomies; remove the C3–C4, C4–C5, and C5–C6 discs; perform the deformity correction; and place an interbody expandable cage and anterior plate between C3 and C6. A third stage was then performed in which the posterior fusion was extended to T9, the temporary rods were removed, and permanent stabilizing rods were secured.

8.3 Discussion

Initial reports on the surgical treatment of patients with cervical deformities suggest that osteotomies are technically challenging high-risk procedures associated with high complication rates.[21,22] Although a wide variety of cervical osteotomy types have been described in the literature, research on clinical outcomes is composed of a small number of retrospective studies

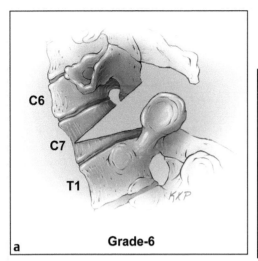

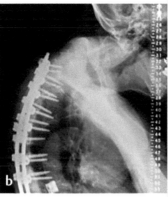

Fig. 8.7 **(a)** Grade 6 osteotomy, closing wedge osteotomy. Pre- **(b,c)** and postoperative images **(d)** showing a patient with a previous T4–ilium fusion who developed a C7 compression fracture and kyphotic deformity, which were treated with a closing wedge osteotomy at C7 with extension of the fusion to C2 (Grade 6, modifier P).

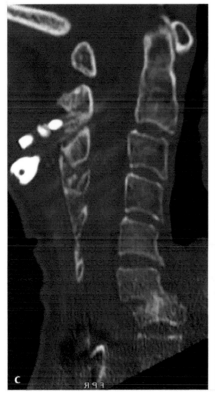

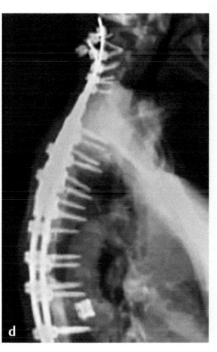

and case series with limited sample sizes. Moreover, the heterogeneity of techniques and their descriptions limits outcome comparisons across studies. Surgeons may have difficulty discerning whether the techniques described and the results reported in a given study apply to their own clinical practices. Recent advancements in surgical techniques, spinal instrumentation, image guidance, neuroanesthesia, and neuromonitoring have considerably improved the safety of patients undergoing complex spine operations. However, clinical research remains ongoing on the effects of these advancements on patient outcomes.

The cervical osteotomy classification system provides a common nomenclature to facilitate effective communication for surgeons and researchers. Analysis of the internal validity of the osteotomy classification system demonstrated high intra- and inter-rater reliability when tested on a group of 11 experienced cervical deformity surgeons.[13] Given that the use of high-grade cervical osteotomies for advanced deformities is relatively uncommon, future research in this area may require multi-institutional participation to have sufficient sample sizes. The use of standardized language will help facilitate collaboration and increase the generalizability of study findings.

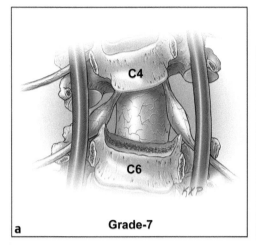

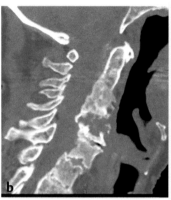

Fig. 8.8 **(a)** Grade 7 osteotomy, vertebral column resection. Pre- **(b, c)** and postoperative images **(d, e)** depicting a patient with erosive arthritis treated with two-level vertebral column resection at C4 and C5 (Grade 7, modifier PAP).

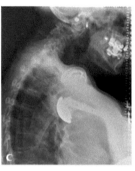

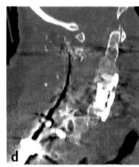

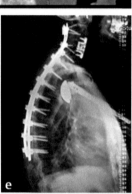

References

[1] Belanger TA, Milam RA, IV, Roh JS, Bohlman HH. Cervicothoracic extension osteotomy for chin-on-chest deformity in ankylosing spondylitis. J Bone Joint Surg Am. 2005; 87(8):1732–1738

[2] Deviren V, Scheer JK, Ames CP. Technique of cervicothoracic junction pedicle subtraction osteotomy for cervical sagittal imbalance: report of 11 cases. J Neurosurg Spine. 2011; 15(2):174–181

[3] Gertzbein SD, Harris MB. Wedge osteotomy for the correction of post-traumatic kyphosis. A new technique and a report of three cases. Spine. 1992; 17 (3):374–379

[4] Kawahara N, Tomita K, Baba H, Kobayashi T, Fujita T, Murakami H. Closing-opening wedge osteotomy to correct angular kyphotic deformity by a single posterior approach. Spine. 2001; 26(4):391–402

[5] McMaster MJ. Osteotomy of the cervical spine in ankylosing spondylitis. J Bone Joint Surg Br. 1997; 79(2):197–203

[6] Mehdian S, Arun R. A safe controlled instrumented reduction technique for cervical osteotomy in ankylosing spondylitis. Spine. 2011; 36(9):715–720

[7] Steinmetz MP, Stewart TJ, Kager CD, Benzel EC, Vaccaro AR. Cervical deformity correction. Neurosurgery. 2007; 60(1) Suppl 1:S90–S97

[8] Stewart TJ, Steinmetz MP, Benzel EC. Techniques for the ventral correction of postsurgical cervical kyphotic deformity. Neurosurgery. 2005; 56(1) Suppl:191–195, discussion 191–195

[9] Wollowick AL, Kelly MP, Riew KD. Pedicle subtraction osteotomy in the cervical spine. Spine. 2012; 37(5):E342–E348

[10] Tokala DP, Lam KS, Freeman BJ, Webb JK. C7 decancellisation closing wedge osteotomy for the correction of fixed cervico-thoracic kyphosis. Eur Spine J. 2007; 16(9):1471–1478

[11] Kim HJ, Piyaskulkaew C, Riew KD. Anterior cervical osteotomy for fixed cervical deformities. Spine. 2014; 39(21):1751–1757

[12] Simmons ED, DiStefano RJ, Zheng Y, Simmons EH. Thirty-six years experience of cervical extension osteotomy in ankylosing spondylitis: techniques and outcomes. Spine. 2006; 31(26):3006–3012

[13] Ames CP, Smith JS, Scheer JK, et al. International Spine Study Group. A standardized nomenclature for cervical spine soft-tissue release and osteotomy for deformity correction: clinical article. J Neurosurg Spine. 2013; 19(3):269–278

[14] Schwab F, Blondel B, Chay E, et al. The comprehensive anatomical spinal osteotomy classification. Neurosurgery. 2015; 76 Suppl 1:S33–S41, discussion S41

[15] Smith-Petersen MN, Larson CB, Aufranc OE. Osteotomy of the spine for correction of flexion deformity in rheumatoid arthritis. Clin Orthop Relat Res. 1969; 66(66):6–9

[16] Geck MJ, Macagno A, Ponte A, Shufflebarger HL. The Ponte procedure: posterior only treatment of Scheuermann's kyphosis using segmental posterior shortening and pedicle screw instrumentation. J Spinal Disord Tech. 2007; 20 (8):586–593

[17] Briggs H, Keats S, Schlesinger PT. Wedge osteotomy of the spine with bilateral intervertebral foraminotomy; correction of flexion deformity in five cases of ankylosing arthritis of the spine. J Bone Joint Surg Am. 1947; 29(4):1075–1082

[18] O'Shaughnessy BA, Liu JC, Hsieh PC, Koski TR, Ganju A, Ondra SL. Surgical treatment of fixed cervical kyphosis with myelopathy. Spine (Phila Pa 1976). 2008; 33:771–778

[19] Bruneau M, Cornelius JF, Marneffe V, Triffaux M, George B. Anatomical variations of the V2 segment of the vertebral artery. Neurosurgery. 2006; 59(1) Suppl 1:ONS20–ONS24, discussion ONS20–ONS24

[20] Scheer JK, Tang JA, Buckley JM, et al. Biomechanical analysis of osteotomy type and rod diameter for treatment of cervicothoracic kyphosis. Spine. 2011; 36(8):E519–E523

[21] Etame AB, Wang AC, Than KD, La Marca F, Park P. Outcomes after surgery for cervical spine deformity: review of the literature. Neurosurg Focus. 2010; 28 (3):E14

[22] Smith JS, Ramchandran S, Lafage V, et al. International Spine Study Group. Prospective multicenter assessment of early complication rates associated with adult cervical deformity surgery in 78 patients. Neurosurgery. 2016; 79 (3):378–388

9 Technique of Low-Grade Osteotomies for Semirigid Deformities

Philippe Bancel

Abstract

Cervical deformity can occur in all three planes, but kyphosis remains the most common type. It has been demonstrated that cervical deformity, with its consequences (imbalance, neurologic disability), can have major impact on health-related quality of life. Clinical examination should include assessment of global and local alignment, pain and neurologic symptoms, and flexibility of the cervical spine. Radiographic evaluation should include objective assessment of regional and global alignment parameters, as well as deformity flexibility. If possible, magnetic resonance imaging should be obtained in order to evaluate for evidence of neural compromise. Computed tomographic imaging can be useful for detailed bony assessment, including general anatomy, anomalies, and evidence of posterior facet arthrodesis. Angiography can be used to assess the course of the vertebral arteries and for evidence of variant anatomy. Otolaryngologist's evaluation may be useful in guiding approach side for anterior procedures, especially in the setting of previous anterior surgery. For some cervical deformities, an anterior cervical approach with low-grade osteotomies (partial or total uncinate resection) can enable deformity correction, as well as decompression of the spinal cord and nerve roots, while avoiding the greater risks of complications that can be associated with higher-grade osteotomies. Low-grade cervical osteotomies are accomplished via an anterior approach for discectomy and medial and lateral exposure of the bilateral uncinate processes. Vertebral arteries are protected by spatulas inserted laterally after a blunt dissection close to the bone. A partial or complete resection of the uncinate processes may be performed using a variety of instruments, including high-speed drill and Kerrison rongeurs. Posterior fixation and arthrodesis with or without osteotomy (in case of facet fusion) may be necessary to increase correction and solidity. This technique decreases perioperative and postoperative risk of complications while providing excellent lordosis restoration and decompression.

Keywords: cervical deformity, anterior cervical approach, low-grade cervical osteotomy, semirigid cervical deformities

9.1 Introduction

Cervical deformity can occur in all three planes, but kyphosis remains the most common type. Kyphosis can progress and become more rigid with abnormal projection of the center of gravity of the head. Affected patients can develop difficulty in maintaining horizontal gaze or upright posture, swallowing dysfunction, respiratory compromise, radiculopathy, and/or myelopathy. Pain can develop and may be attributable to disc and/or facet degeneration, nerve compression, soft-tissue constraints, and muscle strain. Low back pain may also occur, resulting from an attempt to compensate to maintain global alignment. It has been demonstrated that cervical deformity, with its consequences, can have profound impact on health-related quality of life.

9.2 Clinical Presentation

Normally the head is centered over the pelvis in both the sagittal and coronal planes. Clinical examination of the cervical deformity patient should include a visual assessment of global spinal alignment (▶ Fig. 9.1). This analysis of clinical global

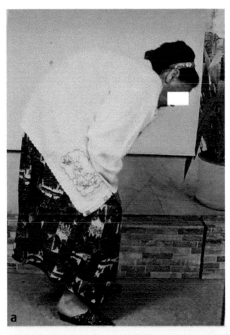
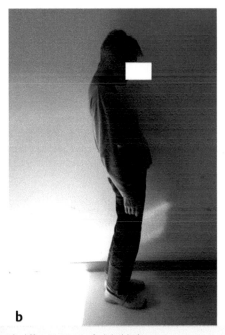
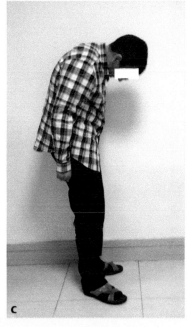

Fig. 9.1 Example of cervical deformities associated with different types of global balance.

balance and assessment of deformity location can prove invaluable in selecting the correct spinal levels for surgery. This has been emphasized by Riew[1] who reported that persistence of an imbalance after correction can lead to failure.

Cervical malalignment can be evaluated clinically through assessment of the chin–sternum distance and chin–brow vertical angle (CBVA), which quantifies horizontal gaze. Clinical assessment of the anterior or posterior projection of the head can be correlated with the tilt angle (measured on lateral radiographs). Vital et al[2] defined this projection as "protraction or retraction."

Flexibility of the cervical deformity can be invaluable for surgical planning. In the standing position, the patient is examined with passive and active extension to assess the extent to which cervical kyphosis can be corrected. In the supine position, the distance between the examination table and the occiput is measured; however, some flexibility may exist above and below the deformity. Koller[3] has described three types of "flexibility" (▶ Fig. 9.2). Clinical examination can be correlated with radiographic measurements of the C2–C7 Cobb angle changes on lateral flexion and extension views. In fused or rigid deformity, there is minimal or no change (<2 degrees). Semirigid deformities have partial correction, while flexible deformities have correction to cervical lordosis.

Overall mobility of the cervical spine is linked to segmental motion across each of the disc spaces and the facets. Pathological processes may induce stiffness. In ankylosing spondylitis, all elements (anterior and posterior) are fused, and the deformity tends to be rigid. In drop head, discs and posterior facets often remain mobile, and these deformities are typically flexible. In semirigid deformities, the disc spaces and uncinates and/or posterior facets may be partially fused, and some correction may be possible in extension.

A thorough neurological examination is also important. This should include an assessment for sensory changes, motor examination in upper and lower extremities, as well as an assessment for evidence of myelopathy.

9.3 Imaging

Full-length standing spine radiographs, including anteroposterior (AP) and lateral views, are necessary to measure the global alignment. AP and lateral cervical incidence can be used to determine the extent of kyphosis and vertebral levels involved and permit measurement of important radiographic parameters, including C2–C7 lordosis, C2–C7 sagittal vertical axis, thoracic kyphosis, lumbar lordosis, pelvic incidence, and pelvic tilt.

Lateral radiographs in maximum flexion and extension can be used to determine rigidity and residual flexibility of the spine above and below the deformity. These radiographs can also be helpful in localizing the area to be treated; EOS imaging, which minimizes radiation exposure and allows a full-body view, can be particularly useful for global deformity assessment. Magnetic resonance imaging (MRI) should be obtained if possible for the assessment of spinal cord and nerve root compression. Alternatively, a CT myelogram can provide similar information if MRI cannot be obtained. CT imaging is important for surgical planning, particularly to analyze whether disc spaces are open (i.e., not fused), presence of osteophytes, and evidence of ossification of the posterior longitudinal ligament. CT is also useful in assessing fusion of the uncus and facets.

The vertebral arteries (VA) can have aberrant anatomy or pathways and may have areas of adhesions, particularly in cases of inflammatory diseases (e.g., rheumatoid arthritis or infection) or in the setting of previous surgery. Surgeons should maintain a low threshold for obtaining angiography (e.g., CT angiogram) to characterize the anatomy and pathways of the VAs, as well as to assess the patency and for evidence of dominant anatomy.

Otolaryngologist's evaluation is indicated particularly if the patient is planned for an anterior cervical approach and especially if the patient has had previous anterior surgery. In the series of Lee and colleagues,[4] previous anterior surgery or multilevel fusions had increased risk for dysphagia and dysphonia. If vocal cord function is normal bilaterally, then a left or right anterior approach can be considered. In the case of previous surgery, some surgeons prefer to avoid scar tissue. However, in the presence of vocal cord paralysis, the approach must be through the scar to avoid injury to the contralateral vocal cord.

9.4 Preoperative Planning

The decision of whether to pursue surgical treatment should include consideration of response to nonsurgical treatments, deformity progression, clinical symptoms, quality-of-life consequences, and patient's preferences. The presence of myelopathy

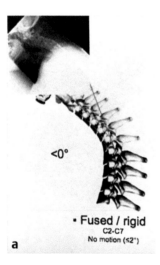

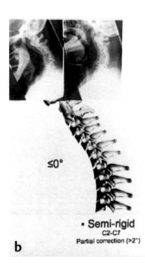

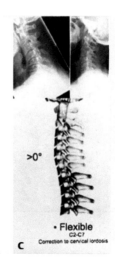

Fig. 9.2 The "three types of cervical flexibility."

a • Fused / rigid
C2-C7
No motion (≤2°)

b • Semi-rigid
C2-C7
Partial correction (>2°)

c • Flexible
C2-C7
Correction to cervical lordosis

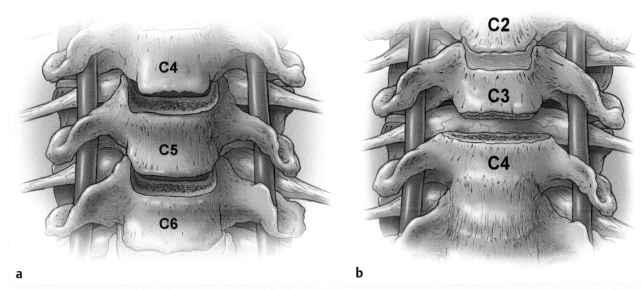

Fig. 9.3 Anterior uncinate osteotomies. (Reproduced with permission from Ames et al.[6])

should favor surgical treatment, especially in cases in which it is severe or demonstrates significant progression. The surgery plan requires localization of the levels of deformity and its extent, measurement of the degree of deformity and prediction of the amount of correction needed, and assessment of the rigidity of the deformity, including the surrounding flexibility of the cervical segments above and below. The plan should also account for the potential need to address neurological compromise, including that resulting from direct compression, instability, or from spinal stretch over kyphotic segments.

9.5 Surgical Technique

Semirigid deformity can be corrected by either anterior or posterior osteotomies. The anterior approach is the preferred technique if preoperative assessment demonstrates isolated anterior fusion. Multilevel anterior cervical discectomy and fusion (ACDF) or corporectomy may ultimately be performed; however, here we will follow, step by step, the uncovertebral joint osteotomy, defined as an osteotomy through the uncovertebral joints and extending next to the transverse foramen bilaterally, as well described by Tan and Riew.[5]

Cervical osteotomy techniques have been described and classified by Ames and colleagues.[6] Their classification of osteotomies and soft-tissue releases includes seven anatomical grades of resection that represent progressively greater degrees of bony removal and potential destabilization. Since the surgical procedure for a given case may involve combinations of resection types, the highest grade of osteotomy is designated as the "major osteotomy," while lower grades of osteotomy are designated as "minor osteotomies." In this classification, complete resection of the uncovertebral joints is classified as a Grade 4 osteotomy (▶ Fig. 9.3).

Prior to surgery, the patient can be placed in halo-traction at bedside with the addition of muscle relaxants, in order to try to reduce the deformity. Lateral radiographs can demonstrate the

amount of reduction obtained. We more frequently use a halo than Gardner-Wells tongs, since this technique allows us to manipulate the head more easily during surgery. Surgery is done under general anesthesia. Depending on the deformity, sometime intubation orally is impossible, and can only be done through nasal passage (▶ Fig. 9.4). The patient is placed in a supine position, but in the setting of rigid kyphosis the head may not rest on the table and may require pillows for support.

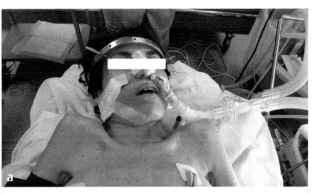

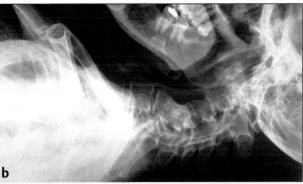

Fig. 9.4 Halo-head traction and nasal intubation tube.

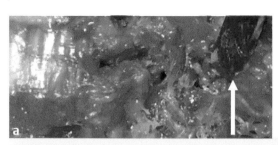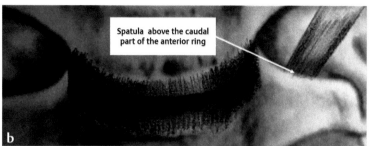

Fig. 9.5 Exposure of the anterior ring of the foramen transversarium; the spatula dissects over the cranial border. (Spatula shows the upper part of the anterior ring.)

Under anesthesia, we measure the distance between the occipital protuberance and the table, as well as the chin–sternum distance, and assess spinal alignment with lateral views under fluoroscopy. Sometimes partial reduction of the deformity is obtained, when the patient relaxes under general anesthesia. Cervical traction is applied (2–3 kg) through the halo, and arterial pressure is maintained around 80 mm Hg (particularly in the case of spinal cord compression). The neck is prepared and draped in the usual sterile fashion, and a Smith–Robinson approach is used, for which we prefer a vertical incision for deformity correction. A right or left approach may be used depending on the deformity, history of previous surgery, vocal cord function, and surgeon's preference. In the case of a coronal deformity (scoliosis), we prefer to approach on the convex side, allowing for more space and easier correction.

An anterior approach for significant cervical can be challenging and demanding. Application of traction during surgery and even for several days prior to surgery for semirigid curves can help partially reduce the deformity and provide improved operating access. In this chapter, we discuss osteotomies for two situations, semirigid and rigid deformities of the subaxial cervical spine generally based on the technique of Tan and Riew.[5]

The anterior cervical spine is exposed, and the longus colli muscles are detached and retracted bilaterally. This dissection may create bleeding, for which we use cautery and surgical wax. A major step is to localize the uncinate, which can be achieved through blunt dissection close to the bone, using a 2- or 4-mm spatula, lateral to the uncinate. The costal process (anterior ring of the foramen transversarium) is used as a landmark to identify the fused disc space, since the disc space and uncinate are just medial to the cranial border of the costal process (▶ Fig. 9.5).

The spatula remains in place during resection, identifying the lateral border of the uncinate, protecting the VA, and guiding the lateral bony resection. In case of concern regarding VA anomalies and in difficult case, we use the VA dissection technique of George.[7, 8] Gradually, the anterior ring of the foramen transversarium is fully exposed, then by a blunt dissection close to the bone, the foramen is penetrated above and below the ring. Using a small Kerrisson punch, we resect the anterior ring. The VA is identified and can be safely excluded from the resection area

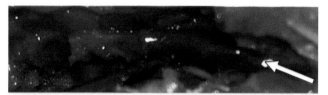

Fig. 9.6 If the anterior ring is resected, the vertebral artery appears in the foramen transversarium and can be followed.

(▶ Fig. 9.6). The VA can be surrounded by a venous complex, which can be addressed with bipolar cautery to avoid bleeding.

At this point, the fused uncinates are exposed and the VAs are excluded. Next, we do not use Caspar pins, as described by Riew, as we find that they overload the operative field due to their convergence, and they tend to impede the passage of the surgeon's hands when releasing the opposite side. Furthermore, Riew used these pins for deformity correction, which we consider potentially risky, particularly in older and osteoporotic patients. In contrast, we implant very laterally, perpendicular to the vertebral body, two 15/10 pins, which increase retraction of the muscles and soft tissue (▶ Fig. 9.7). These pins make an angle which we measure at the beginning of the osteotomy, and the new angle after the osteotomy provides an estimate of the amount of expected correction achieved. Discectomy is then completed down to the longitudinal ligament, after which the uncinates are totally exposed medially and laterally (▶ Fig. 9.8).

The osteotomy is then initiated with a high-speed surgical drill (▶ Fig. 9.9). In the case of a purely kyphotic deformity, bony resection must be absolutely perpendicular to the cervical spine and in the same space as the disc. Any asymmetric resection can induce iatrogenic coronal deformity. Conversely, the resection should be asymmetric, in the case of a mixed coronal and kyphotic deformity. Bony resection is performed down to the posterior longitudinal ligament. Dural lesion must be avoided during this stage.

Resection of the uncus is initially partial. If the uncinates are not totally fused, total resection is not necessary. If the uncinates are fused, an attempt can be made using a Cobb elevator which may be rotated in the disc space, close to the residual uncinate, to produce some "breakage," in order to avoid the need for total resection of the uncinate. The same maneuver can also be done with a vertebral body spreader.

If "mobility" is not obtained, total uncinate resection must be achieved. Importantly, the burr never passes the lateral border of the uncinate. When there remains only a very thin shell of bone, the residual bone can be removed by a very small Kerrisson or curette. Since correction of local kyphosis, by opening the anterior disc space, may induce stenosis of the

foramen, a foraminotomy is recommended to avoid root entrapment.

Once both sides are sufficiently released or totally resected, correction of the kyphosis can be realized. The pillows under the head are removed, and the surgeon applies controlled pressure on the anterior ring of the halo. A Cobb retractor and spreader can help at the same time by opening and distracting the disc space (▶ Fig. 9.10). We do not like to use the two Caspar pins as a means of correction, since the force applied is not biomechanically satisfying, and in old patients these may

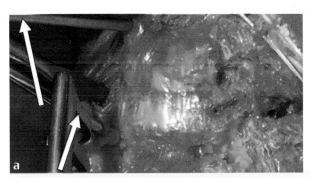
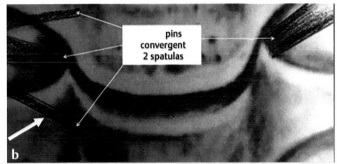

Fig. 9.7 Exposure of the disc space, two very lateral pins are inserted in the vertebral body with an angle of convergence.

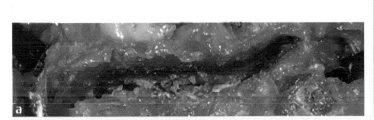
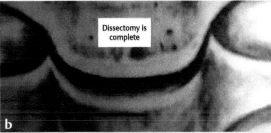

Fig. 9.8 Dissection and exposure of the uncinate.

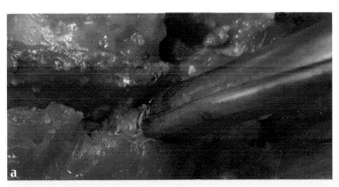
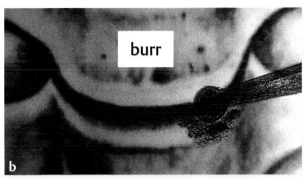

Fig. 9.9 High-speed surgical drill.

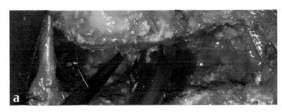
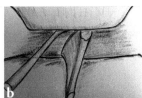

Fig. 9.10 Cobb retractor, by maneuver of rotation, distracts the intervertebral space; the uncinate appears totally resected; the cord is seen deeply in the operative field.

risk vertebral body fracture. The new angle of the pins will reflect the local amount of correction. If the posterior facet joints are not fused and have residual mobility, this will allow easier correction. Even if the facet joints are partially fused, correction can be obtained, thanks to the anterior long lever arm.

At this stage, the risk is not overcorrection (the rest of the spine is flexible) but rather hypocorrection. It is necessary to try to assess the new sagittal alignment. The head must now touch the operative table, and the chin–sternum distance must return to a normal value. Radiographs are done to measure the new Cobb angle. Lordosis is stabilized by increasing the halo traction weight to 9 kg.

If the osteotomies have been realized at multiple levels, large cages can be used. If all corrections have been achieved at a single level, leaving a big gap, we prefer to use iliac crest bone graft, which will be easier to shape and to better adapt to the space. It is important to provide the largest surface area between the graft and the endplate support to avoid pseudarthrosis and subsidence. An anterior plate, bent in lordosis, is applied. Screws are implanted at the upper and lower part of the construct. In old patients with osteoporotic bone, we add a posterior fusion and fixation to help ensure postoperative stability.

If correction is inadequate, the facets are fused, the spine is already fixed posteriorly, or there is a posterior mass of fusion, a second-stage surgery may be necessary to increase correction. In this case, only graft material is placed in the anterior part of the osteotomy in order to leave freedom when additional lordosis is created from the posterior approach. A buttress plate is fixed with only screws above or below just to avoid graft extrusion. Additional lordosis from the posterior approach will induce compression on the posterior part of the anterior graft permitting fusion. Posterior osteotomies can be achieved as described by Ames et al[6] at one or multiple levels with fixation and fusion.

Closure is done with drainage. Theoretically, no external immobilization is needed. Early mobilization and physical therapy are recommended (▶ Fig. 9.11)

9.6 Discussion

The decision-making process can be challenging for semirigid deformities of the cervical spine. The overall goals of surgery are to restore the best local and global alignment and, in the case of myelopathy or radiculopathy, to improve pain and deficit with positive consequences on quality of life. This correction is maintained by fusion and fixation.

Current literature offers little help in surgical planning. In a recent study from the International Spine Study Group,[9] Smith and colleagues concluded that there was a marked lack of consensus for surgery treatment, even for the most simple types of cervical deformities. Kandasamy and Abdullah,[10] Nemani et al,[11] Etame et al,[12] and Han et al[13] have all reviewed the general literature, which primarily consists of retrospective series with mixed etiologies.

Posterior osteotomies were first proposed by Simmons[14] for ankylosing spondylitis. Recently, Smith et al[15] reviewed 23 patients who underwent posteriorly based three-column osteotomy correction and noted an overall complication rate of 56.5%. Posterior correction at the apex of deformity can be realized too. Partial facet resection or total facet resection (Ponte-type) has been proposed, but these osteotomies depend on residual anterior column mobility to obtain the necessary correction. Anterior correction offers another tool, allowing correction, cord and root decompression, spinal reconstruction, and lower complication risks than those often seen with posterior high-grade osteotomies.

Initially, surgeons performed anterior corporectomy and fusion without internal fixation. In the series of Zdeblick and Bohlman,[16] loss of correction was at least 4 degrees, and in the series of Riew et al[17] only 8/18 patients had a decreased degree of kyphosis. With the introduction of cervical plating and screws, better correction has been achieved with lower rates of complications. Some authors have proposed mixed techniques of ACDF and corpectomy; however, corpectomy tends to produce less sagittal correction and imposes a longer segment across which fusion must be achieved.

Anterior osteotomy at one level or mutilevel discectomy is another efficient technique for correction of semirigid cervical spine deformities. Kim and Riew[18] were the first to detail this technique. In the series from Kim and colleagues,[18] the authors reviewed 38 patients who underwent anterior osteotomy for rigid cervical deformity. They demonstrated that anterior osteotomies provided an average of 23 degrees of angular correction and 1.3 cm of translational correction. If performed in combination with Smith–Petersen osteotomies (SPO), they obtained an average angular correction of 33 degrees and translational correction of 3.7 cm, although most of these were performed only for additional stabilization. They did not, furthermore, describe any neurological complications or intraoperative neuromonitoring changes in either group. There were no early or late losses of correction or other complications.

In a more recent study of 61 patients, Kim et al[19] described the amount of correction obtained with different types of osteotomies in the cervical spine when treating cervical deformity. They concluded that posteriorly based osteotomies provided better translational correction than anterior osteotomies (ATOs). The angular correction achieved by one PSO (pedicle subtraction osteotomy) was similar to ATO + SPOs. ATO + SPOs provided equal or better corrections than isolated PSOs, with equal length of stay and less estimated blood loss.

9.7 Conclusion

Anterior cervical osteotomy, classified as "low-grade osteotomy" in the nomenclature of Ames and colleagues, is a very efficient tool for the correction of semirigid cervical spine deformity. This technique decreases perioperative and postoperative risk of complications compared with high-grade posterior osteotomies. A posterior technique with additional release may be helpful in some cases to improve correction and stability.

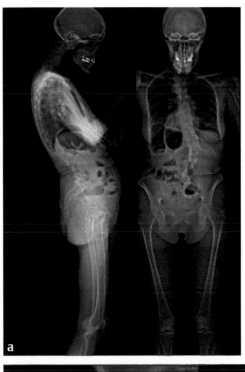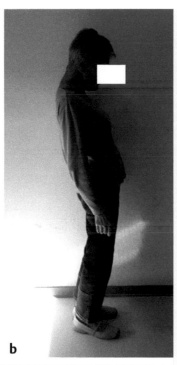

Fig. 9.11 Case presentation (O. Gille's collection): A 60-year-old woman with loss of horizontal gaze, radiculopathy, and neck pain, disability in everyday function. EOS full body shows a lumbar scoliosis associated with high retroversion of the sacrum. (a) Hyperextension of the hips does not allow the patient to restore normal alignment. (b) Lateral cervical radiographs in neutral and extension show a rigid midcervical kyphosis. The facet joints, however, are not fused. (c) Anterior osteotomy at multiple levels with cages and plate permit restoration of cervical lordosis and normal global alignment (d).

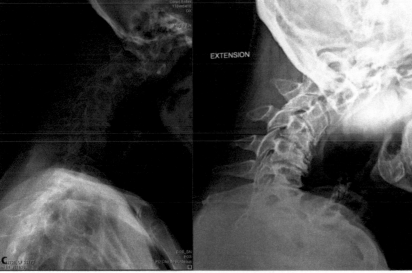

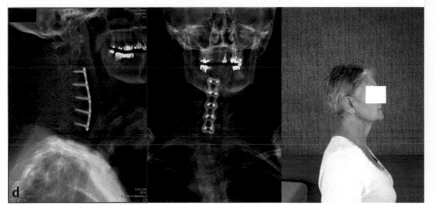

References

[1] Riew KD. Cervical deformity assessment, clinical impact and a new technique for cervical deformities. Conference at the Annual Meeting SFCR; June 1–3, 2017

[2] Vital JM, Senegas L, Yoshida G. Les nouvelles données sur l'équilibre sagittal cervical. Le Rachis. 2016; 4:27–29

[3] Koller H. Cervical spine profile issues- cervical kyphosis. The XVIII CSRS-ES Cadaveric Instructional Course. March 31–April 1, 2016. Barcelona, Spain

[4] Lee MJ, Bazaz R, Furey CG, Yoo J. Risk factors for dysphagia after anterior cervical spine surgery: a two-year prospective cohort study. Spine J. 2007; 7 (2):141–147

[5] Tan LA, Riew KD. Anterior cervical osteotomy: operative technique. Eur Spine J. 2018; 27 Suppl 1:39–47

[6] Ames CP, Smith JS, Scheer JK, et al. International Spine Study Group. A standardized nomenclature for cervical spine soft-tissue release and osteotomy for deformity correction: clinical article. J Neurosurg Spine. 2013; 19(3):269–278

[7] Bancel PH. Abord anterieur de l'artère vertébrale et de la charnière occipito cervicale Pre meeting. Laboratoire d'anatomie - Fer à Moulin Annual meeting SFCR Paris; June 2014

[8] Georges B, Laurian C. Surgical approach to the whole length of the vertebral artery with special reference to the third portion. Acta Neurochir. 1980; 51:259–272

[9] Smith JS, Klineberg E, Shaffrey CI, et al. International Spine Study Group. Assessment of surgical treatment strategies for moderate to severe cervical spinal deformity reveals marked variation in approaches, osteotomies, and fusion levels. World Neurosurg. 2016; 91:228–237

[10] Kandasamy R, Abdullah JM. Cervical spine deformity correction: an overview. World Neurosurg. 2016; 91:640–641

[11] Nemani VM, Derman PB, Kim HJ. Osteotomies in the cervical spine. Asian Spine J. 2016; 10(1):184–195

[12] Etame AB, Than KD, Wang AC, La Marca F, Park P. Surgical management of symptomatic cervical or cervicothoracic kyphosis due to ankylosing spondylitis. Spine. 2008; 33(16):E559–E564

[13] Han K, Lu C, Li J, et al. Surgical treatment of cervical kyphosis. Eur Spine J. 2011; 20(4):523–536

[14] Simmons EH. The surgical correction of flexion deformity of the cervical spine in ankylosing spondylitis. Clin Orthop Relat Res. 1972; 86(86):132–143

[15] Smith JS, Shaffrey CI, Klineberg E, et al. on behalf of the International Spine Study Group. Complication rates associated with 3-column osteotomy in 82 adult spinal deformity patients: retrospective review of a prospectively collected multicenter consecutive series with 2-year follow-up. J Neurosurg Spine. 2017; 27(4):444–457

[16] Zdeblick TA, Bohlman HH. Cervical kyphosis and myelopathy. Treatment by anterior corpectomy and strut-grafting. J Bone Joint Surg Am. 1989; 71 (2):170–182

[17] Riew KD, Hilibrand AS, Palumbo MA, Bohlman HH. Anterior cervical corpectomy in patients previously managed with a laminectomy: short-term complications. J Bone Joint Surg Am. 1999; 81(7):950–957

[18] Kim HJ, Piyaskulkaew C, Riew KD. Anterior cervical osteotomy for fixed cervical deformities. Spine. 2014; 39(21):1751–1757

[19] Kim HJ, Piyaskulkaew C, Riew KD. Comparison of Smith-Petersen osteotomy versus pedicle subtraction osteotomy versus anterior-posterior osteotomy types for the correction of cervical spine deformities. Spine. 2015; 40 (3):143–146

10 Uncovertebral Joint Osteotomy (Anterior Riew Osteotomy) for Correction of Rigid Cervical Spine Deformity

Lee A. Tan, Christopher P. Ames, and K. Daniel Riew

Abstract

Anterior cervical osteotomy is a powerful surgical technique for rigid cervical deformity correction. Compared to cervical pedicle subtraction osteotomy, anterior osteotomy is safer and more versatile in that it can be performed at multiple levels throughout the cervical spine. In this chapter, a step-by-step guide is provided for anterior cervical osteotomy with a discussion on surgical nuances and complication avoidance. Spine surgeons should be familiar with this technique to optimize clinical outcome in patients undergoing rigid cervical deformity correction.

Keywords: cervical deformity, anterior osteotomy, cervical spine, kyphosis, chin-on-chest

10.1 Introduction

Cervical spine deformity can cause significant disability and have negative impact on the quality of life. Patients with deformity in the cervical spine can often present with neck pain, myelopathy, and sensorimotor deficits. Furthermore, patients with severe kyphotic deformity often have difficulty in maintaining horizontal gaze, which can significantly impact the patient's functional status and limit the ability to perform activities of daily living. Surgical correction of cervical deformities can be challenging, especially in the setting of rigid cervical deformities, which often require osteotomies to obtained adequate correction.

Posteriorly based osteotomy such as pedicle subtraction osteotomy is typically limited to the cervicothoracic junction at C7 or T1, due to the presence of vertebral arteries; and PSO can be technically challenging in this region due to the important innervation of cervical nerve roots. In contrast, the anterior Riew osteotomy, defined as osteotomy through the disc space and uncovertebral joints up to the transverse foramen bilaterally, is a powerful deformity correction technique that can be performed throughout the cervical spine.[1] In addition, it can be performed in conjunction with posterior facet release as needed, which allows for significant kyphosis correction in rigid cervical deformity. Furthermore, asymmetrical anterior osteotomy can be utilized in patients with fixed coronal malalignment such as in cases of "ear-on-shoulder" deformity to gain significant coronal correction.

In this chapter, a step-by-step guide for the anterior Riew osteotomy is provided with a discussion of surgical nuances and various pearls for complication avoidance. Anterior Riew osteotomy is a powerful tool for fixed cervical spine deformity correction. Spine surgeons should be familiar with this technique for cervical deformity correction.

10.2 Preoperative Evaluation and Surgical Planning

Preoperative evaluation should include a thorough neurological examination and a comprehensive review of preoperative imaging studies. Any neurological deficits should be clearly documented and correlated with imaging findings to identify potential symptomatic neural compression. Decompression of these neural elements should be included in the overall treatment plan. Neurological exam findings that are not congruent with imaging findings warrant further workup to rule out non–spinal-related etiology such as peripheral neuropathy and various nerve entrapment syndromes. Useful preoperative imaging modalities include AP/lateral/oblique/dynamic cervical X-rays, scoliosis film, computed tomography (CT), and magnetic resonance imaging (MRI). Cervical X-rays are helpful in assessing the severity of deformity, location of the apex, flexibility of the deformity, as well as presence of any bony foraminal stenosis on oblique views. Scoliosis films can provide information regarding global balance, as some cervical deformities are related to concurrent thoracolumbar deformities. CT is very useful in determining location of preexisting bony fusion, and MRI is the modality of choice in assessing neural compression. If MRI is contraindicated, or has too much artifact from existing instrumentation, CT myelogram can be obtained instead.

Relevant radiographic parameters including cervical lordosis, chin–brow vertical angle (CBVA), C2–C7 sagittal vertical axis (SVA), and T1 slope should be measured on preoperative imaging. The desired amount of correction in both sagittal and coronal planes should be determined based on each patient's symptomatology, unique medical circumstances, and individual needs. The flexibility of the deformity can be assessed on lateral dynamic cervical X-rays; thin-cut CT can be obtained to evaluate for the presence of ankylosis anteriorly or posteriorly. If the facets are fused in addition to the anterior column ankylosis, then a posterior facet release and instrumentation are required to gain adequate deformity correction in conjunction with anterior osteotomy.

In patients with previous anterior cervical spine surgery, the vocal cord function should be assessed preoperatively by an otolaryngologist. If vocal cord dysfunction is already present, the cervical spine should be approached from the ipsilateral side as the prior surgery to avoid potential bilateral vocal cord paralysis. If the vocal cord function is normal, then a left-side approach is generally preferred, due to the longer course of the left recurrence laryngeal nerve and the theoretically lower risk of iatrogenic nerve injury. In patients with significant coronal deformity, approaching the cervical spine from the convex side is generally easier. Furthermore, the course of the vertebral arteries must be carefully studied on preoperative imaging studies to avoid inadvertent injury.

Anterior osteotomy can be used to treat rigid deformities in both coronal and sagittal planes, such as "chin-on-chest" and "ear-on-shoulder" deformities. By removing the uncinate processes bilaterally, the anterior spinal column is released and correction of the rigid deformity is then possible. If posterior facet fusion is present, anterior osteotomy can be combined with posterior facet release to achieve deformity correction; this is achieved by placing standalone anterior grafts with one single screw or a buttress plate anteriorly, so that additional correction can be obtained after posterior release.

10.3 Surgical Technique

The patient is brought into the operating room and undergoes general endotracheal intubation. Neuromonitoring is established and baseline signals are obtained in patient with spinal cord compression. In patients with kyphotic deformity, cervical traction with Gardner-Wells tongs (usually 15 lb) can be applied to facilitate intubation and the initial approach to the anterior cervical spine. If the cervical kyphosis is severe, the head may be suspended in the air during the initial positioning; in this situation, folded sheets can be stacked together to help in supporting the head at the beginning of the case. After the anterior osteotomy, the head has to be pushed back toward the table to correct the kyphosis. Therefore, it is critical that it is initially positioned off the table adequately to allow for posterior migration. In general, we position the head such that it is approximately 30 to 40 cm off the table, depending on the magnitude of the deformity. Exposure of the apex of the kyphotic deformity can be challenging, since it is deep in the wound. In patients with cervical spinal cord compression, the mean arterial pressure (MAP) should be kept above 80 mm Hg to maintain adequate cord perfusion not only during intubation but also throughout the procedure.

After positioning the patient supine on the operating table, the neck is prepped and draped in the usual sterile fashion. A microscope is draped and used throughout the case. The anterior cervical spine exposure is obtained via the standard Smith–Robinson approach, and the spinal levels are confirmed with fluoroscopy. The longus colli muscles are detached from their insertion sites bilaterally at the midvertebral body using bipolar cautery, and table-mounted retractors are inserted under the longus colli cuff to maintain exposure. Anterior osteophytes are removed with Leksell rongeurs or a high-speed burr. Caspar pins are placed at the level with intended anterior osteotomy. Two sets of pins can be used if the bone quality is osteoporotic for additional purchase. The pins are placed perpendicular to the anterior plane of the spine, resulting in divergent pins alignment in a kyphotic spine. Additional lordosis can be gained with this pin placement as the pins are distracted after the osteotomy (▶ Fig. 10.1).

The osteotomy is performed using a high-speed 2.5-mm matchstick burr. For kyphotic deformities, bony resection should be kept perpendicular to the cervical spine in the same space as the former disc space to prevent asymmetrical resection in the coronal plane. For mixed coronal and kyphotic deformities, asymmetrical bony resection can be made on purpose to correct both the coronal and sagittal deformities. The dorsal limit of bony resection is up to the posterior longitudinal ligament. The lateral aspect of the bony resection is performed carefully in a step-wise fashion with extreme caution, in order to prevent iatrogenic vertebral artery injury. First, Penfield nos. 4 and 2 dissectors are used to dissect lateral to the uncinate processes. The Penfield no. 2 is then kept in place lateral to the uncinate process during the lateral bony resection to demarcate the lateral border and to protect the vertebral artery (▶ Fig. 10.2). Once the bone is resected close to the lateral border, the remaining thin shell of bone can be broken off using a microcurette. Bilateral anterior foraminotomies are typically performed to prevent nerve root compression when the cervical spine is extended during deformity correction.

After the osteotomy is complete, the anesthesiologist can help remove sheets initially placed under the head one-by-one, while surgeon exerts gentle downward force on the forehead through the sterile drape (▶ Fig. 10.3). In addition, an intervertebral spreader or a Cobb elevator can be placed within the

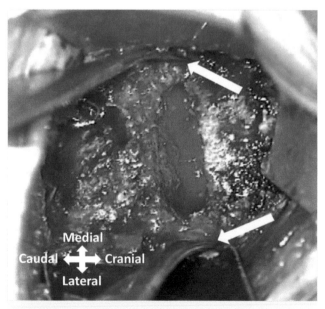

Fig. 10.2 A photograph demonstrating the vertebral arteries protected by using Penfield no. 2 dissectors during resection of the uncinate processes.

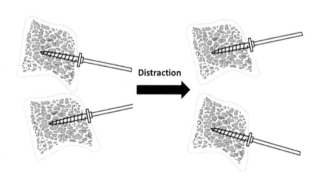

Fig. 10.1 The Caspar pins are placed perpendicular to the anterior surface of the kyphotic cervical spine initially, and distraction of the pins maximizes the amount of lordosis obtained through the anterior osteotomy.

osteotomy site for additional distraction along with the Caspar pins during kyphosis correction (▶ Fig. 10.4). Alternatively, sequentially larger sizes can be used to help open up the disc space. Pushing down gently on the forehead provides the most biomechanical leverage with the least amount of risk for Caspar pin loosening and vertebral body fracture during kyphosis correction. Partial kyphosis correction can often be obtained even if there was prior posterior instrumentation, since most cervical rods will be bent into less kyphosis with this maneuver. Even with a solid posterior fusion with 3.5-mm titanium rods, it is often possible to get partial correction of the deformity, as the fusion mass and the posterior instrumentation will flex a few degrees. However, if 3.5-mm cobalt chromium rods were utilized posteriorly and there is a solid fusion, one can get only minimal correction after the anterior osteotomy and the rest of the correction has to be done posteriorly. When the head touches the operating table, the anterior part of the kyphosis correction is then complete. If additional kyphosis correction is necessary, one can ask the anesthesiology team to place folded sheets under the shoulders to lift the head off of the table such that it can be pushed further posteriorly. Cervical traction with Gardner-Wells tongs can be increased to 25 lb to maintain the correction if needed.

Next, bone graft is inserted into the distracted osteotomy site. Since the bone edges in the osteotomy site are usually cancellous, there is a high chance of graft subsidence; thus, it is important to fit the largest bone graft possible into the

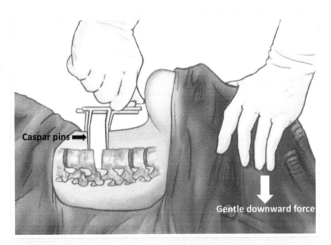

Fig. 10.3 An illustration showing correction cervical kyphosis by pushing down on the forehead taking advantage of large moment provided by the long lever arm, while simultaneously distracting with Caspar pins.

osteotomy site to provide the maximum amount of surface area possible for endplate support. If adequate deformity correction has been obtained, then an anterior cervical plate with fixed angle screws is placed; if additional posterior correction is required, then a trapezoid-shape bone graft (contacting the anterior but not the posterior aspect of the osteotomy site) is used, so that further lordosis can be achieved with posterior compression. A buttress plate or an interference screw is used to prevent graft extrusion during the posterior portion of the procedure when the patient is prone (▶ Fig. 10.5). More commonly, we now tend to use a standalone cage fixed with a single screw, which keeps the cage in place and allows for further correction posteriorly.

After hemostasis is obtained, the wound is closed in the standard fashion with a Penrose drain. A Penrose drain is preferred over a closed-suction drain, as it will never occlude. Since the drainage will wet the dressing and make a mess, we use an abdominal pad, which wicks the blood away from the skin and keeps it drier than cotton dressings. Posterior instrumentation and fusion is generally preferred to augment the anterior osteotomy in our practice. If posterior fixation is not done immediately following anterior osteotomy, then a halo or a rigid brace is recommended until the posterior procedure is possible. If the deformity has been adequately corrected anteriorly, the posterior instrumentation is placed simply to maintain the correction. However, if after the anterior procedure there is residual deformity, then one has to perform a posterior Smith–Petersen osteotomy(ies) to further correct the deformity. This is a simple procedure that has been adequately described elsewhere in this book. Even with an anterior correction, it is quite easy to place the cervicothoracic junction in too much kyphosis. One can avoid this by making sure that the spinous processes between C6 and T5 (or the lowest instrumented vertebra) are no more than 5 to 7 mm apart from the adjacent one. If the interspinous process distance is greater than 5 to 7 mm apart, we use spinous process cables or a third rod attached to laminar screws to compress them together.

10.4 Postoperative Care and Complications

The patient is typically extubated immediately after surgery, if the duration of the anterior retraction time is less than 3 hours. If the retraction time for the anterior procedure is much longer than 3 hours, then airway edema may result; so, we often keep the patient intubated overnight and perform a cuff-leak test

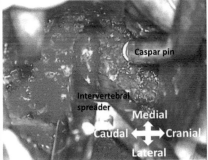
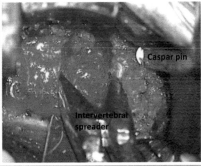

Fig. 10.4 An intraoperative photograph demonstrating an intervertebral spreader is inserted into the disc space (left) to distract open the disc space after anterior osteotomy (right).

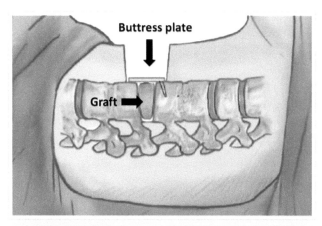

Fig. 10.5 An illustration showing a buttress plate with a single screw to prevent graft extrusion.

prior to extubating the patient. The Penrose drain is typically removed on postoperative day 1 or 2. We leave it until the dressing remains dry for an 8-hour shift. All patients start physical therapy on postoperative day 1, and are placed in a cervical orthosis to hasten bony fusion. If the anterior and posterior fixation was solid, a soft collar is used. If not, then we use a hard collar.

Complications from the anterior cervical approach may include dysphagia, vocal cord paralysis, tracheal/esophageal injury, vertebral artery injury, spinal cord or nerve root injury, cerebral spinal fluid leak, pseudoarthrosis, instrumentation failure, graft subsidence, and wound infection. Dysphagia is a common complaint immediately after surgery in patients after anterior cervical procedures. Fortunately, it is usually transient and most patients' symptoms resolve with time. A short course of steroids can also help in improving dysphagia symptoms. Wound-related complications are rare for anterior-only procedures, but can occur with much higher frequency if posterior cervical approach is utilized. This risk of infection can be decreased by minimizing the potential dead space in the wound by closing meticulously in multiple myofascial layers, and with using intrawound vancomycin powder. Pseudoarthrosis can occur with multilevel anterior-only construct, but the risk of pseudoarthrosis is very small if the construct is augmented with posterior instrumentation and fusion. The mortality rates can range from 3.1 to 6.7%, while major medical complications can range from 3.1 to 44.4%, and neurological complications can occur in about 13.5% of cases.[2] Despite the complications,[3] the patient satisfaction rates were high. Careful preoperative planning, prudent patient selection, meticulous surgical technique, and optimized postoperative care help minimize complications associated with cervical deformity correction.

10.5 Conclusion

Anterior osteotomy is a powerful tool for the correction of fixed cervical spine deformities. Even patients with severe "chin-on-chest" or "ear-on-shoulder" deformities can be safely and effectively treated with this technique. Spine surgeons should be familiar with this technique during treatment of cervical spine deformity.

References

[1] Kim HJ, Piyaskulkaew C, Riew KD. Anterior cervical osteotomy for fixed cervical deformities. Spine. 2014; 39(21):1751–1757

[2] Etame AB, Wang AC, Than KD, La Marca F, Park P. Outcomes after surgery for cervical spine deformity: review of the literature. Neurosurg Focus. 2010; 28 (3):E14

[3] Smith JS, Ramchandran S, Lafage V, et al. Prospective multicenter assessment of early complication rates associated with adult cervical deformity surgery in 78 patients. 2016; 79(3):378–388

11 Cervical Pedicle Subtraction Osteotomy for Correction of Sagittal Deformities

Winward Choy, Darryl Lau, Cecilia L. Dalle Ore, Heiko Koller, Sang Hun Lee, and Christopher P. Ames

Abstract

Cervical deformities can lead to pronounced symptoms and significant disability in patients. The correction of cervical deformities poses unique challenges as compared to deformities in the more rigid thoracic spine. The optimal surgical approach, extent of osteotomy, and levels involved depend on a number of anatomical and deformity-specific considerations. Extensive osteotomies, such as pedicle subtraction osteotomy (PSO), may be warranted. Preoperative imaging should include standing scoliosis X-rays in the patient's comfortable position, computed tomography (CT) imaging, and magnetic resonance imaging (MRI). Flexion–extension films are warranted to evaluated rigidity. While global spinal alignment is important, key cervical parameters that should be considered include cervical sagittal vertical axis, cervical lordosis, and T1 slope. The appropriate osteotomy should be selected based on the degree of correction needed and the rigidity of the deformity. Extent of osteotomy is readily described by the Ames Cervical Osteotomy Grade. Grade 6 (PSO) and grade 7 (vertebrectomy) osteotomies offers the greatest correction potential. This chapter concentrates on utility of cervical PSO and describes its technique.

Keywords: cervical, kyphosis, deformity, osteotomy

11.1 Introduction

The majority of cervical deformities in adults are kyphotic, and such sagittal plane deformities can produce pronounced symptoms and significant disability. Cervical deformity may result from a number of pathologies including degenerative changes, fractures, myopathies, inflammatory spondyloarthropathies, and iatrogenic complications such as postlaminectomy kyphosis.[1,2,3,4,5] Patients may suffer from dysphagia, difficulty in maintaining horizontal gaze, and gait impairment that can impair activities of daily living (ADLs).[6] Additionally, associated lengthening and flattening of the cord can cause ischemia and spinal cord injury, resulting in myelopathy. Patients may also experience compensatory severe neck pain and interscapular pain as a result of efforts to maintain horizontal gaze.

The correction of cervical deformities poses unique challenges as compared to deformities in the more rigid thoracic spine. These challenges reflect the complexity of the cervical spine, which has the widest range of motion and is critical for the maintenance of neutral head position and horizontal gaze. A number of different surgical strategies exist for deformity correction, including anterior, posterior, and combined approaches. The optimal surgical approach, extent of osteotomy, and levels involved depend on a number of anatomical and deformity-specific considerations. Extensive osteotomies, such as pedicle subtraction osteotomy (PSO), may be warranted.

Similar to its application in the correction of thoracolumbar deformities, PSO can be highly effective in the correction of sagittal plane deformities in the cervical spine. Historically, Smith-Peterson osteotomies (SPO) or combined anterior-posterior (AP) approaches have been the preferred technique for the correction of cervical deformities.[7,8,9,10] However, in cases of nonmobile, fixed cervical deformities, such as patients with ankylosing spondylitis (AS) or diffuse idiopathic skeletal hyperostosis, three-column osteotomies (PSO and vertebral column resection [VCR]) may be warranted. Unlike SPO, in which resection is limited to the posterior elements of the spine, PSO involves wedge resection of the vertebral body and facet joints (as in SPO). In a PSO, the anterior spinal column functions as a fulcrum, the spinal canal is shortened, and fusion is promoted by bone-on-bone contact. This chapter reviews the preoperative evaluation and surgical management of cervical sagittal deformities, with a focus on the role of cervical PSO.

11.2 Preoperative Evaluation

The goals of surgery in patients with cervical sagittal deformity and malalignment are deformity correction, spinal cord and nerve root decompression, restoration of horizontal gaze, and spinal stabilization through a biomechanically sound construct.[11] Evaluation of both cervical and global spinal alignment is critical for surgical planning. Preoperative evaluation typically comprises standing scoliosis (long-cassette) radiographs that allow for visualization from the external auditory canal to the femoral heads in order to evaluate global and regional sagittal alignment. Flexion and extension X-rays can be used to differentiate rigid versus flexible deformity, ultimately dictating the surgical approach and correction needed. Preoperative computed tomography (CT) and magnetic resonance imaging (MRI) may be used to evaluate vertebral anatomy and spinal cord or nerve root compression.

11.2.1 Cervical Sagittal Alignment and Quality-of-Life Outcomes

The goals of deformity correction are cervical sagittal vertical axis (C2 SVA) less than 40 mm and neutral chin–brow vertical angle (CBVA) evaluated in a fully relaxed C1–C2 position of comfort. Studies examining the correlation between cervical radiographic parameters and health-related quality-of-life (HRQOL) outcomes have been used to guide the extent of correction in cervical deformity surgery. Postoperative C2 SVA and CBVA have been shown to correlate with HRQOL and ADL-related outcomes following deformity correction.[12,13,14] C2 SVA captures regional sagittal plane translation, and is defined as the distance between the plumb line drawn from the odontoid of C2 and the posterior and superior-most point of the C7 vertebral body.[5] Correction should strive to produce postoperative C2 SVA of less than 40 mm.[15] CBVA quantifies horizontal gaze, and is measured by subtending an angle between a vertical line and a line drawn from the patient's chin to brow on clinical photographs. CBVA should be corrected to as close to 10 degrees as possible. Correction of CBVA following cervical deformity surgery has been associated with improved horizontal gaze, ADLs, and gait.[12,13,14] In evaluating the degree of sagittal correction required, the preoperative assessment of cervical radiographic parameters should be performed on X-rays taken in a position of comfort with a fully relaxed C1–C2, rather than a position in which the patient is told to look straight ahead (▶ Fig. 11.1). X-rays taken in the position of comfort often reveals a greater angular correction required by unmasking the true extent of the sagittal imbalance.

In contrast to C2 SVA and CBVA, there is not an established correlation between C2–C7 Cobb angle (CC) and HRQOL.[16,17] In patients undergoing surgery for cervical kyphosis, Lau et al demonstrated increased kyphosis based on Cobb angles was associated with increased neck pain.[18] However, Smith et al did not find a correlation between CC and modified Japanese Orthopedic Association (mJOA) scale in preoperative patients.[16, 17] Similarly, in a prospective, double-blind study, postoperative CC resulting from use of lordotic versus parallel allographs for anterior cervical discectomy and fusion (ACDF) was not correlated with postoperative clinical outcomes.[19] Reasons for the lack of correlation between CC and postoperative outcomes are multifold. Sagittal cervical alignment can be highly variable,[20,21] and normative CC may range from -25 to 44 degrees. Additionally, deformities often do not occur in isolation: structural deformity in one region may produce an abnormal secondary curve in another. Cervical lordosis thus does not necessitate higher HRQOL scores, as it may reflect compensatory changes necessary to maintain sagittal balance and horizontal gaze in patients with thoracolumbar deformity and global sagittal malalignment.[22,23]

The degree of correction should also be guided by subaxial and thoracolumbar alignment.[24] The cervical spine is highly mobile and may undergo reciprocal changes to compensate for sagittal deformities elsewhere in the spine.[23,25,26] T1 slope has been identified as a potential predictor of sagittal balance.[27] T1 slope is the angle between a line parallel to the T1 endplate and a horizontal line. T1 slope serves as a surrogate for compensatory subaxial lordosis required to maintain a balanced center of gravity of the head; increasing T1 slope requires increased

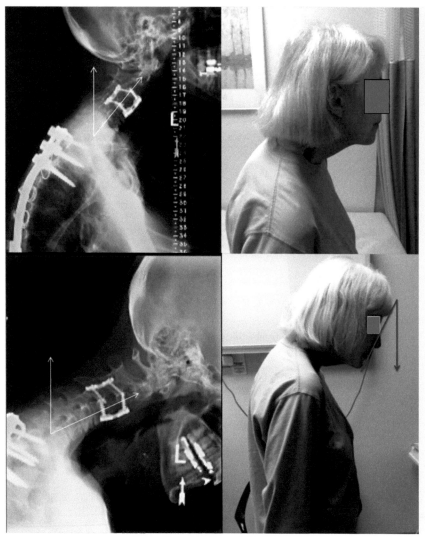

Fig. 11.1 Examples of positioning for evaluation of radiographic parameters. In the top panel, the patient is instructed to look forward. In the bottom panel, the patient is instructed to take a position of comfort, unmasking a larger degree of sagittal imbalance, C2 SVA, and CVBA.

cervical lordosis to maintain sagittal balance and horizontal gaze. T1 slope can be used to assess whether subjacent deformity is contributing to cervical malalignment: sagittal thoracolumbar deformity is likely present in cases with a T1 slope greater than 30 degrees.[28,29] A close relationship exists between T1 slope and C2–C7 Cobb angle such that a difference greater than 17 degrees between these two measurements suggests true cervical deformity even in the presence of deformity of the thoracolumbar spine.

11.3 Surgical Considerations in Cervical Deformity

The extent of deformity correction achieved intraoperatively is dependent on the approach and techniques utilized. Studies have found that 11 to 32 degrees of correction can be obtained with an anterior approach,[30,31,32,33,34] 23 to 54 degrees with a posterior approach,[35,36,37,38,39,40,41,42] and 24 to 61 degrees via a combined approach.[4,43,44] Similar to the management of thoracolumbar deformities, cervical osteotomies ranging from facet joint release to complete vertebrectomy may be employed for the correction of cervical sagittal deformity. Ames et al classified cervical osteotomies into seven categories (▸ Table 11.1), and the appropriate osteotomy should be selected based on the degree of correction needed and the rigidity of the deformity (▸ Fig. 11.2).[7] A Grade 1 osteotomy (or partial facet join resection) is a partial resection of the uncinate joints and/or partial removal of the posterior facets. A Grade 2 osteotomy is a complete facet joint resection, wherein both the inferior and superior articular facets are removed. A Grade 3 osteotomy is a complete corpectomy, including adjacent discs. A Grade 4 osteotomy is a corpectomy with associated complete resection of the uncinate joints laterally to the transverse foramen. A Grade 5 osteotomy is the resection of the posterior elements (lamina, spinous process, and facets), closure of the posterior defect, and controlled fracture of the ankylosed anterior column. A Grade 6 osteotomy is a PSO comprising complete removal of the lamina,

spinous process, facets, and pedicles at the desired level with a closing wedge osteotomy (CWO) in the vertebral body. A Grade 7 osteotomy is a complete vertebrectomy with removal of the vertebral body and uncinate joints anteriorly, and complete removal of the facets, lamina, and spinous process posteriorly.

Characterization of the underlying cause of malalignment, degree of rigidity, and type of deformity is critical in surgical planning. Cervical deformities are either rigid (a deformity that cannot be passively corrected) or flexible (a deformity that is passively correctable). Rigid deformities may be ankylosed. In patients with a cervical kyphosis that is ankylosed anteriorly, an anterior osteotomy followed by posterior decompression and instrumentation is favored. Ventral release alone may not provide adequate decompression, and the deformity cannot be corrected without initial anterior release.[43,45] In patients with rigid cervical kyphosis with ankyloses of the posterior elements, a three-step surgery is required for kyphosis correction. A posterior osteotomy is first performed, followed by anterior release with interbody grafting, followed by posterior instrumentation and fusion. This combined approach—anterior, posterior, anterior—allows for both dorsal and ventral decompression with osteotomies for full release of the ankyloses.

Combinations of multilevel discectomies and corpectomies can be performed through an anterior approach. Use of a sequential interbody dilation technique followed by placement of lordotic cages[18] or by placement of an expandable cage[46] can provide significant kyphosis correction, anterior decompression, and internal fixation by an anterior-only approach. Single-level corpectomy and two-level discectomy can provide up to 5 to 8 degrees[47,48,49] of global cervical correction. In cases of mid-cervical kyphosis, correction can be achieved with a posterior type 2 osteotomy and an anterior type 4 osteotomy. However, anterior approaches carry a unique risk profile with risks for vocal cord injury and dysphagia. Additionally, cases of cervical deformities with fixed posterior elements cannot be correct by an anterior approach alone, and warrant a posterior-anterior-posterior approach.[50,51,52]

Table 11.1 Ames cervical osteotomy grade[7]

Spine type	Cervical osteotomy grade	Technique
Flexible	1	Partial joint resection including partial resection of the uncinate joints and/or partial removal of the posterior facets
Flexible	2	Removal of both the inferior and superior articular facets
Rigid	3	Corpectomy
Rigid	4	Corpectomy with associated complete resection of the uncinate joints laterally to the transverse foramen
Rigid/ankylosed	5	Complete resection of the posterior elements (lamina, spinous process, and facets), closure of the posterior defect, and controlled fracture of the ankylosed anterior column
Rigid/ankylosed	6	PSO (complete removal of the lamina, spinous process, facets, and pedicles at the desired level), followed by creation of a closing wedge osteotomy in the vertebral body
Rigid/ankylosed	7	Complete vertebrectomy (removal of the vertebral body and uncinate joints anteriorly, and complete removal of the facets, lamina, and spinous process posteriorly)

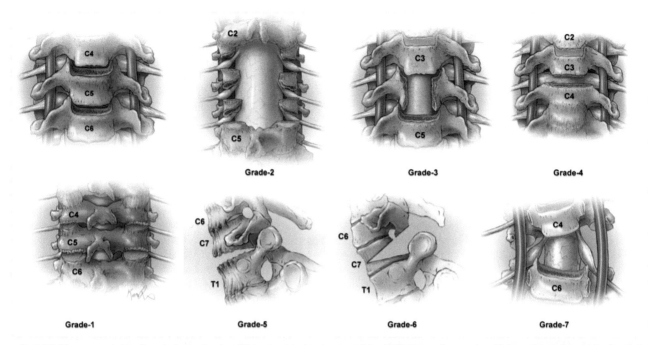

Fig. 11.2 The seven grades of cervical osteotomies offering progressive degrees of destabilization and correction. Please refer to the text for detailed description by grade.

11.3.1 Correction of Cervical Deformities with Pedicle Subtraction Osteotomy

Cervical PSO is most often indicated in cases of severe fixed kyphotic deformities associated with AS, previous cervical surgery, or trauma. PSOs provide a number of advantages as compared to SPOs. PSOs allow for greater extent of sagittal correction, produce superior biomechanical stability, allow for more controlled closure, produce a large bone-on-bone load-bearing interface that promotes fusion and stiffness, and avoid the anterior open wedge defects associated with SPO.[53,54] Compared to studies on the application of PSO in the thoracic and lumbar spine, reports that focus on cervical PSO are limited. PSOs for cervical deformity are most frequently performed in the cervicothoracic junction at C7, T1, T2, or T3.[13,14,40,43,55,56] Reasons for the preferential application of PSO at the cervicothoracic junction are multifold: the canal diameter is smaller in the upper and middle cervical spine, iatrogenic injury at lower cervical levels can spare the upper extremities, and lower cervical PSO allows for avoidance of the vertebral arteries, which enter the transverse foramen at C6.[57,58]

Selection of the lowermost instrumented vertebra (LIV) in cervical deformity correction is aimed at minimizing risk for postoperative distal junctional kyphosis (DJK). The LIV is often in the upper thoracic spine in patients with a normal C2 SVA and mild upper thoracic kyphosis who require a small degree of sagittal correction. In contrast, the LIV should be below the thoracic apex to T9 or lower in patients with significant upper or midthoracic kyphosis, or with global imbalance requiring a cervical PSO.

Traditional Cervical PSO

C7 PSO is performed via a posterior approach. The patient is placed in a prone position and a midline incision is made to expose the cervical and thoracic levels. Subperiosteal dissection is performed to expose the spinous, lateral, and transverse processes of the cervical and thoracic spine. The spine is then instrumented; depending on the construct needed, C2 pedicle screws, C3–C5 lateral mass screws, and thoracic pedicle screws may be placed. The extent of instrumentation depends on patient anatomy and degree of correction needed. Instrumentation can be extended up to C2 to allow for a stronger point of fixation with bicortical screw placement. The caudal extent of instrumentation is determined by the severity of thoracic kyphosis. In patients with normal thoracic curvature, the fusion can end at T3 for three fixation points below the C7 PSO. However, if thoracic kyphosis is pronounced, the fusion may be extended to T5 to involve the thoracic curve apex.[13]

The C7 PSO begins with removal of the caudal portion of the C6 lamina and the cranial portion of the C7 lamina as needed. The C7 lateral mass is resected, and the bilateral C6–C7 and C7–T1 facets are removed. The nerve roots at C7 and C8 are exposed, and the C7 pedicle is skeletonized and removed. Sequential lumbar taps with increasing diameter are used to decancellate the vertebral body through the pedicle osteotomy, and the tapped holes are widened and connected. The C7 lateral and posterior vertebral walls are removed, and a 30-degree osteotomy through the vertebral body is performed with osteotomes and down-pushing curettes. To close the PSO, the patient's head is carefully extended. Following wedge closure, the C7 and C8 nerve roots should be examined to identify possible nerve impingement. After appropriate correction is achieved, the rods are secured with locking caps. It is critical to utilize neuromonitoring data (both somatosensory evoked potentials and motor evoked potentials) throughout the case and particularly during closure of the PSO to prevent iatrogenic injury to the nerve roots and spinal cord. Intraoperative AP and lateral images are obtained to evaluate the degree of correction and overall sagittal alignment of the cervical spine.

Cervical Y-Type Osteotomy

A potential shortcoming of the PSO is the shortening effect on the posterior elements and consequent posterior compression following closure of the wedge osteotomy. This shortening following closure of a C7 PSO can cause root impingement of the C7 and C8 nerve roots. The Y-type osteotomy (YTO)—a modified cervical PSO—was developed to overcome some of the limitations of both CWOs such as the PSO and opening wedge osteotomies (OWOs) such as the SPO, while merging the benefits of each technique.[59] In YTO, the posterior column resection

is similar to a CWO, but the tip of the wedge targets the vertebral midsagittal point. A straight plane is osteotomized anteriorly from this point parallel to the endplates. The plane can also be modified according to the intended center of surgical correction. The YTO reduces the amount of anterior distraction that results from an OWO and reduces the posterior shortening produced by CWO, while enabling significant correction. The correction angle can be increased with YTO in comparison to classic PSO as a result of the correction mechanism, while maintaining balance of posterior shortening and anterior distraction.

Case Presentation

PSO can be successfully and safely performed to produce significant correction of lower cervical deformity. An illustrative case is presented (▶ Fig. 11.3, ▶ Fig. 11.4, ▶ Fig. 11.5). A 47-year-old male with a history of AS presents with chin-on-chest deformity and myelopathy. Preoperative AP X-ray, lateral X-ray, and sagittal CT demonstrate a nonmobile, severe cervical kyphosis

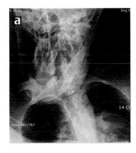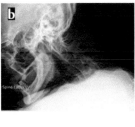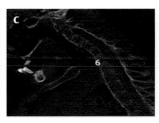

Fig. 11.3 Preoperative AP (**a**) and lateral (**b**) X-rays, and sagittal CT (**c**) of a patient with severe cervical kyphosis with scoliosis, resulting in significant sagittal malalignment.

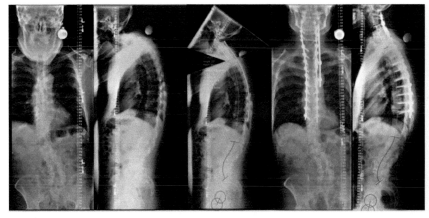

Fig. 11.4 An example of a cervical PSO planning simulation software used to guide deformity correction. Preoperative AP and lateral X-rays are shown on the left. The planned correction shown with a cervical PSO in the center is generated based on standing scoliosis X-rays. AP and lateral films following surgery are shown on the right.

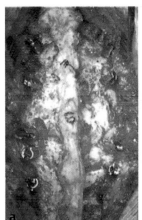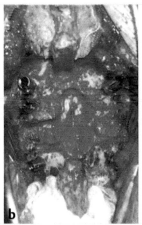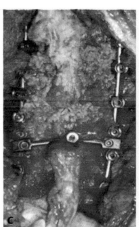

Fig. 11.5 Intraoperative photos of a C6 PSO are shown. Pedicle screws are placed from C3 to T2 (**a**). The vertebral artery is exposed bilaterally following bony removal and soft-tissue dissection. The osteotomy is completed with resection of the pedicles which allows for wide decompression of the nerve roots as shown to prevent compression during wedge closure (**b**). Instrumentation is secured and fusion graft is placed (**c**).

with scoliosis resulting in significant sagittal malalignment (abnormal C2 SVA) and slight coronal imbalance (▶ Fig. 11.3). Preoperative planning software can be utilized to calculate the angle at cervicothoracic junction and simulate the goal of correction based on standing scoliosis X-rays. An example of a preoperative cervical PSO plan used to guide deformity correction is shown in ▶ Fig. 11.4.

The patient underwent C6 PSO and instrumented fusion for deformity correction. Intraoperative photos can be seen in ▶ Fig. 11.3. Pedicle screws from C3 to T2 are inserted. Bony removal and soft-tissue dissection completely exposes the vertebral artery on both sides (▶ Fig. 11.5a). The pedicles are removed and the spinal nerves are decompressed and exposed widely to ensure compression does not occur during closure of the osteotomy (▶ Fig. 11.5b). The C6 foramen is unroofed along the dotted lines following the placement of pedicle screws (▶ Fig. 11.6a), and the right vertebral artery at C6 is dissected (▶ Fig. 11.6b) and isolated. The C6 pedicle is resected (▶ Fig. 11.6c) and the anterior tubercle is released (▶ Fig. 11.6d). The bony surface is decancellated (▶ Fig. 11.6e), and the osteotomy can be closed using the anterior column as a fulcrum. ▶ Fig. 11.6f shows the complete C6 PSO prior to osteotomy reduction providing significant correction. The instrumentation is secured and fusion graft material is laid down (▶ Fig. 11.5c). Cervical PSO instrument set used for such cases can be seen in ▶ Fig. 11.7. Postoperative AP X-ray, lateral X-ray, and sagittal CT demonstrate significant improvement in sagittal balance with restoration of cervical lordosis (▶ Fig. 11.8).

11.4 Postoperative Complications

Surgeries in the cervical spine can result in injury to the vertebral artery, spinal cord, or nerve roots. Rates of postoperative neurological deficits are as high as 23.4% following correction of cervical deformities.[57,60] Additionally, complications can also include cerebrospinal fluid leaks and wound infections/dehiscence. In a recent prospective multicenter study of 78 patients undergoing correction of adult cervical deformity, Smith et al reported that 43.6% of patients had at least one complication. The most common complications were dysphagia in 11.5% of patients, wound infections in 6.4%, C5 palsy in 6.4%, and respiratory failure in 5.1%. Complications were highest following

combined AP approaches (79.3%) and posterior-only approaches (68.4%), and lowest in the anterior-only group (27.3%).[56] In a review of literature comprising 14 studies and 399 patients, Etame et al reported mortality rates of 3.1 to 6.7% and rates of medical complications between 3.1 and 44.4% following surgery for symptomatic cervical and cervicothoracic kyphosis.[61]

Reports of complications specific to cervical PSO are limited to small retrospective studies. In a review of 11 patients who underwent cervicothoracic PSO, Deviren et al reported no intraoperative or neurological complications. Postoperatively, there were two pneumonias, one dysphagia, and one rod fracture at 4 months.[13] In a series of eight patients who underwent PSO for cervicothoracic kyphosis, Samudrala et al reported two patients with transient hand numbness and weakness. One patient had right upper extremity weakness that required reoperation to decompress the nerve root.[55] Tokala et al reported mild C8 radiculopathy in three and deep wound infections in two out of seven patients following C7 PSO for cervicothoracic kyphosis. The C8 radiculopathy was transient and resolved within 4 weeks.[40] In a study of 23 patients undergoing VCR or PSO for cervicothoracic deformities, Smith et al reported neurological deficits in 17.4%, wound infection in 8.7%, and DJK in 8.7%.[56] Three patients required reoperation for DJK, nerve root decompression, and implant prominence.

11.5 Conclusion

Cervical sagittal deformities can be particularly debilitating as a result of pain, neurological deficits, and impaired horizontal gaze. Correction of cervical deformity, as indicated by improved C2 SVA and CBVA, is critical in improving quality-of-life measures and neurological outcomes. The goals of deformity correction are C2 SVA less than 40 mm and neutral CBVA evaluated in a fully relaxed C1–C2 position. A number of osteotomies are available and may be warranted in patients with severe or rigid deformity. The cervicothoracic PSO is a powerful and effective tool in the correction of severe kyphotic cervical deformities and has been demonstrated to produce significant improvements in C2 SVA, cervical Cobb angle, and CBVA and corresponding improvements in HRQOL. However, a number of complications following cervical PSO

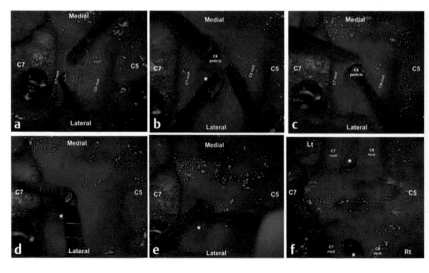

Fig. 11.6 Vertebral artery release during a C6 PSO is shown. After placement of pedicle screws, the C6 foramen is unroofed along the dotted lines (a), and the right vertebral artery at C6 is completely dissected (b). The C6 pedicle is resected (c) and the anterior tubercle is released (d). The bony surface is then decancellated to promote bony fusion (e). The complete C6 PSO prior to osteotomy reduction is shown in (f). The asterisk marks the vertebral artery trajectory.

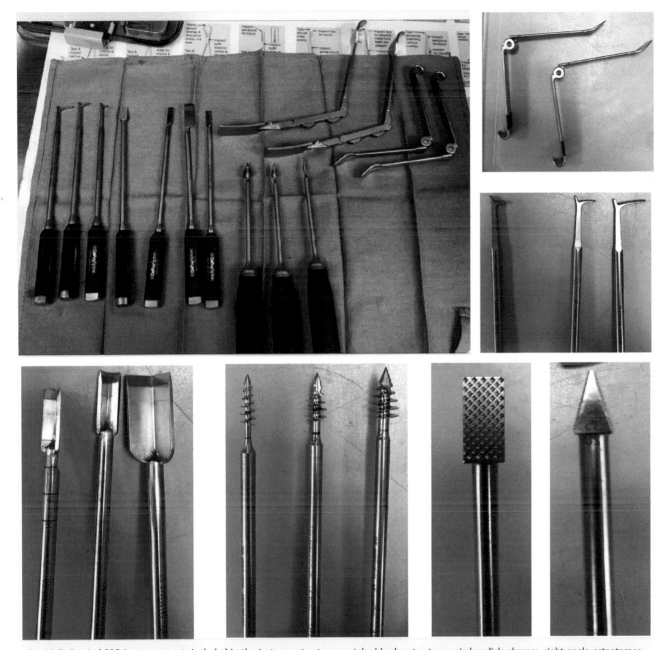

Fig. 11.7 Cervical PSO instrument set. Included in the instrument set are vertebral body retractors, spiral pedicle shavers, right angle osteotomes, central impactors, wedge-shaped rasp/shaver.

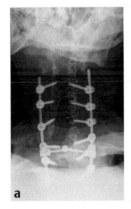
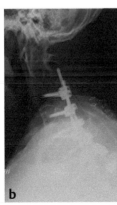
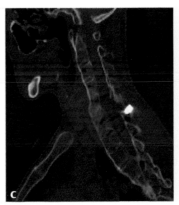

Fig. 11.8 Postoperative AP (**a**) and lateral (**b**) X-rays, and sagittal CT (**c**) show restoration of cervical lordosis following completion of the osteotomy.

have been reported and surgeon experience in PSO and SPO is useful. With careful preoperative planning and consideration of spinal biomechanics, cervical PSO and related osteotomies can improve the quality of life of patients with severe sagittal deformities.

References

[1] Albert TJ, Vacarro A. Postlaminectomy kyphosis. Spine. 1998; 23(24):2738–2745

[2] Kaptain GJ, Simmons NE, Replogle RE, Pobereskin L. Incidence and outcome of kyphotic deformity following laminectomy for cervical spondylotic myelopathy. J Neurosurg. 2000; 93(2) Suppl:199–204

[3] Steinmetz MP, Stewart TJ, Kager CD, Benzel EC, Vaccaro AR. Cervical deformity correction. Neurosurgery. 2007; 60(1) Supp1 1:S90–S97

[4] O'Shaughnessy BA, Liu JC, Hsieh PC, Koski TR, Ganju A, Ondra SL. Surgical treatment of fixed cervical kyphosis with myelopathy. Spine. 2008; 33 (7):771–778

[5] Ames CP, Blondel B, Scheer JK, et al. Cervical radiographical alignment: comprehensive assessment techniques and potential importance in cervical myelopathy. Spine. 2013; 38(22) Suppl 1:S149–S160

[6] Griegel-Morris P, Larson K, Mueller-Klaus K, Oatis CA. Incidence of common postural abnormalities in the cervical, shoulder, and thoracic regions and their association with pain in two age groups of healthy subjects. Phys Ther. 1992; 72(6):425–431

[7] Ames CP, Smith JS, Scheer JK, et al. International Spine Study Group. A standardized nomenclature for cervical spine soft-tissue release and osteotomy for deformity correction: clinical article. J Neurosurg Spine. 2013; 19(3):269–278

[8] Law WA. Osteotomy of the cervical spine. J Bone Joint Surg Br. 1959; 41-B:640–641

[9] Urist MR. Osteotomy of the cervical spine; report of a case of ankylosing rheumatoid spondylitis. J Bone Joint Surg Am. 1958; 40-A(4):833–843

[10] Simmons EH. The surgical correction of flexion deformity of the cervical spine in ankylosing spondylitis. Clin Orthop Relat Res. 1972; 86(86):132–143

[11] Tan LA, Riew KD, Traynelis VC. Cervical spine deformity-part 3: posterior techniques, clinical outcome, and complications. Neurosurgery. 2017; 81 (6):893–898

[12] Suk KS, Kim KT, Lee SH, Kim JM. Significance of chin-brow vertical angle in correction of kyphotic deformity of ankylosing spondylitis patients. Spine. 2003; 28(17):2001–2005

[13] Deviren V, Scheer JK, Ames CP. Technique of cervicothoracic junction pedicle subtraction osteotomy for cervical sagittal imbalance: report of 11 cases. J Neurosurg Spine. 2011; 15(2):174–181

[14] Kim KT, Lee SH, Son ES, Kwack YH, Chun YS, Lee JH. Surgical treatment of "chin-on-pubis" deformity in a patient with ankylosing spondylitis: a case report of consecutive cervical, thoracic, and lumbar corrective osteotomies. Spine. 2012; 37(16):E1017–E1021

[15] Tang JA, Scheer JK, Smith JS, et al. ISSG. The impact of standing regional cervical sagittal alignment on outcomes in posterior cervical fusion surgery. Neurosurgery. 2012; 71(3):662–669, discussion 669

[16] Bao H, Varghese J, Lafage R, et al. Principal radiographic characteristics for cervical spinal deformity: a health-related quality-of-life analysis. Spine. 2017; 42(18):1375–1382

[17] Smith JS, Lafage V, Ryan DJ, et al. Association of myelopathy scores with cervical sagittal balance and normalized spinal cord volume: analysis of 56 preoperative cases from the AOSpine North America Myelopathy study. Spine. 2013; 38(22) Suppl 1:S161–S170

[18] Lau D, Ziewacz JE, Le H, Wadhwa R, Mummaneni PV. A controlled anterior sequential interbody dilation technique for correction of cervical kyphosis. J Neurosurg Spine. 2015; 23(3):263–273

[19] Villavicencio AT, Babuska JM, Ashton A, et al. Prospective, randomized, double-blind clinical study evaluating the correlation of clinical outcomes and cervical sagittal alignment. Neurosurgery. 2011; 68(5):1309–1316, discussion 1316

[20] Le Huec JC, Demezon H, Aunoble S. Sagittal parameters of global cervical balance using EOS imaging: normative values from a prospective cohort of asymptomatic volunteers. Eur Spine J. 2015; 24(1):63–71

[21] Abelin-Genevois K, Idjerouidene A, Roussouly P, Vital JM, Garin C. Cervical spine alignment in the pediatric population: a radiographic normative study of 150 asymptomatic patients. Eur Spine J. 2014; 23(7):1442–1448

[22] Ha Y, Schwab F, Lafage V, et al. Reciprocal changes in cervical spine alignment after corrective thoracolumbar deformity surgery. Eur Spine J. 2014; 23 (3):552–559

[23] Smith JS, Shaffrey CI, Lafage V, et al. International Spine Study Group. Spontaneous improvement of cervical alignment after correction of global sagittal balance following pedicle subtraction osteotomy. J Neurosurg Spine. 2012; 17 (4):300–307

[24] Hwang SW, Samdani AF, Tantorski M, et al. Cervical sagittal plane decompensation after surgery for adolescent idiopathic scoliosis: an effect imparted by postoperative thoracic hypokyphosis. J Neurosurg Spine. 2011; 15(5):491–496

[25] Protopsaltis TS, Scheer JK, Terran JS, et al. International Spine Study Group. How the neck affects the back: changes in regional cervical sagittal alignment correlate to HRQOL improvement in adult thoracolumbar deformity patients at 2-year follow-up. J Neurosurg Spine. 2015; 23(2):153–158

[26] Oh T, Scheer JK, Eastlack R, et al. International Spine Study Group. Cervical compensatory alignment changes following correction of adult thoracic deformity: a multicenter experience in 57 patients with a 2-year follow-up. J Neurosurg Spine. 2015; 22(6):658–665

[27] Lee SH, Kim KT, Seo EM, Suk KS, Kwack YH, Son ES. The influence of thoracic inlet alignment on the craniocervical sagittal balance in asymptomatic adults. J Spinal Disord Tech. 2012; 25(2):E41–E47

[28] Knott PT, Mardjetko SM, Techy F. The use of the T1 sagittal angle in predicting overall sagittal balance of the spine. Spine J. 2010; 10(11):994–998

[29] Protopsaltis T, Schwab F, Bronsard N, et al. International Spine Study Group. The T1 pelvic angle, a novel radiographic measure of global sagittal deformity, accounts for both spinal inclination and pelvic tilt and correlates with health-related quality of life. J Bone Joint Surg Am. 2014; 96(19):1631–1640

[30] Zdeblick TA, Bohlman HH. Cervical kyphosis and myelopathy. Treatment by anterior corpectomy and strut-grafting. J Bone Joint Surg Am. 1989; 71 (2):170–182

[31] Herman JM, Sonntag VK. Cervical corpectomy and plate fixation for postlaminectomy kyphosis. J Neurosurg. 1994; 80(6):963–970

[32] Steinmetz MP, Kager CD, Benzel EC. Ventral correction of postsurgical cervical kyphosis. J Neurosurg. 2003; 98(1) Suppl:1–7

[33] Ferch RD, Shad A, Cadoux-Hudson TA, Teddy PJ. Anterior correction of cervical kyphotic deformity: effects on myelopathy, neck pain, and sagittal alignment. J Neurosurg. 2004; 100(1) Suppl Spine:13–19

[34] Song KJ, Johnson JS, Choi BR, Wang JC, Lee KB. Anterior fusion alone compared with combined anterior and posterior fusion for the treatment of degenerative cervical kyphosis. J Bone Joint Surg Br. 2010; 92(11):1548–1552

[35] McMaster MJ. Osteotomy of the cervical spine in ankylosing spondylitis. J Bone Joint Surg Br. 1997; 79(2):197–203

[36] Abumi K, Shono Y, Taneichi H, Ito M, Kaneda K. Correction of cervical kyphosis using pedicle screw fixation systems. Spine. 1999; 24(22):2389–2396

[37] Belanger TA, Milam RA, IV, Roh JS, Bohlman HH. Cervicothoracic extension osteotomy for chin-on-chest deformity in ankylosing spondylitis. J Bone Joint Surg Am. 2005; 87(8):1732–1738

[38] Simmons ED, DiStefano RJ, Zheng Y, Simmons EH. Thirty-six years experience of cervical extension osteotomy in ankylosing spondylitis: techniques and outcomes. Spine. 2006; 31(26):3006–3012

[39] Langeloo DD, Journee HL, Pavlov PW, de Kleuver M. Cervical osteotomy in ankylosing spondylitis: evaluation of new developments. Eur Spine J. 2006; 15 (4):493–500

[40] Tokala DP, Lam KS, Freeman BJ, Webb JK. C7 decancellisation closing wedge osteotomy for the correction of fixed cervico-thoracic kyphosis. Eur Spine J. 2007; 16(9):1471–1478

[41] Gerling MC, Bohlman HH. Dropped head deformity due to cervical myopathy: surgical treatment outcomes and complications spanning twenty years. Spine. 2008; 33(20):E739–E745

[42] Lee SH, Kim KT, Suk KS, Kim MH, Park DH, Kim KJ. A sterile-freehand reduction technique for corrective osteotomy of fixed cervical kyphosis. Spine. 2012; 37(26):2145–2150

[43] Mummaneni PV, Dhall SS, Rodts GE, Haid RW. Circumferential fusion for cervical kyphotic deformity. J Neurosurg Spine. 2008; 9(6):515–521

[44] Nottmeier EW, Deen HG, Patel N, Birch B. Cervical kyphotic deformity correction using 360-degree reconstruction. J Spinal Disord Tech. 2009; 22(6):385–391

[45] Hann S, Chalouhi N, Madineni R, et al. An algorithmic strategy for selecting a surgical approach in cervical deformity correction. Neurosurg Focus. 2014; 36(5):E5

[46] Perrini P, Gambacciani C, Martini C, Montemurro N, Lepori P. Anterior cervical corpectomy for cervical spondylotic myelopathy: reconstruction with ex-

pandable cylindrical cage versus iliac crest autograft. A retrospective study. Clin Neurol Neurosurg. 2015; 139:258–263

[47] Burkhardt JK, Mannion AF, Marbacher S, et al. A comparative effectiveness study of patient-rated and radiographic outcome after 2 types of decompression with fusion for spondylotic myelopathy: anterior cervical discectomy versus corpectomy. Neurosurg Focus. 2013; 35(1):E4

[48] Lin Q, Zhou X, Wang X, Cao P, Tsai N, Yuan W. A comparison of anterior cervical discectomy and corpectomy in patients with multilevel cervical spondylotic myelopathy. Eur Spine J. 2012; 21(3):474–481

[49] Oh MC, Zhang HY, Park JY, Kim KS. Two-level anterior cervical discectomy versus one-level corpectomy in cervical spondylotic myelopathy. Spine. 2009; 34(7):692–696

[50] Singh K, Marquez-Lara A, Nandyala SV, Patel AA, Fineberg SJ. Incidence and risk factors for dysphagia after anterior cervical fusion. Spine. 2013; 38 (21):1820–1825

[51] Zeng JH, Zhong ZM, Chen JT. Early dysphagia complicating anterior cervical spine surgery: incidence and risk factors. Arch Orthop Trauma Surg. 2013; 133(8):1067–1071

[52] Bazaz R, Lee MJ, Yoo JU. Incidence of dysphagia after anterior cervical spine surgery: a prospective study. Spine. 2002; 27(22):2453–2458

[53] Chin KR, Ahn J. Controlled cervical extension osteotomy for ankylosing spondylitis utilizing the Jackson operating table: technical note. Spine. 2007; 32 (17):1926–1929

[54] Scheer JK, Tang JA, Buckley JM, et al. Biomechanical analysis of osteotomy type and rod diameter for treatment of cervicothoracic kyphosis. Spine. 2011; 36(8):E519–E523

[55] Samudrala S, Vaynman S, Thiayananthan T, et al. Cervicothoracic junction kyphosis: surgical reconstruction with pedicle subtraction osteotomy and Smith-Petersen osteotomy. Presented at the 2009 Joint Spine Section Meeting. Clinical article. J Neurosurg Spine. 2010; 13(6):695–706

[56] Smith JS, Shaffrey CI, Lafage R, et al. ISSG. Three-column osteotomy for correction of cervical and cervicothoracic deformities: alignment changes and early complications in a multicenter prospective series of 23 patients. Eur Spine J. 2017; 26(8):2128–2137

[57] Wollowick AL, Kelly MP, Riew KD. Pedicle subtraction osteotomy in the cervical spine. Spine. 2012; 37(5):E342–E348

[58] Kim HJ, Nemani VM, Daniel Riew K. Cervical osteotomies for neurological deformities. Eur Spine J. 2015; 24 Suppl 1:S16–S22

[59] Koller H, Koller J, Mayer M, Hempfing A, Hitzl W. Osteotomies in ankylosing spondylitis: where, how many, and how much? Eur Spine J. 2018; 27 Suppl 1:70–100

[60] Etame AB, Than KD, Wang AC, La Marca F, Park P. Surgical management of symptomatic cervical or cervicothoracic kyphosis due to ankylosing spondylitis. Spine. 2008; 33(16):E559–E564

[61] Etame AB, Wang AC, Than KD, La Marca F, Park P. Outcomes after surgery for cervical spine deformity: review of the literature. Neurosurg Focus. 2010; 28 (3):E14

12 Cervical Opening Wedge Osteotomy

Lee A. Tan and Christopher P. Ames

Abstract

Posterior cervical osteotomies are powerful techniques utilized by spine surgeons to correct rigid cervical spinal deformity. Two main types of posterior osteotomy include the Smith-Petersen osteotomy (SPO) and pedicle subtraction osteotomy (PSO). The "opening wedge" osteotomy (OWO) is a modified technique from the standard SPO by creating an osteoclastic fracture during posterior osteotomy closure to achieve kyphosis correction. This chapter provides a detailed step-by-step technical guide for performing a cervical OWO at C7, with a discussion of surgical pearls and complication avoidance.

Keywords: opening wedge, osteotomy, cervical spine, cervical deformity, deformity correction

12.1 Introduction

Posterior cervical osteotomies are powerful surgical techniques utilized by spine surgeons to treat rigid cervical spinal deformity. Two main types of posterior osteotomy include the Smith-Petersen osteotomy (SPO) and pedicle subtraction osteotomy (PSO). The SPO was originally described by Smith-Petersen in 1945 in the lumbar spine for the treatment of kyphotic deformity.[1] This technique involved bony resection of the posterior elements including the spinous process, lamina, and bilateral facet joints, along with removal of underlying ligamentum flavum and complete bilateral foraminotomies that skeletonize exiting nerve roots. Complete and thorough central and foraminal decompression are essential at the osteotomy site to prevent spinal cord and nerve root compression during osteotomy closure.

In 1958, Urist modified the original SPO technique and performed the first cervical "opening wedge" osteotomy (OWO) at C7 to treat a patient with rigid cervical kyphotic deformity due to ankylosing spondylitis.[2] The OWO differs from the standard SPO by way of an osteoclastic fracture that is created during posterior osteotomy closure and kyphosis correction, in which an "opening wedge" is created anteriorly with lengthening of the anterior spinal column. In 1972, Simmons[3] had reported a series of 11 patients who underwent cervical OWO for correction of rigid cervical kyphotic deformity in the setting of ankylosing spondylitis. He positioned the patient in the sitting position with halo traction to stabilize the head and neck, and the operation was performed under local anesthesia. This allowed real-time monitoring of the patient's neurological status and immediate detection of potential neurological deficits during osteotomy closure. In 2006, Simmons et al[4] published an updated series of 131 patients undergoing cervical OWO in the sitting position and demonstrated that the sitting position with local anesthesia was safe and allowed for controlled deformity correction.

In contrast, the PSO technique was first introduced by Thomasen in 1985.[5] He describe performing lumbar PSOs in 11 patients with rigid kyphotic deformity due to ankylosing spondylitis. In contrast to SPO, PSO required removal of additional bony elements including the pedicles, a wedge of the vertebral body, and a portion of the lateral and posterior vertebral walls. This technique allowed more angular correction and better fusion due to the lack of an open gap in the anterior column; thus, it is also known as "closing wedge" osteotomy (CWO). In 2007, Tokala et al[6] first reported performing cervical PSO at C7 in series of eight patients with fixed cervicothoracic kyphosis. Several other clinical series of cervical PSO have been reported,[7,8,9] including a series of 11 patients from the author's home institution. In most cases, both the opening and closing wedge cervical osteotomies are performed at C7 due to the relatively wide spinal canal at C7–T1, the mobility of the spinal cord and eighth cervical nerves in this region, the preservation of reasonable hand function in the event of C8 nerve root injury, and the absence of vertebral artery in the C7 transverse process for most patients.

In this chapter, we provide a detailed step-by-step technical guide for performing a cervical OWO at C7, with a discussion of surgical pearls and complication avoidance. The techniques for cervical PSO (CWO) are discussed in detail elsewhere in this book.

12.2 Indication and Preoperative Evaluation

Cervical OWO is typically performed for fixed kyphotic cervical deformities often due to ankylosing spondylitis. These patients often have impaired ability to maintain horizontal gaze, dysphagia, and pain and neurological deficits. Traditionally, the opening wedge cervical osteotomy was performed under local anesthesia with the patient awake in the sitting position in a halo vest. This was done partly due to difficulty with intubation for these patients, but another advantage for local anesthesia is the ability to have real-time patient feedback on neurological functions intraoperatively.[2,3] However, with the advancement in modern anesthesia techniques and intraoperative neuromonitoring, posterior cervical osteotomies can be safely performed with general anesthesia in the prone position in experienced hands.[7,10]

Preoperative imaging study should include dynamic cervical X-rays, scoliosis films, magnetic resonance imaging (MRI), and computed tomography (CT) of the cervical spine. Any compression of neural elements should be noted and decompression should be planned as part of the overall procedure. Any vascular anomaly involving the vertebral artery should be noted. Various cervical radiographic parameters should be measured and the desired amount of correction should be determined. Specifically, the chin–brow vertical angle (CBVA) is the parameter often used to calculate the amount of kyphosis correction needed (▶ Fig. 12.1).

Suk et al[11] recommended a CBVA range of -10 to +10 degrees for optimized horizontal gaze. Another study by Song et al[12] suggested a postoperative CVBA between +10 and +20 degrees (i.e., slight flexion) had best overall results with both indoor and outdoor activities. We prefer a neutral or slight flexion head tilt as it balances appearance and function, which maximizes clinical outcome and patient satisfaction. Overcorrection

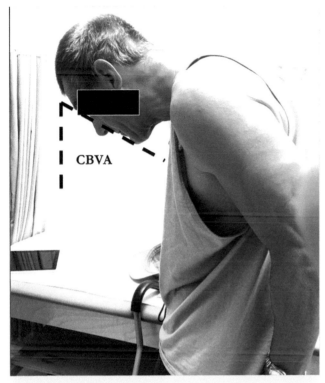

Fig. 12.1 A clinical photograph demonstrating the CBVA measurement.

of cervical kyphosis can impair the patient's ability to perform activities such as cooking, walking, and toileting, which all require downward line of vision.

12.3 Operative Technique

12.3.1 Positioning

The patient is brought into the operating room and undergoes general endotracheal anesthesia. Neuromonitoring and adequate vascular access are established. The open Jackson table is used for positioning, and the head is secured with either a Mayfield head frame or a dual-vector cervical traction system with Gardner-Wells tongs. The patient is then placed prone on a Jackson table with a chest bolster, anterior iliac crest pads, and several pillows for leg support. The head is secured using either Mayfield head clamp (▶ Fig. 12.2) or Gardner-Wells tongs with 15 pounds of weight and dual-vector cervical traction (▶ Fig. 12.3). The operating table is positioned with maximum amount of reverse Trendelenburg to offset the cervicothoracic kyphosis so that the surgical field is more horizontal, and this position also helps to reduce intraoperative blood loss as venous blood volume pools in the legs and the abdomen.

12.3.2 Exposure

The region of cervical and upper thoracic spine is exposed in the standard fashion. The lateral masses in the cervical spine

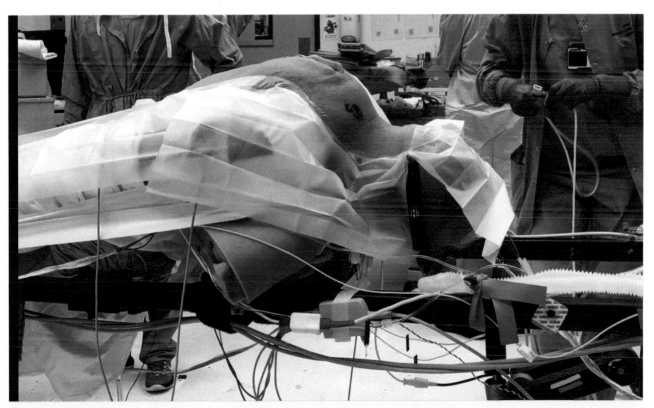

Fig. 12.2 A photograph demonstrating patient positioning with Mayfield head clamp on a Jackson table.

and transverse processes of the thoracic spine are exposed in their entirety to facilitate lateral mass and pedicle screw placement. The proximal extent of the dissection depends on the planned uppermost level of instrumentation. Every effort should be made to preserve the occipitoatlantal and atlantoaxial joints if possible, since these two levels account for about 50% the total range of motion in the cervical spine. If the cervical spine is already completely ankylosed, the instrumentation can be extended to the occiput because of the strong bony fixation that can be obtained around the external occipital protuberance. It is preferable to have three to four levels of fixation points distal to the osteotomy site; therefore, the distal part of the construct typically ends at either T3, T4, or T5. If there is coexisting thoracolumbar deformity, the caudal end of exposure may need to extend into the lower thoracic or even lumbosacral spine. Meticulous hemostasis is necessary to minimize blood loss during exposure.

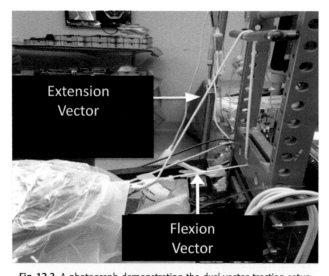

Fig. 12.3 A photograph demonstrating the dual-vector traction setup with Jackson table.

12.3.3 Instrumentation

After exposure, the instrumentation is placed above and below the C7 OWO site. C2 fixation can be achieved using either pedicle, pars, or translaminar screws if needed. Lateral mass screws are placed bilaterally at C3, C4, and C5, and pedicle screws are placed bilaterally at T2, T3, and T4. Screws at either C6 or T1 can be placed depending on whether more proximal or distal fixation points are needed. If a C6 lateral mass screw is used, the T1 pedicle screw is left out, and vice versa, as there is often not enough room for both screws after osteotomy closure.

With modern instrumentation systems, especially those with an articulated or hinged rod, it is possible to use a single rod to connect the upper cervical spine to the upper thoracic spine. This avoids the need for connectors and allows the surgeon to place screws at every level of the spine. It is important to place the screws in a straight line, which makes the placement of rods significantly easier and avoids the need for bending the rod in both the sagittal and coronal planes. Accessory rods can be used across osteotomy site to minimize the risk of rod fracture.

12.3.4 Opening Wedge Osteotomy

To begin the C7 OWO, a complete C7 laminectomy is performed. The lamina and spinous process are removed, which should be used as local bone graft later. Partial laminectomies of the C6 inferior lamina and the T1 superior lamina are also performed to prevent compression of the spinal cord after osteotomy closure. The spinous processes of C6 and T1 vertebrae are left intact if possible.

Next, the C7–T1 facet joints are removed bilaterally using a combination of the Leksell rongeur and high-speed burr, including the inferior articular process of C7 and the superior articular process of T1. The T1 pedicles must also be clearly exposed so that there is no overhanging facet cranial to the pedicle, which may compress the C8 root during osteotomy closure. The C7 pedicle is also removed using high-speed burr and Leksell rongeur to prevent compression of the C8 nerve root during osteotomy closure (▶ Fig. 12.4). The C8 nerve roots are completely

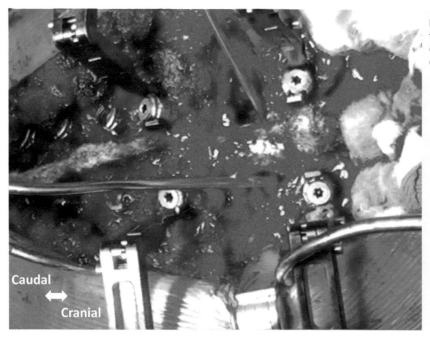

Fig. 12.4 An intraoperative photo demonstrating the amount of bony resection of posterior elements for opening wedge osteotomy prior to osteoclasis and osteotomy closure.

exposed, clearly visible and free of compression. Hemostasis is then achieved in preparation for osteotomy closure and correction of the deformity.

12.3.5 Osteotomy Closure

The rod is bent to desired curve and then fixed to the thoracic pedicle screws. The surgeon then pulls on the Mayfield clamp or the Gardner-Wells tongs to extend the neck (▶ Fig. 12.4). Following extension of the neck and osteoclasis, the C7 and C8 roots must be carefully examined for any signs of impingement. Further bony resection may be necessary if the C7 and C8 roots are not completely free. Often, a temporary rod is placed across the osteotomy site to prevent subluxation or premature osteotomy closure.

As the head is progressively extended to close the osteotomy site, the rod should engage the screw heads of the previously placed cervical lateral mass screws. Locking caps are placed to secure the rod to the screws as the head is extended. Alternative, hinged rods can be used to facilitate osteotomy closure (▶ Fig. 12.5). Once the deformity is corrected, neuromonitoring signals are checked to ensure that there has been no change.

Lateral X-rays are then obtained to assess the amount of correction and the overall alignment of the cervical spine. To ensure arthrodesis, local autograft from the bony resections performed at C7 as well as from the lateral mass of C6 and T1

are often used. The spinous process of C7 is split in the sagittal plane and placed along the sides of the decorticated C6 and T1 spinous processes and cabled into position. If a gap remains between the C6 lateral mass and T1, a spinous process from the upper thoracic spine can provide adequate local bone to fill the void. Finally, the defect between the C6 and T1 laminae is covered with the remaining local bone, including the bone dust created by the use of the high-speed burr.

12.3.6 Wound Closure

The posterior wound closure must be meticulous and is performed in multiple layers to minimize potential dead space, maximize tissue coverage, reduce infection, decrease wound dehiscence, and optimize cosmesis. If there is excessive amount of redundant tissue after deformity correction, an ellipse of full-thickness skin can be cut out to eliminate the redundancy. Surgical drains are usually left in place and hemostasis is assured as each layer is closed. Postoperatively, patients can be immobilized with a hard cervical collar to facilitate fusion.

12.4 Clinical Pearls

One potential issue with OWO is the translation that may occur during osteotomy closure due the opening wedge created and during osteoclasis and kyphosis correction (▶ Fig. 12.6), which

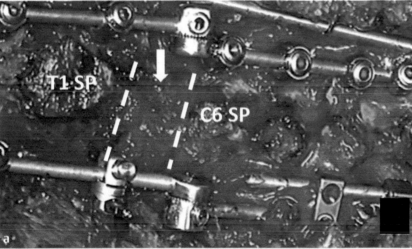
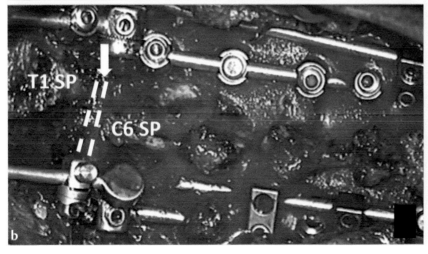

Fig. 12.5 Intraoperative photos demonstrating osteotomy **(a)** preclosure and **(b)** postclosure utilizing hinged rods. SP, spinous process.

makes OWO inherently less stable compared to CWO. In patients with concomitant cervical and thoracic hyperkyphosis (▶ Fig. 12.7), additional osteotomy may be needed in the thoracolumbar spine in order to achieve adequate deformity correction (▶ Fig. 12.8).

Scheer et al[15] performed a biomechanical study comparing stability of OWO versus CWO, and they demonstrated significantly increased stiffness across the osteotomy site in specimen with CWO (▶ Fig. 12.9). One strategy to address the anterior gap in OWO is to perform additional anterior cervical interbody fusion after posterior deformity correction, which helps to minimize risk for pseudoarthrosis. However, this may not be necessary in patients with ankylosing spondylitis, as these patients often fused with posterior-only constructs, but adding anterior column support may minimize the risk for rod fractures before bony fusion takes place.

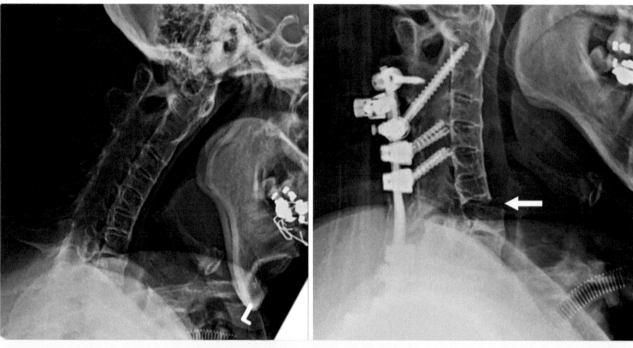

Fig. 12.6 Pre- and postoperative X-rays demonstrating opening wedge osteotomy kyphotic for deformity correction in a patient with ankylosing spondylitis (*arrow* demonstrating translation that can occur with OWO).

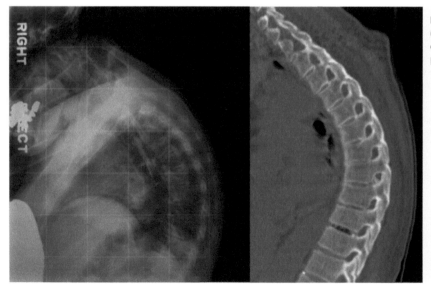

Fig. 12.7 Preoperative lateral X-rays (left) and CT (right) demonstrating rigid cervical kyphotic deformity with concomitant thoracic hyperkyphosis.

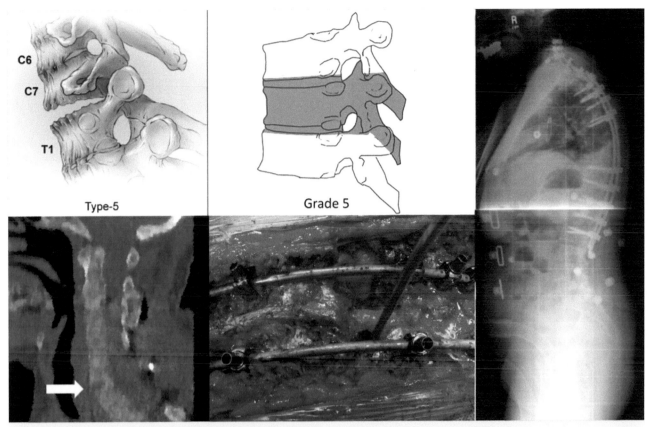

Fig. 12.8 An illustration (left top) and postoperative CT (left bottom) demonstrating C7 OWO (type 5 cervical osteotomy),[13] which was performed in conjunction with T4 vertebral column resection (Grade 5 thoracolumbar osteotomy,[14] middle panels), to treat a patient with concomitant cervical and thoracic hyperkyphosis; postoperative X-ray (right) demonstrated good deformity correction.

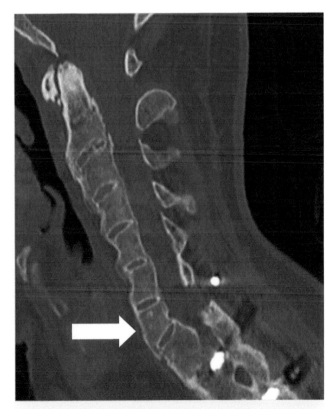

Fig. 12.9 A postoperative CT demonstrating solid fusion without any anterior column gap or translation in a patient with C7 PSO (closing wedge osteotomy) 1 year after surgery.

12.5 Conclusion

OWO is a powerful tool in the treatment of fixed cervical deformity. Spine surgeons should keep this technique in their armamentarium during evaluation and treatment of rigid cervical spine deformities.

References

[1] Smith-Petersen MN, Larson CB, Aufranc OE. Osteotomy of the spine for correction of flexion deformity in rheumatoid arthritis. J Bone Joint Surg. 1945; 27(4):1–11

[2] Urist MR. Osteotomy of the cervical spine; report of a case of ankylosing rheumatoid spondylitis. J Bone Joint Surg Am. 1958; 40-A(4):833–843

[3] Simmons EH. The surgical correction of flexion deformity of the cervical spine in ankylosing spondylitis. Clin Orthop Relat Res. 1972; 86(86):132–143

[4] Simmons ED, DiStefano RJ, Zheng Y, Simmons EH. Thirty-six years experience of cervical extension osteotomy in ankylosing spondylitis: techniques and outcomes. Spine. 2006; 31(26):3006–3012

[5] Thomasen E. Vertebral osteotomy for correction of kyphosis in ankylosing spondylitis. Clin Orthop Relat Res. 1985(194):142–152

[6] Tokala DP, Lam KS, Freeman BJC, Webb JK. C7 decancellisation closing wedge osteotomy for the correction of fixed cervico-thoracic kyphosis. Eur Spine J. 2007; 16(9):1471–1478

[7] Wollowick AL, Kelly MP, Riew KD. Pedicle subtraction osteotomy in the cervical spine. Spine. 2012; 37(5):E342–E348

[8] Deviren V, Scheer JK, Ames CP. Technique of cervicothoracic junction pedicle subtraction osteotomy for cervical sagittal imbalance: report of 11 cases. J Neurosurg Spine. 2011; 15(2):174–181

[9] Khan SN, Braaksma B, An HS. Cervical pedicle subtraction osteotomy for fixed flexion deformities. Orthopedics. 2012; 35(6):484–489

[10] Tan LA, Riew KD, Traynelis VC. Cervical spine deformity-part 3: posterior techniques, clinical outcome, and complications. Neurosurgery. 2017; 81 (6):893–898

[11] Suk K-S, Kim K-T, Lee S-H, Kim J-M. Significance of chin-brow vertical angle in correction of kyphotic deformity of ankylosing spondylitis patients. Spine. 2003; 28(17):2001–2005

[12] Song K, Su X, Zhang Y, et al. Optimal chin-brow vertical angle for sagittal visual fields in ankylosing spondylitis kyphosis. Eur Spine J. 2016; 25(8):2596–2604

[13] Ames CP, Smith JS, Scheer JK, et al. International Spine Study Group. A standardized nomenclature for cervical spine soft-tissue release and osteotomy for deformity correction: clinical article. J Neurosurg Spine. 2013; 19(3):269–278

[14] Schwab F, Blondel B, Chay E, et al. The comprehensive anatomical spinal osteotomy classification. Neurosurgery. 2014; 74(1):112–120, discussion 120

[15] Scheer JK, Tang JA, Buckley JM, et al. Biomechanical analysis of osteotomy type and rod diameter for treatment of cervicothoracic kyphosis. Spine. 2011; 36(8):E519–E523

13 Cervical Pedicle Screw Fixation

Sang Hun Lee, Corinna C. Zygourakis, and Christopher P. Ames

Abstract

Since the 1990s, several case series have demonstrated favorable outcomes with cervical pedicle screw fixation. Cervical pedicle screw fixation can provide more rigid fixation via a posterior-only approach compared to more conventional posterior stabilization options (e.g., cervical lateral mass screws) and even anterior-posterior combined techniques. Despite the biomechanical advantages, the small size and higher medial angle of cervical pedicles predispose to lateral pedicle breaches and resultant vertebral artery and nerve root injury. Although the risks of cervical pedicle screw placement have been mitigated by novel surgical techniques, expanded clinical experience, and navigation-assisted technologies, these risks cannot be completely prevented. Successful cervical pedicle screw placement can be accomplished with careful preoperative planning, thorough knowledge of local anatomy, and potentially navigation-assisted technology. Although cervical pedicle screws are not the standard of care for posterior cervical stabilization, this technique can be a useful option to provide more rigid stabilization, correct spinal deformity, and save the number of fusion segments in appropriately selected cases. In this chapter, we review the biomechanical and anatomical characteristics, surgical technique, and clinical outcomes of cervical pedicle screw fixation. Finally, we describe clinical settings in which cervical pedicle screw fixation is helpful and advantageous.

Keywords: cervical pedicle screw, lateral mass screw, posterior cervical stabilization, posterior cervical fixation, cervical deformity, cervical kyphosis, vertebral artery injury, navigation

13.1 History and Background

Starting with the early clinical series of Roy-Camille in the 1960s[1,2,3,4,5,6] and gaining popularity in the 1980s, pedicle screw fixation has been used in the thoracolumbar spine for mechanical stabilization, deformity correction, and fusion. Thoracolumbar pedicle fixation was initially applied to the treatment of traumatic conditions and extended to degenerative disease, tumor, and spinal deformity afterward. Thoracolumbar pedicle screw fixation is now widely accepted as the main stabilization method for various spinal conditions.[1,2,5,7]

Cervical pedicle fixation was first described at C2 for a hangman's fracture by LeConte in 1964[8] and Borne et al in 1984.[9] However, it was not until the early 1990s that the method was clinically applied to the subaxial cervical spine by Abumi et al.[10,11,12]

In 1994, Abumi et al reported the first clinical case series using subaxial cervical pedicle screws in the setting of trauma.[10] Since then, the same group has published several case series with cervical pedicle screws for various spinal conditions.[11,12,13,14,15,16,17,18] During the 1990s, multiple reports on

anatomic characteristics, entry points, and biomechanical properties of cervical pedicle screws were published. Over the past two decades, research on cervical pedicle screw fixation has expanded to include drill-guide or navigation-assisted methods to minimize the risks and improve outcomes with clinical pedicle screws.

In this chapter, we review the biomechanical and anatomical characteristics, surgical technique, and clinical outcomes of cervical pedicle screw fixation. Finally, we describe clinical settings in which cervical pedicle screw fixation is helpful and advantageous.

13.2 Pros and Cons of Cervical Pedicle Screw Fixation

Cervical pedicle screws follow a trajectory from the lateral mass through the pedicle into the vertebral body. As a result, their main advantage is more rigid fixation than other types of cervical fixation, such as wiring, plating, or lateral mass screws.[19,20,21,22,23,24,25,26] This can allow for more stable fixation and correction, particularly in cervical deformity cases (e.g., one-stage posterior correction of cervical kyphosis). In addition, cervical pedicle screws may be advantageous in patients with osteoporotic bone or highly unstable spines after severe trauma or radical tumor excision. Furthermore, cervical pedicle screw placement may provide a wider fusion bed than lateral mass screws, given the entry of the pedicle screw is located lateral to the entry point for lateral mass screws.

Despite these advantages, there are several drawbacks that have prevented widespread acceptance and utilization of cervical pedicle screws. First and foremost is the risk of vertebral artery injury.[27,28,29,30] Cervical pedicles have smaller diameters and a higher medial convergence angle than those of the thoracolumbar spine. As a result, these anatomical characteristics predispose to lateral pedicle wall violation when placing cervical pedicle screws. In the majority of patients, the vertebral artery passes through the transverse foramen immediately lateral to the pedicle from C3 to C6 in the subaxial cervical spine. Although the majority of unilateral vertebral artery injury is asymptomatic, severe posterior cranial infarction may occur even with unilateral vertebral artery injury if the patient has insufficient collateral flow through their posterior circulation.[29,30]

In addition, due to the smaller size of cervical pedicles and foramina, cranial or caudal pedicle wall violation is more likely to cause nerve root injury than in the thoracolumbar spine. As a result of these anatomic complexities, as well as the medicolegal environment in many places and a steep learning curve, many surgeons have shied away from cervical pedicle screw placement and instead performed anterior-posterior combined surgery with traditional lateral mass screws when stronger fixation is warranted.

13.3 Biomechanical Characteristics of Cervical Pedicle Screw Fixation

The first biomechanical study on cervical pedicle screws was performed by Kotani et al in 1994.[19] They found that transpedicular cervical fixation provides greater stability than conventional anterior and/or posterior wiring fixation in multilevel constructs under axial, torsional, and flexion loading in a calf cadaveric model.

Since then, several biomechanical studies have compared the pullout strength of cervical pedicle to that of lateral mass screws. In 2004, Kothe et al showed that cervical pedicle screw fixation has significantly higher initial flexion/extension stability as well as stability after cyclic loading compared to lateral mass screw fixation.[20] Johnston et al confirmed these results and demonstrated significantly less screw loosening and higher pullout strength in cervical pedicle compared to lateral mass screws.[31]

In a more recent study in 2014, Ito et al found that the mean pullout strength of cervical pedicle screws was nearly four times greater than the mean pullout strength of lateral mass screws (762 vs. 191 N) after torsion loading, and two times greater after flexion/extension loading (571 vs. 289 N).[32] Duff et al showed that a 360-degree reconstruction model (corpectomy spacer with anterior plating and posterior lateral mass screws from C3 to C7) provided only slightly greater stability compared to C3 and C7 posterior-only fixation with pedicle screws.[24]

These biomechanical reports are limited in that they are cadaveric studies that do not consider dynamic stabilizing factors. However, with its three-column fixation, cervical pedicle screw does appear to provide greater stability than lateral mass screws and may therefore be justified in patients with poor bone quality or highly unstable conditions that require more rigid fixation than the usual clinical settings.

13.4 Anatomical Considerations for Cervical Pedicle Screw Placement

13.4.1 Cervical Spine Pedicles

Cervical Pedicle Anatomy

In 1991, Panjabi et al described in detail the anatomical dimensions of the subaxial cervical spine, including pedicle width, height, cross-sectional area, and medial and sagittal angles.[33] Since then, several other studies have attempted to quantify the dimensions and angulations of cervical pedicles using cadavers or computed tomography (CT) images. Common findings from these studies are as follows:

- The width and height of the subaxial cervical pedicles are smallest at C3 and gradually increase down to C7.
- The medial angle of the pedicle is greatest at C3 (approximately 45 degrees; range: 42–55 degrees) and gradually decreases down to C7 (approximately 32 degrees; range: 24–48 degrees).
- The sagittal angle changes from a cranial orientation at C3 and C4 (3–15 degrees), to an almost neutral orientation at C5, to a caudal orientation at C6 and C7 (0–11 degrees).[34,35,36,37,38,39]

Despite these general principles, it is essential to examine and measure the cervical pedicles on preoperative imaging given the extensive variability in individual spines.

Rao et al reported the mean width and height at all subaxial levels were sufficiently large to accommodate standard 3.5-mm pedicle screws in 98% of the young, healthy volunteers enrolled in a normative CT study.[38] Pedicle widths smaller than 4 mm were rare exceptions (1.7% of the pedicles) and generally observed in women. In general, cervical pedicle screw fixation is not recommended in young children,[40] unless preoperative imaging shows sufficient size of their pedicles for appropriate fixation.

Another important anatomic characteristic of the cervical pedicles is in their 3D structure.[36,40,41] They have an elliptical to triangular cross-sectional shape, with a medial wall that is 1.4 to 3.6 times thicker than the lateral wall, similar to the thoracolumbar spine. This is yet another reason that lateral wall violation is more likely than medial wall violation for cervical pedicle screws and may predispose to vertebral artery injury.

Entry Points

Many researchers have published various cervical screw entry points in the literature. In 1994, Jeanneret et al recommended an "entry point 3 mm beneath the facet joint on the vertical line in the middle of the articular mass'" with an average 45-degree medial angle[35]. Common recommendations from the subsequent studies are as follows:

- The entry point should be close to the bony notch below the facet joint in the cranial-caudal plane, furthest away at C7 and getting gradually closer at C3.
- In the medial-lateral plane, the entry point should be the most lateral at C3 and gradually move medially by C7. However, it should not be in the medial half of the lateral mass.[34,35,36,37,38]

Perhaps most importantly, like pedicle screw trajectory, length, and diameter, the entry point should be individualized to local anatomy and measurements on preoperative images.

13.4.2 Vertebral Artery and Nerve Roots in Subaxial Cervical Spine

The vertebral artery arises from the subclavian artery and enters the transverse foramen at the C6 level in more than 90 to 92% of patients. However, in some patients, the vertebral artery may enter the foramen at an abnormal level: specifically, C5, C4, and C7 in order of frequency in the literature.[27,42,43] The following points about the course of the vertebral artery in the cervical spine should be noted:

- The course is not always straight; it may be tortuous following degenerative changes in the cervical spine.
- The location of the vertebral artery within the transverse foramen is anterior and medial, instead of central.
- There may be a significant difference in flow/diameter of the right and left vertebral arteries, with one side extremely small or even absent. If one side is known to be dominant from preoperative imaging, the surgeon should be extremely careful to avoid vertebral artery injury on that side during surgery.

Anatomical studies show that, unlike lumbar nerve roots, cervical nerve roots pass through the foramina closer to the inferior than superior pedicle in the sagittal plane.[44] In the coronal plane, the nerve root exit angle is largest at C3 (where it is approximately 90 degrees) and gradually decreases to C6 and C7.[44] The cervical nerve root overlies the intervertebral disc level at C4–C5 and traverses the proximal part of the intervertebral disc at the C5–C6 and C6–C7 levels. These findings imply that superior pedicle wall violation is more likely than inferior wall violation to produce nerve root symptoms in the cervical spine.[45]

13.5 Cervical Pedicle Fixation Techniques

13.5.1 Abumi's Technique and Modifications

Abumi's Original Technique

In their initial article,[10] Abumi et al described the cervical pedicle screw entry point as "slightly lateral to the center of the articular mass and close to the posterior margin of the superior articular surface," with a medial angulation of 30 to 40 degrees. For safe insertion of pedicle screws, they made their entry point with a high-speed burr, 3 to 4 mm in diameter. This allowed them to bury their screw anchor heads, and also to visualize the entrance of the pedicle with a "funnel" technique, similar to that described in thoracic pedicle screw placement. They used fluoroscopy to confirm the sagittal location of the entry point and trajectory angle.

Modified "Funnel" Techniques

Several modifications of cervical screw placement technique have been reported since 2012,[46,47,48] and mirror the development of new cervical implant technologies. For example, Lee et al described a "key slot" technique which is a modified entry hole that creates a slot in the coronal plane and a triangular shape in the axial plane based on the pedicle medial angle. This technique may avoid the bony defect produced by the Abumi's "funnel" and fits better with modern polyaxial screw heads.[46]

Authors' Preferred Technique

Preoperative Examination

To check for vertebral artery abnormal course and dominance, we obtain vascular-enhanced CT scans on all patients prior to cervical pedicle fixation surgery. We also use these preoperative CT scans to measure the convergence angle and the minimum diameter of the pedicle in the axial plane at each instrumented cervical vertebra (▶ Fig. 13.1). We select the length of the screw so that it passes into the anterior one-third of the vertebral body on preoperative imaging. If patients have a pedicle diameter less than 3.5 mm or a pedicle convergence angle greater than 50 degrees, we do not perform cervical pedicle screw fixation at these levels.

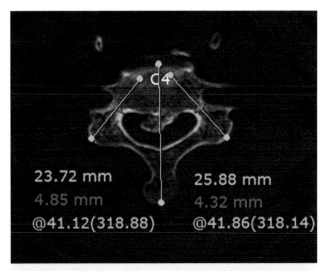

Fig. 13.1 Preoperative measurement of the pedicle diameter, medial convergence angle, and screw length on the axial CT.

Insertion Technique

To find the correct trajectory, we target the virtual pedicle entry point, which is on the line perpendicular to the pedicle's axis (▶ Fig. 13.2a). We begin by creating a key slot–shaped entry on the medial half of the lateral mass with a 3-mm matchstick burr. The key-slot entry shape is a rectangle in the coronal plane (▶ Fig. 13.2b) and a right-angled triangle in the axial plane (▶ Fig. 13.2c). The apex of the triangle is the virtual pedicle inlet, and the oblique side of the triangle is the pedicle's axis (▶ Fig. 13.2a, c). In the sagittal plane, the depth of the drilled entry point is two-thirds of the lateral mass thickness (▶ Fig. 13.2d).

The exact width, depth, and angle of the slot are adjusted according to the individual anatomy of the cervical vertebra on preoperative CT images. When a surgeon is first learning to place cervical pedicle screws, he or she may confirm the location of the entry point and screw trajectory in the sagittal plane with lateral fluoroscopy. With practice and experience, cervical pedicle screw placement is possible without fluoroscopic guidance.

After drilling the key slot–shaped entry, we gently probe the pedicle as close to the medial wall as possible with a 15-degree curved awl. After probing to an approximate 2-cm depth, we confirm the lack of pedicle breach using a ball-tip probe. If we detect a pedicle breach, we change the screw trajectory or skip this level. After confirming there is no pedicle breach, we sequentially drill, tap, and insert the screw in the usual fashion.

A screw with a head that is located on the lateral margin of the lateral mass with a tip that is medial to the uncovertebral joint on plain radiographs is considered to be in the safest position. A screw tip positioned laterally to the uncovertebral joint or a head located out of the lateral mass is expected to increase the risk of pedicle breach[49] (▶ Fig. 13.3).

13.5.2 Foraminotomy-Assisted Technique

In 1998, Albert et al[50] described their "laminoforaminotomy" technique for lower cervical pedicle screws. They recommended

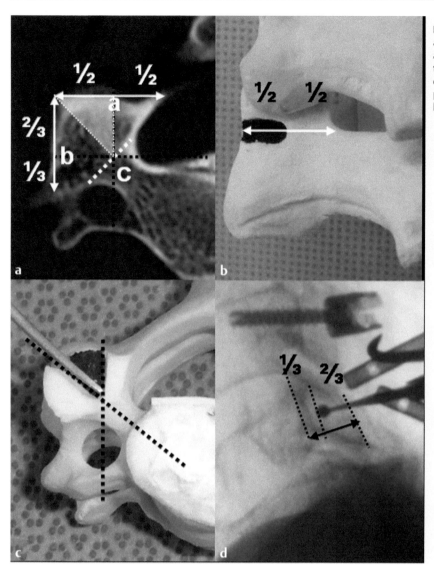

Fig. 13.2 Cutting burr (3 mm). The entry shape is a rectangle in the coronal plane (**a**) and a right-angled triangle in the axial plane (**b**). The apex of the triangle is the virtual pedicle inlet and the oblique side is the pedicle's axis (**c**). In the sagittal plane, the drilled entry depth is two-thirds of the lateral mass thickness, as seen on fluoroscopy (**d**).

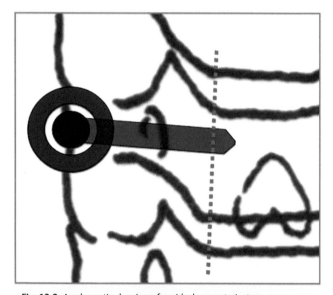

Fig. 13.3 A schematic drawing of an ideal screw trajectory on an anterior-posterior radiograph. A screw with a head that is located on the lateral margin of the lateral mass with its tip medial to the uncovertebral joint is considered to be in the safest position. A screw tip positioned laterally to the uncovertebral joint area or a screw head located out of the lateral mass is expected to increase the risk of pedicle breach.

direct pedicle medial wall palpation via a C6–C7 laminoforaminotomy. Since then, several authors have reported similar modifications using foraminotomies to place cervical pedicle screws.[47,48,51]

The foraminotomy is a simple method to visualize the medial pedicle wall and is helpful for cervical pedicle screw fixation in C7 or T1. It is also possible to perform foraminotomies for pedicle screw placement in the midcervical spine. However, it may take more operative time, requiring greater bony removal and higher blood loss, from C3 to C5 because these levels have greater pedicle medial angles and lateral mass anterior-posterior dimensions than the C6–C7 level.

13.5.3 Navigation-Assisted Technique (▶ Fig. 13.4)

In an effort to enhance accuracy and safety, computer-assisted navigation techniques have been applied to cervical pedicle screw placements. Several cadaveric studies in the 2000s demonstrated improved accuracy with navigation-assisted cervical pedicle screw placement compared to conventional techniques.[52,53,54,55] In 2003, Kotani et al reported the first clinical outcomes which showed significantly improved accuracy with navigation-assisted cervical pedicle screw placement: 1.2

versus 6.7% pedicle wall breach rates compared to the conventional freehand technique.[52] Since this report, many clinical case series using different types of intraoperative navigation systems (3D fluoroscopy, O-arm, intraoperative CT, etc.) have confirmed these findings.[54,55,56,57,58,59,60,61,62,63] Taken together, these studies suggest that navigation-assisted pedicle screw placement is more accurate than the freehand technique, although there is no clear difference in terms of neurovascular complications and reoperation rates. However, we recommend navigation-assisted cervical pedicle screw placement especially

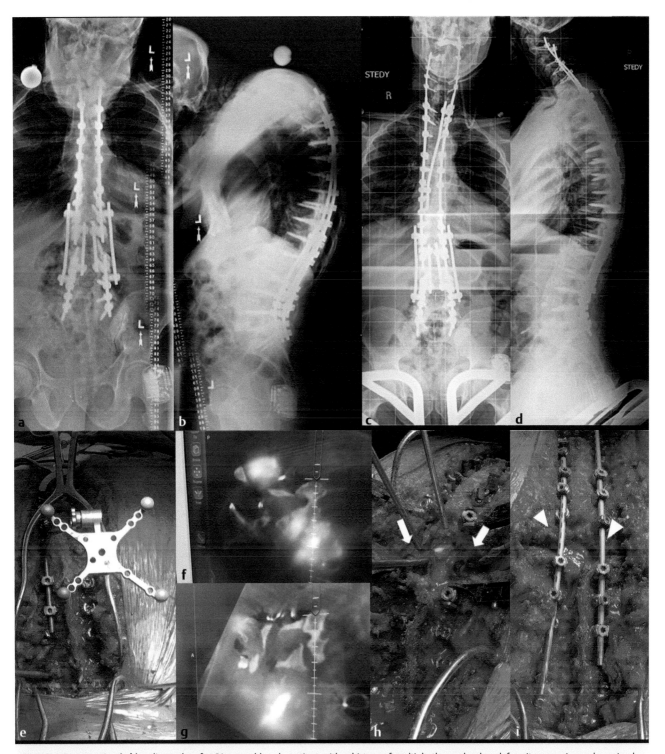

Fig. 13.4 Preoperative **(a,b)** radiographs of a 61-year-old male patient with a history of multiple thoracolumbar deformity surgeries and proximal junctional kyphosis at T3. A posterior vertebral column resection (PVCR) was performed at T3 with extension of fusion up to C2. Postoperative radiographs show significant improvement of sagittal balance **(c,d)**. Cervical pedicle screws were inserted for cervical spine fixation using the O-arm and Stealth navigation-assisted technique **(e-g)**. **(h,i)** The bony gap after T3 PVCR (*arrows* in **h**) was closed after reduction and rod assembly (*arrowheads* in **i**).

13.5.4 Drill and Screw-Guide Template-Assisted Technique

The use of templates based on a patient's individual anatomy have been developed to avoid the high financial and time cost of navigation equipment, the learning curve of using navigation technology, and the additional radiation exposure for the patient. Initial efforts in the 2000s used a custom-made guiding device or CT film template, but more recently in the 2010s, 3D remodeling software and printing systems have been applied to cervical pedicle screw placement.[64,65,66,67] Clinical case series show good accuracy of templates comparable to those of surface landmark–guided or navigation-guided cervical pedicle screw placement.

13.6 Clinical Series and Outcomes

In the first case series, Abumi et al treated 13 patients with traumatic conditions using cervical pedicle screws, reporting satisfactory clinical outcomes without pseudarthrosis or other major complications.[10] Abumi and coworkers have reported good neurological and radiographic outcomes in several consecutive case series using cervical pedicle screw fixation for nontraumatic cervical spine pathology including kyphosis, spondylotic myelopathy, ossification of the posterior longitudinal ligament, rheumatoid arthritis, and metastatic tumors (▶ Table 13.1).

Other groups have confirmed the favorable outcomes and low complication rates of cervical pedicle screw placement.[46,51,56,57,59,69,71,72,73,74] One study proposed that cervical pedicle screw placement is a good fixation option for cervical fractures involving both the lateral mass and pedicle in order to minimize the necessary points of fixation.[17] Rajasekaran et al reported good outcomes in a cohort of pediatric patients (mean age = 9.7 years old) requiring craniovertebral junction stabilization, suggesting cervical pedicle screw fixation may be an option in children as well.[68] Watanabe et al demonstrated an 81% fusion rate with posterior-only cervical pedicle screw fixation in athetoid cerebral palsy patients.[70] In summary, the literature suggests the cervical pedicle screw fixation technique can be applied to nearly any clinical condition requiring posterior fixation of the cervical spine.

13.7 Accuracy and Complications

The accuracy of cervical pedicle screw placement has been extensively assessed by numerous authors. However, it is not easy to compare results between series as they often use variable diagnostic criteria for pedicle breaches (▶ Table 13.1). In Abumi's first case series, the authors found 3 cortical breaches out of 52 screws (5.8%), based on postoperative CT scans.[10] Consecutive studies from the same authors report pedicle breach rates ranging from 4.7 to 6.9%.

In the literature, the incidence of noncritical pedicle breach (< 50% of screw diameter exposed) ranges from 14.8 to 20%, and critical pedicle breach (> 50% of screw diameter exposed) ranges from 4.1 to 9%. On average, 60 to 70% of pedicle perforation is in the lateral direction and approximately 30% is in the medial direction. In addition, several studies demonstrate learning curves of cervical pedicle screw placement. More specifically, the incidence of critical pedicle breach decreases significantly after the initial 15 to 25 cases.[46,69,71]

Fortunately, most cases of the misplaced cervical pedicle screws described in the literature are asymptomatic. However, the most serious complication of cervical pedicle wall breach is vertebral artery injury due to a lateral breach, followed by cervical nerve root injury due to a superior or inferior breach. Spinal cord injury is less common as the cervical pedicle medial wall is thicker, medial breaches are rare, and there is a lot of space between the medial pedicle wall and the spinal cord itself.

In 2000, the first comprehensive study by Abumi et al on cervical pedicle screw complications reported 3 patients with neurovascular complications (1.7% of the patients; 0.4% of 669 total cervical pedicle screws in 180 patients).[68] Kast et al found 2 patients with critical screw breaches resulting in neurological symptoms out of 94 pedicle screws placed in 26 patients (2.1% of screws; 7.7% of patients).[67] Yukawa et al reported one vertebral artery injury (0.16%) and one radiculopathy (0.16%) out of 620 cervical pedicle screws in 114 patients.[73] In 2012, Nakashima et al reported three nerve root injuries (3.6%) and two vertebral artery injuries (2.4%) out of 84 patients undergoing cervical pedicle screw fixation for nontraumatic pathology.[69] Up until 2018, only two cases of cerebellar and/or brainstem stroke due to cervical pedicle screw misplacement have been reported in the English literature.[29,30]

In a systematic review by Yoshihara et al, perioperative neurological and biomechanical complication rates (including pseudarthrosis) are similarly low for cervical pedicle and lateral mass screws, but vertebral artery injuries are significantly more common with cervical pedicle screw placement.[76]

13.8 Clinical Applications of Cervical Pedicle Fixation

In this section, we present several broad categories of clinical applications for cervical pedicle screw fixation. Indications can be expanded depending on the individual patient's bone quality, fusion levels, and local anatomy.

13.8.1 Rigid Fixation for Weak Bone

As several biomechanical studies indicate, cervical pedicle screw fixation provides better fixation strength not only immediately postoperatively but also later after repetitive cyclic loading. One can therefore avoid an anterior-posterior combined surgery by placing strong three-column stabilization via posterior cervical pedicle screws alone. This is particularly advantageous in patients with severe osteoporosis (mean T-score at femoral neck of -4.5 in ▶ Fig. 13.5 example), rheumatoid arthritis, destructive arthropathies, chronic steroid usage, or other pathologies that predispose to weak bone.

Table 13.1 Clinical case series report accuracy of cervical pedicle screw placement using various techniques and pedicle breach criteria

Authors	Number of patients/ screws	Placement technique	Accuracy criteria	Pedicle breach rate	Complications	Other
Abumi et al (2000)[71]	180/667	Fluoroscopy-guided, freehand	Pedicle breach or no breach	6.7%	Radiculopathy (2) VAI (1)	
Yoshimoto et al (2005)[72]	27/134	Fluoroscopy-guided, freehand	No breach Partial: < 1/2 screw diameter Complete: > 1/2 screw diameter	Partial: 7.4% Complete: 3.7%	None	Breach rate decreased from 12 to 7% after the first 18 cases
Kast et al (2006)[67]	36/94	Mixed: navigation-assisted, freehand	Correct: < 1 mm violation Minor: < 25% of transverse foramen Major: > 25%	Correct: 70% Minor: 21% Major: 9%	Radiculopathy (3)	More common pedicle perforation at C3 and C4 Perforation rate decreased from 13 to 4% after the first 20 cases
Ito et al (2008)[57]	50/176	3D fluoroscopy navigation-guided	Grade 1: no breach Grade 2: < 2 mm Grade 3: > 2 mm	Grade 2: 2.8% Grade 3: 0%	None	
Yukawa et al (2009)[7,3]	144/417	Fluoroscopy axial view–guided technique	Exposure: < 50% of screw diameter Perforation: > 50%	Exposure: 9.2% Perforation: 3.9%	Radiculopathy (1) VAI (1)	
Ishikawa et al (2010)[56]	21/108	O-arm-based navigation	Grade 0: no exposure Grade 1: < 2 mm Grade 2: 2–4 mm Grade 3: < 4 mm	Grade 1: 8.3% Grade 2: 2.8% Grade 3: 0	None	
Lee et al (2012)[46]	50/277	Fluoroscopy-guided freehand (modified Abumi technique)	Grade 0 Grade 1: < 25% screw diameter exposure Grade 2: 25–50% Grade 3: > 50%	Grade 1: 12.6% Grade 2: 7.6% Grade 3: 2.2%	None	Breach rate decreased from 20 to 2.7% after the first 10 cases
Nakashima et al (2012)[69]	84/390	Mixed: fluoroscopy-guided, freehand, navigation-assisted	Grade 1: < 50% of screw diameter Grade 2: > 50%	Grade 1: 15.4% Grade 2: 4.1%	Radiculopathy (3) VAI (2)	High breach rate in cervical kyphosis and cerebral palsy patients
Hojo et al (2014)[55]	283/1065	Fluoroscopy-guided, freehand	Grade 1: < 50% of screw exposure Grade 2: > 50%	Grade 1: 9.6% Grade 2: 5.3%	VAI (2)	High perforation rate in rheumatoid patients.
Uehara et al (2014)[60]	129/579	Navigation-assisted	Grade 1: no breach Grade 2: < 50% of screw diameter Grade 3: > 50%	Grade 2: 13.3% Grade 3: 6.7%	None	Breach is more common at C3–C5
Kaneyama et al (2015)[65]	20/80	Patient-specific drill guide template		Class 0: no breach Class 1: < 50% screw diameter exposure Class 2: > 50% Class 3: complete exposure	Class 1: 2.5% No class 2 or 3	3D printing technique

Abbreviation: VAI, vertebral artery injury.
Note: No VAI in the case series reported was symptomatic.

13.8.2 One-Stage Correction of Rigid or Flexible Kyphosis

Abumi et al reported a successful outcome for a one-stage correction of flexible kyphosis by approximately 23 degrees with cervical pedicle screw fixation and reduction.[13] The authors have also applied the one-stage technique for correction of a semi-rigid kyphosis (▶ Fig. 13.6).

13.8.3 Stable Fixation with Osteotomy for Severe Fixed Deformities

Unlike flexible kyphosis, fixed deformities in patients with ankylosing spondylitis, diffuse idiopathic skeletal hyperostosis, or surgically fused segments often require osteotomies performed either anteriorly, posteriorly, or via a combin anterior-posterior approach. As shown in the case of a C7 pedicle

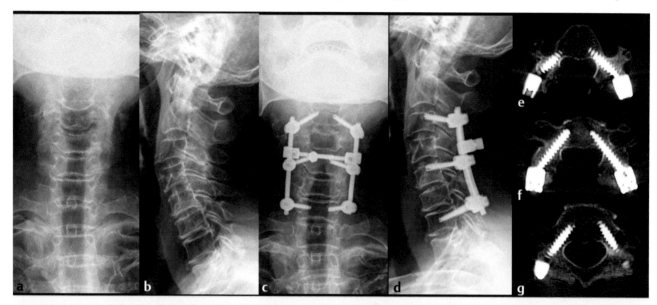

Fig. 13.5 A 78-year-old female with multilevel cervical spondylotic myelopathy and history of severe osteoporosis (mean T-score at femur neck of -4.5) underwent posterior laminectomy and fusion from C3 to C7. Preoperative **(a,b)** and postoperative radiographs **(c,d)** are shown. Cervical pedicle screws were successfully placed at C3, C5, and C7 **(e–g)** without pedicle wall perforation.

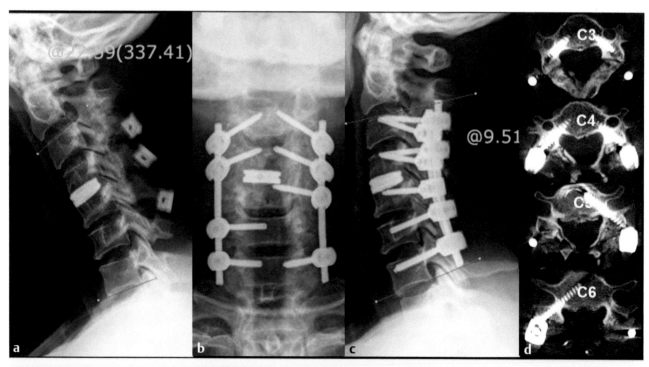

Fig. 13.6 Preoperative cervical spine lateral radiograph **(a)** of a 49-year-old female with myelopathy and semi-rigid postlaminoplasty kyphosis. Posterior decompression with one-stage correction of kyphosis was performed with subaxial pedicle screw fixation from C3 to C7 **(b, c)**. Postoperative axial CT images show all cervical pedicle screws are placed accurately without pedicle wall breach **(d)**.

subtraction osteotomy in ▶ Fig. 13.7, transpedicular fixation may provide more stable fixation and preserve the deformity correction with less incidence of screw loosening and a need for a smaller number of fused levels.

13.8.4 Minimal Segment Fixation to Preserve Maximum Cervical Motion

There has been no research to determine how many fusion levels can be avoided if one uses cervical pedicle screws instead of

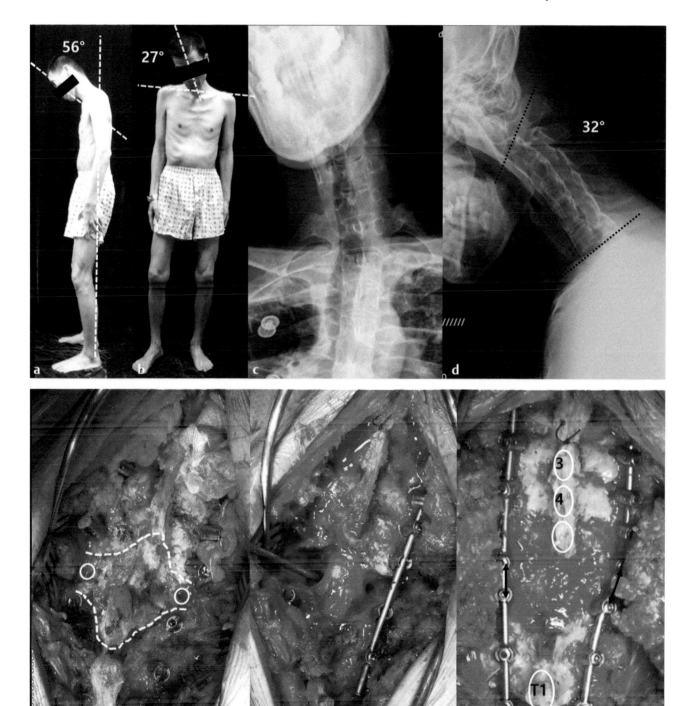

Fig. 13.7 Preoperative clinical pictures (a,b) and radiographs (c,d) of a 36-year-old male patient with ankylosing spondylitis show both sagittal and coronal plane cervical deformity. He underwent a pedicle subtraction osteotomy (PSO) at C7. After placement of cervical and thoracic pedicle screws (e) (C7 pedicle and imaginary osteotomy line were marked, involving the lower C6, entire C7, and upper T1 laminae), the PSO gap was closed with 3D plane correction (f) and local bone autograft (g).

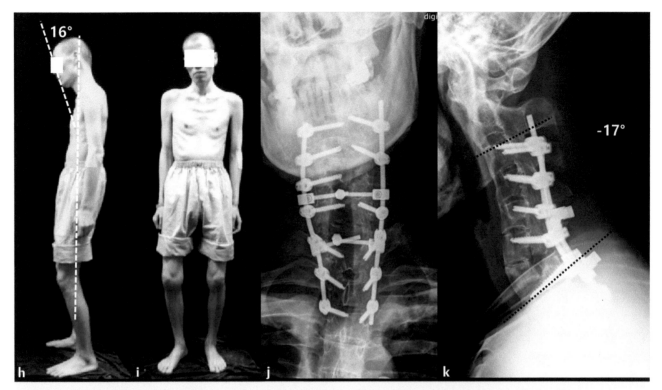

Fig 13.7 (*Continued*) The postoperative clinical pictures (**h,i**) and radiographs (**j,k**) show significant correction of the cervical deformity.

lateral mass screws. However, in select cases, cervical pedicle screw fixation can help decrease the number of fused levels and help maintain mobile segments, as demonstrated in ▶ Fig. 13.8.

13.8.5 Salvage of Lateral Mass Fixation Loss or Bone Defect by Lateral Mass Screw Loosening

Loosening of lateral mass screws occurs commonly due to intraoperative lateral mass fracture during screw insertion, nonunion, and adjacent segment failure. Revision of a lateral mass screw with a bigger diameter lateral mass screw is an option (i. e., revision of a loosened 3.5-mm screw with a 4-mm screw), or conversion into a different method (i.e., failed Magerl technique to Roy-Camille technique). But the resulting biomechanical fixation strength may still be insufficient. The easiest method is often to skip that level and extend the fixation. However, when this is not an option, conversion of the lateral mass to a pedicle screw may be a reasonable alternative, as shown in ▶ Fig. 13.9.

13.8.6 Hybrid Fixation: Lateral Mass Screws on One Side, Pedicle Screws on the Other

When a vertebral artery is injured and/or occluded by trauma (e.g., transverse foramen fracture), severely atrophic, or absent, the other side vertebral artery should be preserved extremely carefully. Risky procedures including dissection and pedicle screw instrumentation should be avoided on the side of the only remaining or dominant vertebral artery. One can therefore perform a hybrid fixation construct, with safer lateral mass screws on the side of the good artery, and more aggressive pedicle fixation on the side of the injured artery, as demonstrated in ▶ Fig. 13.10.

13.9 Conclusion

Since the 1990s, several case series have demonstrated favorable outcomes with cervical pedicle screw fixation. Cervical pedicle screw fixation can provide more rigid fixation via a posterior-only approach compared to more conventional posterior stabilization options (e.g., cervical lateral mass screws) and even anterior-posterior combined techniques. However, despite these biomechanical advantages, the small size and greater medial angle of cervical pedicles predispose to vertebral artery and nerve root injury. Although the risks of cervical pedicle screw placement have been mitigated by novel surgical techniques, expanded clinical experience, and navigation-assisted technologies, these risks cannot be completely prevented.

Successful cervical pedicle screw placement can be accomplished with careful preoperative planning, thorough knowledge of local anatomy, and potentially navigation-assisted technology. Although cervical pedicle screws are not the standard of care for posterior cervical stabilization, this technique can be a useful option to provide more rigid stabilization, correct spinal deformity, and save the number of fusion segments in appropriately selected cases.

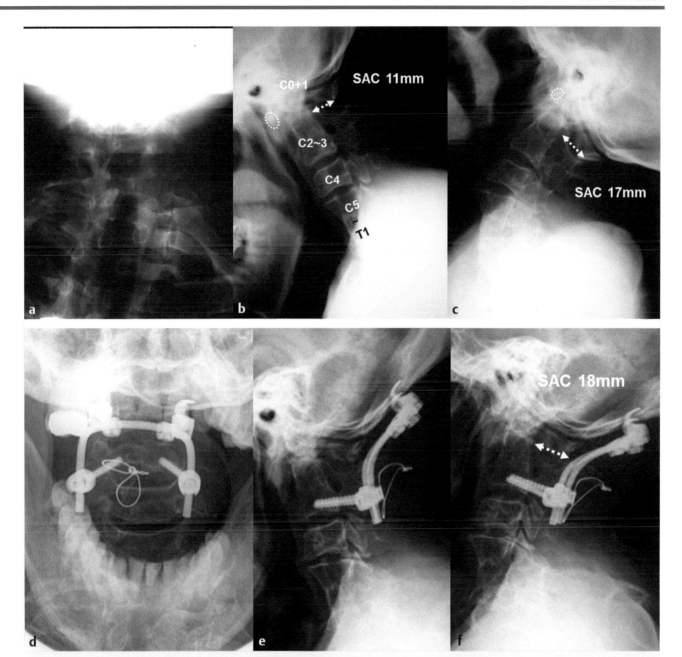

Fig. 13.8 Preoperative anterior-posterior **(a)**, flexion **(b)**, and extension **(c)** lateral cervical spine radiographs of a 55-year-old male with cervical myelopathy. He has a history of Klippel–Feil syndrome (occiput to C1, C2 to C3, and C5 to T1 are fused congenitally) and radiographic atlantoaxial instability. C1–C2, C3–C4, and C4–C5 are the only mobile cervical segments. To preserve maximum mobile segments, C3 pedicle screws were placed. At 7-year follow-up, the radiographs show minimal degenerative changes with segmental motion on flexion–extension radiographs **(d–f)**.

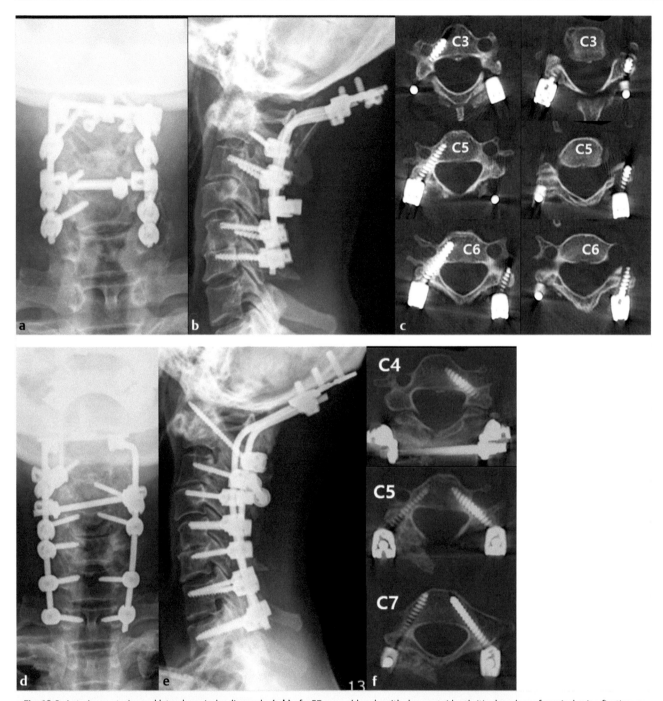

Fig. 13.9 Anterior-posterior and lateral cervical radiographs (**a,b**) of a 57-year-old male with rheumatoid arthritis show loss of cervical spine fixation as well as occipital plate loosening, following an occiput to C6 fusion 3 months earlier. On the CT images, pedicle screws on the right side are intact but the lateral mass screws on the left side are loose (**c**). The patient underwent revision occipital fixation, a conversion of loose lateral mass to pedicle screws on the left side, and additional cervical pedicle screw fixation down to T1 (**d–f**).

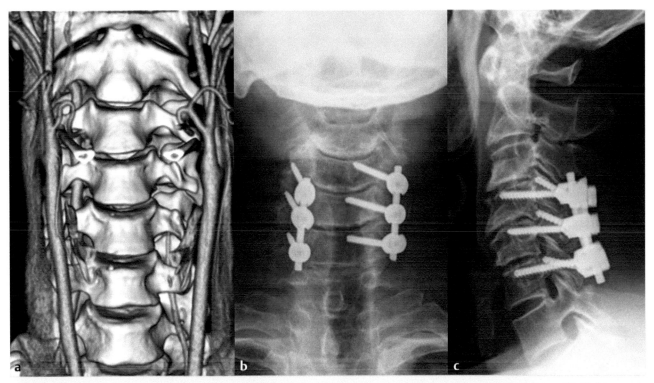

Fig. 13.10 A preoperative 3D CT angiogram of a 23-year-old male with C4–C5 facet dislocation and posterior ligament injury at C5–C6 shows complete occlusion of the left vertebral artery (a). He underwent posterior reduction and instrumented fusion C4 to C6 (b,c). To avoid damage to the remaining right vertebral artery, lateral mass screws were placed on the right side, and pedicle screws were inserted on the left side.

References

[1] Boucher HH. A method of spinal fusion. J Bone Joint Surg Br. 1959; 41-B (2):248–259

[2] Harrington PR. Treatment of scoliosis. Correction and internal fixation by spine instrumentation. J Bone Joint Surg Am. 1962; 44-A:591–610

[3] Harrington PR, Tullos HS. Spondylolisthesis in children. Observations and surgical treatment. Clin Orthop Relat Res. 1971; 79(79):75–84

[4] Roy-Camille R, Saillant G, Mazel C. Internal fixation of the lumbar spine with pedicle screw plating. Clin Orthop Relat Res. 1986(203):7–17

[5] Steffee AD, Biscup RS, Sitkowski DJ. Segmental spine plates with pedicle screw fixation. A new internal fixation device for disorders of the lumbar and thoracolumbar spine. Clin Orthop Relat Res. 1986(203):45–53

[6] Aebi M, Etter C, Kehl T, Thalgott J. Stabilization of the lower thoracic and lumbar spine with the internal spinal skeletal fixation system. Indications, techniques, and first results of treatment. Spine. 1987; 12(6):544–551

[7] Suk SI, Lee CK, Kim WJ, Chung YJ, Park YB. Segmental pedicle screw fixation in the treatment of thoracic idiopathic scoliosis. Spine. 1995; 20(12):1399–1405

[8] LeConte P. Fracture et luxation des deux premieres vertebres cervicales. In: Judet R, ed. Luxation Congenitale de la Hanche Fractures du Cou-de-pied Rachis Cervical Actualites de Chirurgie Orthopedique de l'Hospital Raymond-Poincare. Vol. 3. Paris: Masson et Cie; 1964:147–166

[9] Borne GM, Bedou GL, Pinaudeau M. Treatment of pedicular fractures of the axis. A clinical study and screw fixation technique. J Neurosurg. 1984; 60 (1):88–93

[10] Abumi K, Itoh H, Taneichi H, Kaneda K. Transpedicular screw fixation for traumatic lesions of the middle and lower cervical spine: description of the techniques and preliminary report. J Spinal Disord. 1994; 7(1):19–28

[11] Abumi K, Takada T, Shono Y, Kaneda K, Fujiya M. Posterior occipitocervical reconstruction using cervical pedicle screws and plate-rod systems. Spine. 1999; 24(14):1425–1434

[12] Abumi K, Ito M, Kaneda K. Surgical treatment of cervical destructive spondyloarthropathy (DSA). Spine. 2000; 25(22):2899–2905

[13] Abumi K, Kaneda K, Shono Y, Fujiya M. One-stage posterior decompression and reconstruction of the cervical spine by using pedicle screw fixation systems. J Neurosurg. 1999; 90(1) Suppl:19–26

[14] Abumi K, Shono Y, Kotani Y, Kaneda K. Indirect posterior reduction and fusion of the traumatic herniated disc by using a cervical pedicle screw system. J Neurosurg. 2000; 92(1) Suppl:30–37

[15] Abumi K, Shono Y, Taneichi H, Ito M, Kaneda K. Correction of cervical kyphosis using pedicle screw fixation systems. Spine. 1999; 24(22):2389–2396

[16] Abumi K, Kaneda K. Pedicle screw fixation for nontraumatic lesions of the cervical spine. Spine. 1997; 22(16):1853–1863

[17] Kotani Y, Abumi K, Ito M, Minami A. Cervical spine injuries associated with lateral mass and facet joint fractures: new classification and surgical treatment with pedicle screw fixation. Eur Spine J. 2005; 14(1):69–77

[18] Oda I, Abumi K, Ito M, et al. Palliative spinal reconstruction using cervical pedicle screws for metastatic lesions of the spine: a retrospective analysis of 32 cases. Spine. 2006; 31(13):1439–1444

[19] Kotani Y, Cunningham BW, Abumi K, McAfee PC. Biomechanical analysis of cervical stabilization systems. An assessment of transpedicular screw fixation in the cervical spine. Spine. 1994; 19(22):2529–2539

[20] Kothe R, Rüther W, Schneider E, Linke B. Biomechanical analysis of transpedicular screw fixation in the subaxial cervical spine. Spine. 2004; 29 (17):1869–1875

[21] Kowalski JM, Ludwig SC, Hutton WC, Heller JG. Cervical spine pedicle screws: a biomechanical comparison of two insertion techniques. Spine. 2000; 25 (22):2865–2867

[22] Rhee JM, Kraiwattanapong C, Hutton WC. A comparison of pedicle and lateral mass screw construct stiffness at the cervicothoracic junction. Spine. 2005; 30:E636–E640

[23] Bozkus H, Ames CP, Chamberlain RH, et al. Biomechanical analysis of rigid stabilization techniques for three-column injury in the lower cervical spine: a biomechanical study. Spine. 2005; 30(8):915–922

[24] Duff J, Hussain MM, Klocke N, et al. Does pedicle screw fixation of the subaxial cervical spine provide adequate stabilization in a multilevel vertebral body fracture model? An in vitro biomechanical study. Clin Biomech (Bristol, Avon). 2018; 53:72–78

[25] Hostin RA, Wu C, Perra JH, Polly DW, Akesen B, Wroblewski JM. A biomechanical evaluation of three revision screw strategies for failed lateral mass fixation. Spine. 2008; 33(22):2415–2421

[26] Jones EL, Heller JG, Silcox DH, Hutton WC. Cervical pedicle screws versus lateral mass screws. Anatomic feasibility and biomechanical comparison. Spine. 1997; 22(9):977–982

[27] Neo M, Fujibayashi S, Miyata M, Takemoto M, Nakamura T. Vertebral artery injury during cervical spine surgery: a survey of more than 5600 operations. Spine. 2008; 33(7):779–785

[28] Neo M, Sakamoto T, Fujibayashi S, Nakamura T. The clinical risk of vertebral artery injury from cervical pedicle screws inserted in degenerative vertebrae. Spine. 2005; 30(24):2800–2805

[29] Onishi E, Sekimoto Y, Fukumitsu R, Yamagata S, Matsushita M. Cerebral infarction due to an embolism after cervical pedicle screw fixation. Spine. 2010; 35(2):E63–E66

[30] Zhang J, Xu R, Li Z, Zha W. Cerebral infarction due to malposition of cervical pedicle screw: A case report. Medicine (Baltimore). 2018; 97(7):e9937

[31] Johnston TL, Karaikovic EE, Lautenschlager EP, Marcu D. Cervical pedicle screws vs. lateral mass screws: uniplanar fatigue analysis and residual pullout strengths. Spine J. 2006; 6(6):667–672

[32] Ito Z, Higashino K, Kato S, et al. Pedicle screws can be 4 times stronger than lateral mass screws for insertion in the midcervical spine: a biomechanical study on strength of fixation. J Spinal Disord Tech. 2014; 27(2):80–85

[33] Panjabi MM, Duranceau J, Goel V, Oxland T, Takata K. Cervical human vertebrae. Quantitative three-dimensional anatomy of the middle and lower regions. Spine. 1991; 16(8):861–869

[34] Ebraheim NA, Xu R, Knight T, Yeasting RA. Morphometric evaluation of lower cervical pedicle and its projection. Spine. 1997; 22(1):1–6

[35] Jeanneret B, Gebhard JS, Magerl F. Transpedicular screw fixation of articular mass fracture-separation: results of an anatomical study and operative technique. J Spinal Disord. 1994; 7(3):222–229

[36] Karaikovic EE, Daubs MD, Madsen RW, Gaines RW, Jr. Morphologic characteristics of human cervical pedicles. Spine. 1997; 22(5):493–500

[37] Karaikovic EE, Kunakornsawat S, Daubs MD, Madsen TW, Gaines RW, Jr. Surgical anatomy of the cervical pedicles: landmarks for posterior cervical pedicle entrance localization. J Spinal Disord. 2000; 13(1):63–72

[38] Rao RD, Marawar SV, Stemper BD, Yoganandan N, Shender BS. Computerized tomographic morphometric analysis of subaxial cervical spine pedicles in young asymptomatic volunteers. J Bone Joint Surg Am. 2008; 90(9):1914–1921

[39] Shin EK, Panjabi MM, Chen NC, Wang JL. The anatomic variability of human cervical pedicles: considerations for transpedicular screw fixation in the middle and lower cervical spine. Eur Spine J. 2000; 9(1):61–66

[40] Vara CS, Thompson GH. A cadaveric examination of pediatric cervical pedicle morphology. Spine. 2006; 31(10):1107–1112

[41] Panjabi MM, Shin EK, Chen NC, Wang JL. Internal morphology of human cervical pedicles. Spine. 2000; 25(10):1197–1205

[42] Eskander MS, Drew JM, Aubin ME, et al. Vertebral artery anatomy: a review of two hundred fifty magnetic resonance imaging scans. Spine. 2010; 35(23):2035–2040

[43] Zhao L, Xu R, Hu T, Ma W, Xia H, Wang G. Quantitative evaluation of the location of the vertebral artery in relation to the transverse foramen in the lower cervical spine. Spine. 2008; 33(4):373–378

[44] Uğur HC, Attar A, Uz A, et al. Surgical anatomic evaluation of the cervical pedicle and adjacent neural structures. Neurosurgery. 2000; 47(5):1162–1168, discussion 1168–1169

[45] Tanaka N, Fujimoto Y, An HS, Ikuta Y, Yasuda M. The anatomic relation among the nerve roots, intervertebral foramina, and intervertebral discs of the cervical spine. Spine. 2000; 25(3):286–291

[46] Lee SH, Kim KT, Abumi K, Suk KS, Lee JH, Park KJ. Cervical pedicle screw placement using the "key slot technique": the feasibility and learning curve. J Spinal Disord Tech. 2012; 25(8):415–421

[47] Jo DJ, Seo EM, Kim KT, Kim SM, Lee SH. Cervical pedicle screw insertion using the technique with direct exposure of the pedicle by laminoforaminotomy. J Korean Neurosurg Soc. 2012; 52(5):459–465

[48] Tofuku K, Koga H, Komiya S. Cervical pedicle screw insertion using a gutter entry point at the transitional area between the lateral mass and lamina. Eur Spine J. 2012; 21(2):353–358

[49] Lee SH, Kim KT, Suk KS, et al. Assessment of pedicle perforation by the cervical pedicle screw placement using plain radiographs: a comparison with computed tomography. Spine. 2012; 37(4):280–285

[50] Albert TJ, Klein GR, Joffe D, Vaccaro AR. Use of cervicothoracic junction pedicle screws for reconstruction of complex cervical spine pathology. Spine. 1998; 23(14):1596–1599

[51] Ludwig SC, Kramer DL, Vaccaro AR, Albert TJ. Transpedicle screw fixation of the cervical spine. Clin Orthop Relat Res. 1999(359):77–88

[52] Kotani Y, Abumi K, Ito M, Minami A. Improved accuracy of computer-assisted cervical pedicle screw insertion. J Neurosurg. 2003; 99(3) Suppl:257–263

[53] Richter M, Cakir B, Schmidt R. Cervical pedicle screws: conventional versus computer-assisted placement of cannulated screws. Spine. 2005; 30(20):2280–2287

[54] Takahashi J, Shono Y, Nakamura I, et al. Computer-assisted screw insertion for cervical disorders in rheumatoid arthritis. Eur Spine J. 2007; 16(4):485–494

[55] Hojo Y, Ito M, Suda K, Oda I, Yoshimoto H, Abumi K. A multicenter study on accuracy and complications of freehand placement of cervical pedicle screws under lateral fluoroscopy in different pathological conditions: CT-based evaluation of more than 1,000 screws. Eur Spine J. 2014; 23(10):2166–2174

[56] Ishikawa Y, Kanemura T, Yoshida G, Ito Z, Muramoto A, Ohno S. Clinical accuracy of three-dimensional fluoroscopy-based computer-assisted cervical pedicle screw placement: a retrospective comparative study of conventional versus computer-assisted cervical pedicle screw placement. J Neurosurg Spine. 2010; 13(5):606–611

[57] Ito Y, Sugimoto Y, Tomioka M, Hasegawa Y, Nakago K, Yagata Y. Clinical accuracy of 3D fluoroscopy-assisted cervical pedicle screw insertion. J Neurosurg Spine. 2008; 9(5):450–453

[58] Reinhold M, Bach C, Audigé L, et al. Comparison of two novel fluoroscopy-based stereotactic methods for cervical pedicle screw placement and review of the literature. Eur Spine J. 2008; 17(4):564–575

[59] Richter M, Amiot LP, Neller S, Kluger P, Puhl W. Computer-assisted surgery in posterior instrumentation of the cervical spine: an in-vitro feasibility study. Eur Spine J. 2000; 9 Suppl 1:S65–S70

[60] Uehara M, Takahashi J, Ikegami S, et al. Screw perforation features in 129 consecutive patients performed computer-guided cervical pedicle screw insertion. Eur Spine J. 2014; 23(10):2189–2195

[61] Ishikawa Y, Kanemura T, Yoshida G, et al. Intraoperative, full-rotation, three-dimensional image (O-arm)-based navigation system for cervical pedicle screw insertion. J Neurosurg Spine. 2011; 15(5):472–478

[62] Hlubek RJ, Bohl MA, Cole TS, et al. Safety and accuracy of freehand versus navigated C2 pars or pedicle screw placement. Spine J. 2018; 18(8):1374–1381

[63] Miyamoto H, Uno K. Cervical pedicle screw insertion using a computed tomography cutout technique. J Neurosurg Spine. 2009; 11(6):681–687

[64] Ryken TC, Owen BD, Christensen GE, Reinhardt JM. Image-based drill templates for cervical pedicle screw placement. J Neurosurg Spine. 2009; 10(1):21–26

[65] Kaneyama S, Sugawara T, Sumi M. Safe and accurate midcervical pedicle screw insertion procedure with the patient-specific screw guide template system. Spine. 2015; 40(6):E341–E348

[66] Bundoc RC, Delgado GG, Grozman SAM. A novel patient-specific drill guide template for pedicle screw insertion into the subaxial cervical spine utilizing stereolithographic modelling: an in vitro study. Asian Spine J. 2017; 11(1):4–14

[67] Kast E, Mohr K, Richter HP, Börm W. Complications of transpedicular screw fixation in the cervical spine. Eur Spine J. 2006; 15(3):327–334

[68] Rajasekaran S, Kanna PR, Shetty AP. Safety of cervical pedicle screw insertion in children: a clinicoradiological evaluation of computer-assisted insertion of 51 cervical pedicle screws including 28 subaxial pedicle screws in 16 children. Spine. 2012; 37(4):E216–E223

[69] Nakashima H, Yukawa Y, Imagama S, et al. Complications of cervical pedicle screw fixation for nontraumatic lesions: a multicenter study of 84 patients. J Neurosurg Spine. 2012; 16(3):238–247

[70] Watanabe K, Hirano T, Katsumi K, et al. Surgical outcomes of posterior spinal fusion alone using cervical pedicle screw constructs for cervical disorders associated with athetoid cerebral palsy. Spine. 2017; 42(24):1835–1843

[71] Abumi K, Shono Y, Ito M, Taneichi H, Kotani Y, Kaneda K. Complications of pedicle screw fixation in reconstructive surgery of the cervical spine. Spine. 2000; 25(8):962–969

[72] Yoshimoto H, Sato S, Hyakumachi T, Yanagibashi Y, Masuda T. Spinal reconstruction using a cervical pedicle screw system. Clin Orthop Relat Res. 2005 (431):111–119

[73] Yukawa Y, Kato F, Ito K, et al. Placement and complications of cervical pedicle screws in 144 cervical trauma patients using pedicle axis view techniques by fluoroscope. Eur Spine J. 2009; 18(9):1293–1299

[74] Tauchi R, Imagama S, Sakai Y, et al. The correlation between cervical range of motion and misplacement of cervical pedicle screws during cervical posterior spinal fixation surgery using a CT-based navigation system. Eur Spine J. 2013; 22(7):1504–1508

[75] Yoshimoto H, Sato S, Hyakumachi T, Yanagibashi Y, Kanno T, Masuda T. Clinical accuracy of cervical pedicle screw insertion using lateral fluoroscopy: a radiographic analysis of the learning curve. Eur Spine J. 2009; 18(9):1326–1334

[76] Yoshihara H, Passias PG, Errico TJ. Screw-related complications in the subaxial cervical spine with the use of lateral mass versus cervical pedicle screws: a systematic review. J Neurosurg Spine. 2013; 19(5):614–623

14 Upper Thoracic Osteotomy for Cervical Deformity

Sang Hun Lee, Khaled M. Kebaish, and Paul D. Sponseller

Abstract

Upper thoracic osteotomy for cervical deformity correction is less common than cervical or thoracolumbar osteotomy. Most cervical deformities are not rigid and have an apex in the mid or lower cervical spine segment, allowing correction within the cervical spine. However, upper thoracic osteotomy is a treatment option for rigid or fixed cervicothoracic kyphosis, upper thoracic kyphosis with high T1 slope and/or high thoracic inlet angle, and cervical deformity combined with upper thoracic proximal junctional kyphosis after thoracolumbar fusion. When planning upper thoracic osteotomy, evaluating the rigidity of the deformity is critical. Three-column osteotomy, including pedicle subtraction osteotomy or vertebral column resection, is required for most fixed or rigid deformities that cannot be corrected by flexion–extension position, supine position, or skeletal traction. Posterior column osteotomies, including multilevel Smith-Petersen osteotomies, are used to correct pediatric proximal junctional kyphosis and deformities that are not fixed or completely ankylosed. A fused spine (fused surgically or spontaneously by ankylosing spondylitis or diffuse idiopathic skeletal hyperostosis) does not need traction and requires three-column osteotomy. In this chapter, we describe various techniques for treating cervical deformity by using upper thoracic osteotomy.

Keywords: cervical deformity, pedicle subtraction osteotomy, Smith-Petersen osteotomy, spinal osteotomy, upper thoracic osteotomy, vertebral column resection

14.1 Introduction and Literature Review

Upper thoracic osteotomy, which is less common than cervical and thoracolumbar osteotomy, can be performed for correction of cervicothoracic junction (CTJ) kyphosis and proximal junctional kyphosis (PJK) after thoracolumbar fusion. Osteotomy at the upper thoracic spine may provide more effective correction of sagittal balance than cervical osteotomy in selected cases and may be performed from T1 to T5, depending on the deformity.[1,2,3,4]

The definition of the CTJ varies. It is typically considered the region from C7 to T1 but can be extended to include C6–T4.[5,6,7,8] Compared with kyphotic deformity in the cervical spine, CTJ kyphosis causes greater sagittal imbalance of the cervical spine and more severe clinical problems, including chronic neck pain, inability to achieve a horizontal gaze, and difficulty maintaining hygiene and swallowing. Conventional approaches to CTJ kyphosis correction are lengthening of the anterior column and/or shortening of the posterior column. Although the anterior approach to the cervical spine is easier and safer (to avoid spinal cord and nerve root injuries), access is challenging because of the complex vascular and bony anatomy of the CTJ. In addition, the anterior approach may be impossible in patients with severe kyphotic deformity in the CTJ.

Another indication for upper thoracic osteotomy is PJK. Patients with previous thoracolumbar fusion extending to the upper thoracic spine may have PJK and an associated variable degree of cervical spine deformity caused by global sagittal imbalance, spinal compensation mechanisms, underlying cervical spine conditions, and flexibility of the cervical spine. In these cases, upper thoracic osteotomy can correct PJK and the secondary cervical deformity.

There are few studies of upper thoracic osteotomy. In addition, there is no consensus on the optimal osteotomy level (lower cervical or upper thoracic spine) and method (three-column osteotomy, including pedicle subtraction osteotomy [PSO]; vertebral column resection [VCR]; or posterior column osteotomy [multilevel Smith-Petersen osteotomy, SPO]).

The first case series on upper thoracic osteotomy was reported by Samudrala et al in 2010.[3] They reported the outcomes of osteotomy for surgical correction of CTJ kyphosis. Their cases consisted of PSO at T1 in five patients, at C7 in one patient, at T2–T3 in one patient, and anterior-posterior surgery in one patient. They reported a mean correction of 36 degrees, with excellent clinical outcomes.

McClendon et al[2] reported a mean correction of 31 degrees for proximal junctional angles after multilevel SPO for PJK of the upper thoracic spine. Their series consisted of multilevel SPO in six cases and VCR in one case.

In a 2015 multicenter study, Theologis et al[4] compared lower cervical osteotomy with upper thoracic osteotomy (T1-T5) for CTJ deformity in 48 patients. They performed PSO or VCR in 24 patients each, C7 osteotomy in 15 patients, and upper thoracic osteotomy in 33 patients (at T1 in 4 patients, T2 in 7, T3 in 9, T4 in 9, and T5 in 4). They reported significant improvements in cervical sagittal vertical axis (SVA), cervical lordosis (CL), Neck Disability Index score, and Scoliosis Research Society domains in both groups, with no significant differences between groups. Reoperation rates were also similar between groups. Indications were not specified. The mean correction of the C2-T1 angle was 44 degrees in the C7 PSO group and 26 degrees in the upper thoracic osteotomy group. Compared with the C7 PSO group, the upper thoracic group had significantly higher changes in T1 slope (20 vs. 3.6 degrees) and SVA correction (2.5 vs. -1.3 cm).

14.2 Indications for Upper Thoracic Osteotomy for Cervical Deformity

Traditionally, the ideal level of osteotomy was considered to be the apex of the deformity. However, spinal osteotomy outside the deformity may be considered for the following reasons: (1) to achieve safer correction at a level where the spinal canal is wider (e.g., C7 or T1 PSO instead of C5 or C6 PSO) or at the level of cauda equina rather than a level of the spinal cord (e.g., L2 or L3 PSO instead of T11, T12, or higher PSO); (2) to achieve more correction angle with the same amount of bone resection (e.g., larger correction angle in SVA at L3 or L4 vs. L1 or L2); or (3) to achieve correction when the deformity involves a transitional area such as the cervicothoracic, thoracolumbar, or lumbosacral segments.

Osteotomy in the upper thoracic spine (between T1 and T5) is less commonly indicated than osteotomy in the cervical spine because the apex of cervical deformity is typically at the mid or lower cervical spine segments, and correction is possible within the cervical spine given most cervical deformity is not fixed. However, osteotomy in the upper thoracic spine is an option in the following cases: (1) rigid or fixed cervical deformities with upper thoracic kyphosis (TK), high T1 slope, and/or high thoracic inlet angle (TIA); and (2) cervical deformity combined with upper thoracic PJK in patients with thoracolumbar fusion.

In this chapter, we will discuss evaluation of upper thoracic spinal alignment, surgical planning for upper thoracic osteotomy, and surgical techniques.

14.3 Evaluation of Upper Thoracic Spine Alignment

14.3.1 Global Spinal Alignment and Fusion Status of the Cervical Spine

All patients should undergo detailed preoperative radiographic imaging studies, including standing 36-inch anteroposterior and lateral radiographs, as well as routine cervical, thoracic, and lumbar spine radiographs. An additional lateral radiograph including the chin–brow line is needed for patients with severe sagittal imbalance. Computed tomography (CT) and magnetic resonance imaging (MRI) are necessary to evaluate ossification, fusion, and possible spinal canal stenosis with foraminal stenosis. Like all cervical spine deformities, global spinal alignment, including C7 SVA and chin–brow vertical angle (CBVA) should be evaluated. If the cervical deformity is not fixed, C7 SVA and CBVA are less important because compensatory changes will occur in the cervical spine after corrective osteotomy. However, when the patient's cervical spine has been fused surgically or by ankylosing spondylitis or diffuse idiopathic skeletal hyperostosis, measuring the preoperative CBVA is critical. Overcorrection of the cervical deformity can result in an upward gaze, which is less favorable than undercorrection for activities of daily living such as eating, reading, and walking down stairs.[9]

14.3.2 Thoracic Kyphosis, T1 Slope, and Cervicothoracic Angle

TK, typically measured from the T4 upper endplate to the T12 lower endplate, is one of the baseline angles of thoracic spine alignment. The normal range for TK is 20 to 70 degrees, depending on the patient's age and lumbopelvic alignment, including lumbar lordosis (LL), pelvic incidence (PI), and sacral slope.[10,11] T1 slope is the angle created by the upper endplate of T1 and the horizontal plane; it is one of the most important parameters, providing the mechanical base of the cervical spine. Patients with a high T1 slope require more CL to obtain a horizontal gaze, and vice versa. Normal values range from 22 to 31 degrees.[12,13]

Cervicothoracic angle (CTA) includes both lordotic segments of the lower cervical spine and kyphotic segments of the upper thoracic spine. Normal values of CTA, which is measured from the C6 upper endplate to the T4 lower endplate, have been reported as ranging from 3.9 to 7.2 degrees, with a mean of 4.9 degrees of kyphosis in the middle-aged population; CTA can increase to 23 degrees in those older than 75 years.[7,8]

If a patient has cervical kyphosis with normal T1 slope, the deformity is located within the cervical spine. When the cervical deformity is combined with a high T1 slope, high TK, and a kyphotic CTA, an upper thoracic osteotomy is a good option for correction of the deformities in the cervical and thoracic spine (▶ Fig. 14.1a,b). If the deformity shows a high T1 slope, high TK, and a normal CTA, it means the apex of the deformity is in the midthoracic spine. Midthoracic osteotomy below T5 may be considered (▶ Fig. 14.1). However, if the deformity shows high T1 slope but normal TK, it means the deformity is located in the thoracolumbar or lumbar spine, which is an indication for thoracolumbar osteotomy (see Chapter 15).

14.3.3 T1 Slope minus Cervical Lordosis, C2–C7 SVA, Thoracic Inlet Angle, and Neck Tilting

Based on the concept of T1 slope, T1 slope minus CL (or C2–C7 angle) is another parameter that reflects the balance between CL and T1 slope to provide information on cervical spine sagittal balance.[12,13,14] It is similar to the concept of PI minus LL in lumbopelvic balance. In the same way that high PI requires a more lordotic lumbar spine to achieve sagittal balance, high T1 slope requires more CL to achieve a horizontal gaze and balanced SVA. Several studies report the ideal value of T1 slope minus CL as 15 degrees and define cervical spine deformity as T1 slope minus CL greater than 20 degrees.[12,14] C2–C7 SVA influences health-related quality-of-life and patient-reported outcomes after surgical treatment. C2–C7 SVA less than 4 cm is associated with disability according to the Neck Disability Index (▶ Fig. 14.2).[12,14,15]

Although many studies have analyzed the importance of T1 slope to cervical spine alignment, there are several alignment parameters unexplained by T1 slope alone. First, T1 slope is the angle between the upper end of T1 and the horizontal plane, but is not a constant parameter because it is influenced by global posture. When the patient is sitting, leaning, supine, or prone, TK and T1 slope cannot be used as a predictive parameter for CL. In other words, T1 slope, like sacral slope, is a changing parameter rather than a constant parameter.

Anatomically and biomechanically, the cervical spine and cranium are placed on the TIA, a bony circle without range of motion consisting of the T1 vertebral body, the first ribs on both sides, and the upper part of the sternum. The sagittal balance of the cranium and cervical spine, integral to maintaining an upright posture and horizontal gaze, is influenced by the shape and orientation of the TIA in a similar manner to PI in the pelvis. Moreover, important musculature of the neck, including sternocleidomastoid, scalenes, and strap muscles, inserts on the thoracic inlet and several other important cervical paraspinal muscles. TIA is a constant parameter, unaltered by changes in TK. Normal TIA is 70 to 80 degrees.[8,13,16]

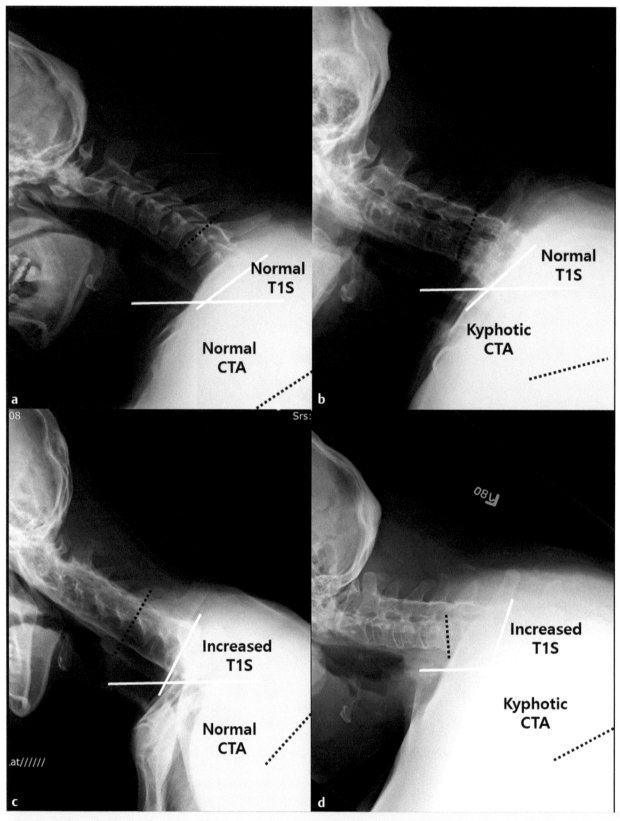

Fig. 14.1 Radiographs showing four types of fixed cervical kyphosis with similar chin–brow vertical angle and C2–C7 sagittal vertical axis, with different T1 slope (T1S) and cervicothoracic angle (CTA). **(a)** Patient shows normal T1S and CTA. **(b)** Patient shows normal T1S and kyphotic CTA. **(c)** Patient shows increased T1S and normal CTA. **(d)** Patient shows increased T1S and kyphotic CTA. Surgical treatment strategies would differ in the four patients on the basis of T1S and CTA, even though they have similar chin–brow vertical angles and C2–C7 sagittal vertical axis.

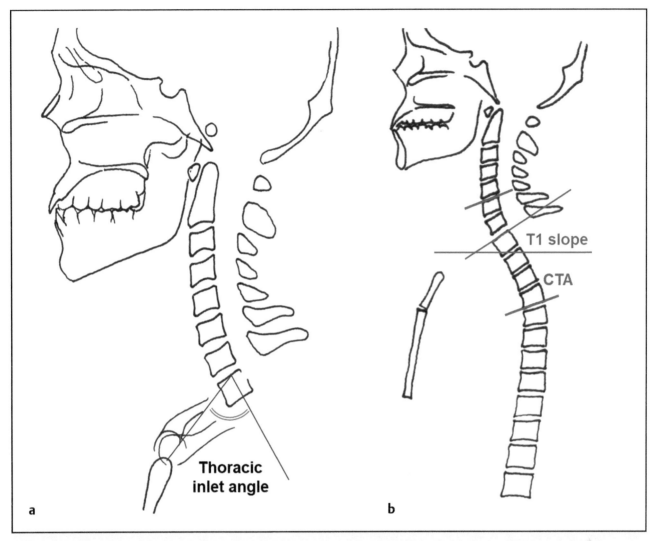

Fig. 14.2 Schematic drawing of radiographic measurements of **(a)** thoracic inlet angle and **(b)** T1 slope and cervicothoracic angle (CTA).

Upper thoracic osteotomy is an appropriate surgical option for patients with a high TIA and kyphotic CTA. Lower cervical osteotomy is a better option for patients with a normal TIA and kyphotic CTA (▸ Fig. 14.3).

14.4 Surgical Planning for Upper Thoracic Osteotomy

14.4.1 The Apex of Deformity

Cervical deformities with a kyphotic CTA that have an apex between the lower cervical spine and the upper thoracic spine (C6–T4) are candidates for upper thoracic osteotomy. If the deformity has a high TIA and the apex is located at the upper thoracic spine (T1–T4), osteotomy around the apex is a good

strategy. When the apex is located at the lower cervical spine or normal T1 slope and TIA, lower cervical osteotomy is a better option (▸ Fig. 14.4).

14.4.2 Rigidity of the Deformity

Three-column osteotomy, which may include PSO or VCR, is required for most fixed or rigid deformities that are not corrected by position changes on flexion–extension views or supine transtable lateral radiographs. Skeletal traction using Gardner-Wells tongs is a good option for evaluating the flexibility of the deformity before making a treatment decision. Traction starts with a small amount of weight, approximately 5 pounds, and gradually increases up to 15 to 20 pounds for 2 to 3 days as tolerated. Successful correction is possible with PSO, including multilevel SPO for deformities that are reducible with

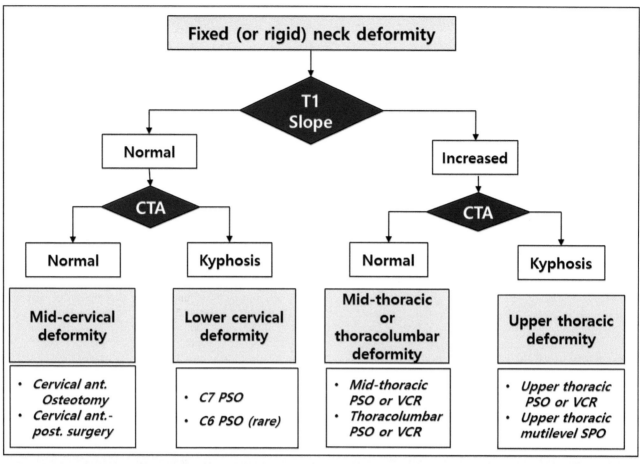

Fig. 14.3 A flowchart for surgical strategy to treat rigid neck deformity using T1 slope and cervicothoracic angle (CTA), which is measured from the C6 upper endplate to the T4 lower endplate. Ant., anterior; post., posterior; PSO, pedicle subtraction osteotomy; SPO, Smith-Petersen osteotomy; VCR, vertebral column resection.

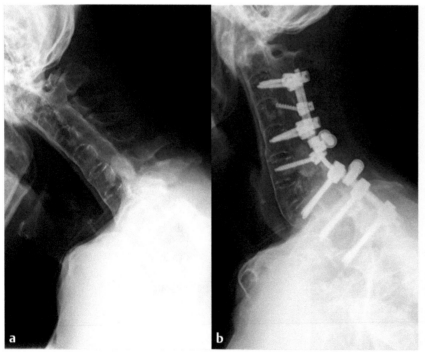

Fig. 14.4 (a) Preoperative and **(b)** postoperative cervical spine lateral radiographs of a 57-year-old man with ankylosing spondylitis who underwent C7 pedicle subtraction osteotomy.

skeletal traction, deformities without complete ankylosis, and most pediatric PJK cases. A spine that has been fused surgically or spontaneously does not need traction, and correction is impossible without three-column osteotomy.

14.4.3 Estimation of the Required Correction Angle

Reconstruction to normalize CL, C2–C7 SVA, and T1 slope is the goal; however, normative values vary. Correction of CTA to a normal value of 5 to 10 degrees is another indicator of a successful correction. Preoperative estimation of the posterior column resection length and vertebral body wedge resection angle is required. The CBVA is one of the most important angles to consider in patients with a spine fused from the occiput to the lower cervical spine. Undercorrection of up to 10 to 15 degrees is desirable to improve functioning for activities of daily living. When the patient has mobile segments from the occiput to C2, CBVA is less important because the upper cervical segments can compensate for the changes of subaxial cervical spine alignment caused by fusion.

Although mean correction angles are reportedly 30 to 40 degrees in PSO and approximately 10 degrees per segment in SPO,[1,4,17,18,19] they vary according to segmental ossification, flexibility, and extent of bone resection. Angle of correction may be adjusted according to the intraoperative radiographs by compression between the segments or additional resection of the posterior column or vertebral bodies.

14.4.4 Extent of Fusion

Upper thoracic osteotomy typically requires fixation up to the lower cervical spine, at least three vertebrae above and below the osteotomy. For patients with osteoporosis, more segmental fixation is mandatory to avoid fixation failure; however, the upper cervical spine (occiput to C2) should be preserved as much as possible to allow neck motion and compensate for the changes in subaxial cervical spine alignment. In patients with a fused spine, extension of the previous fusion is sufficient.

14.4.5 Fixation Methods

Lateral mass, pedicle, or translaminar screws are used for lower cervical spine fixation. Lateral mass screws are the easiest and the most common fixation method. Pedicle screw fixation is an option even at the subaxial cervical spine, but is less commonly performed because of technical difficulty (small pedicle diameter and larger medial angle, approximately 45 degrees) and risk of vertebral artery injury.[17,18] In many cases, C7 pedicle screw fixation is possible with minimal risk of vertebral artery injury because approximately 95% of vertebral arteries enter the transverse foramen at the level of C6. Translaminar screw fixation can be applied to C2 with small pedicles and high-riding vertebral arteries. In some patients with small pedicles, translaminar screws at C7 and the upper thoracic spine are a useful fixation method or salvage technique.

14.5 Surgical Techniques

14.5.1 Pedicle Subtraction Osteotomy at T1

General anesthesia is standard for patients undergoing CTJ deformity surgery. However, bronchoscopy-guided intubation with the patient in a conscious state may be required in those with severe kyphosis. Spinal cord monitoring with somatosensory evoked potentials, transcranial motor-evoked potentials, and free-running electromyography is used routinely. Mayfield skull clamps (Integra LifeSciences, Plainsboro, NJ) or Gardner-Wells tongs can be used for head fixation. Patient positioning (prone on the operating table) is the same as that used for cervical osteotomy. Many surgeons prefer the arms-on-side position. The sterile skin drape should cover the occiput to low thoracic spine for possible extension of fusion. After positioning, an intraoperative lateral radiograph is necessary to confirm cervicothoracic spine alignment. Adjustment of the head and neck position may be required if the radiograph shows inappropriate alignment (▶ Fig. 14.5a,b).

A midline skin incision is made and followed by subperiosteal dissection of the paraspinal muscles to expose the spinous processes, laminae, facet joints, transverse processes, and part of the first ribs. Exposure may be extended three to five levels above and below the intended osteotomy level. Before the osteotomy is performed, pedicle screws and/or lateral mass screws are placed at the appropriate adjacent levels, excluding the level of PSO. We prefer to place pedicle screws at C2, C7, and thoracic levels and to use lateral mass screws in the other subaxial cervical vertebrae. Subaxial cervical pedicle screw fixation, from C3 to C6, may be considered for patients with severe osteoporosis or for those in whom as many motion segments as possible must be preserved with more rigid fixation (▶ Fig. 14.5). For subaxial pedicle screw fixation, location of the bilateral vertebral arteries and presence of abnormal vertebral arteries should be evaluated. In addition, measurement of pedicle dimensions and angles with preoperative CT images is necessary.

The first step is to perform laminectomies, starting with complete T1 laminectomy and extending to the lower 50% of the C7 and upper 50% of T2 laminae. The lateral margins of the laminectomy are on the laminar-facet junction. Wide laminectomies toward the cephalad-caudal direction are necessary to avoid spinal cord impingement when more correction angle is required. Corresponding ligamentum flava should be removed accordingly. Complete bilateral facetectomies are performed above and below the pedicle to expose the cranial and caudal intervertebral foramina and nerve roots.

The next step is resection of the bilateral transverse process at the base using osteotomes or a bone scalpel at the junction of the transverse process and facet. After removal of the transverse process, the first rib will be exposed, which should be removed approximately 2 to 3 cm distal to the rib head–vertebral body junction, before pedicle resection. This is a unique part of T1 PSO because the C8 and T1 nerve roots are overwrapping the first rib to form the inferior trunk of the brachial

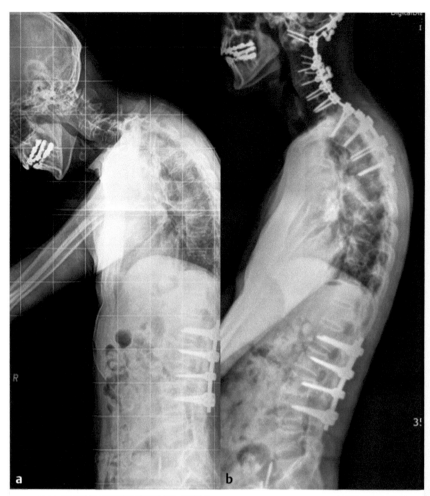

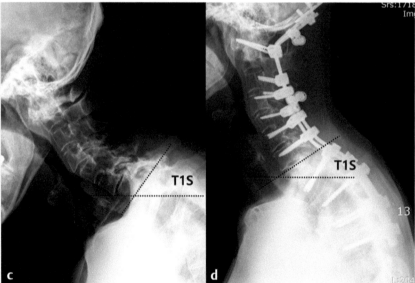

Fig. 14.5 (a) Preoperative and (b) postoperative standing whole-spine radiographs of a 47-year-old patient with ankylosing spondylitis and rheumatoid cervical spine conditions. After T1 pedicle subtraction osteotomy, high T1 slope (T1S) and thoracic inlet angle are corrected, and C7 sagittal vertical axis and chin–brow vertical angle are improved. (c) The patient had rheumatoid cervical spine lesions, including fixed C1–C2 subluxation, basilar invagination, subaxial subluxation at C6–C7 and C7–T1, high T1S, high thoracic inlet angle, and increased C2–C7 sagittal vertical axis. (d) The patient underwent C1 ring resection, C1–C2 intraarticular fusion with vertical distraction, and T1 pedicle subtraction osteotomy. T1S improved from 50 to 35 degrees.

plexus immediately distal to the first rib (▶ Fig. 14.6). If the first rib is not removed sufficiently, the C8 and T1 nerve root could be impinged by the remnant of the first rib after closing the osteotomy.

Removal of the pedicles, vertebral body decancellation, and reduction of the PSO are almost identical to those performed for PSO at other thoracic levels after the first rib resection. A high-speed burr is used to thin the pedicle wall to facilitate pedicle wall resection using osteotomes or rongeurs. Variable-sized straight and reversed-angle curettes are used to remove the cancellous bone inside the vertebral body. The posterior wall can be crushed using impactors or reversed-angle curettes. The lateral wall of the vertebral body should be removed in a tapered wedge (a blunt osteotome is helpful for gentle closure

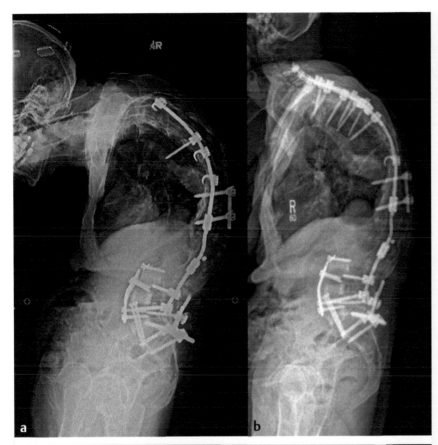

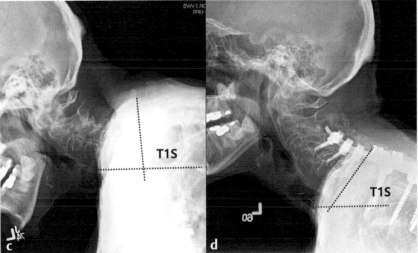

Fig. 14.6 **(a)** Radiographs of a 69-year-old woman with a history of multiple thoracolumbar spine deformity surgeries to correct severe upper thoracic and neck deformity. **(b)** After T2 pedicle subtraction osteotomy, T1 slope (T1S) improved from 95 to 55 degrees. Horizontal gaze was possible after surgical correction of her upper thoracic deformity.

of the osteotomy). The anterior wall may be left intact to create a greenstick fracture. In a vertebra with a thick, strong anterior wall, the surgeon may need to make a fracture using a blunt osteotome or Cobb elevator. To limit cancellous bleeding, homeostatic agents such as thrombin with a collagen sponge are useful (▶ Fig. 14.7).

During resection of the pedicle and vertebral body, temporary rod fixation is required to provide stability from the other side. This is critical to prevent inadvertent translation or subluxation of the spinal column before a controlled gradual reduction of the deformity. Using irrigation-coupled bipolar cautery is safer than regular bipolar or Bovie electrocautery because a sudden jerky motion caused by electrical irritation may result

in unintended fracture and subluxation at the final stage of the osteotomy.

Although several reduction methods have been reported, including manual reduction, malleable rods, and mechanical reduction frame and hinged rod techniques, manual reduction is the most commonly used method for gradual, gentle reduction.[18,20,21,22] Our preferred technique is a freehand sterile reduction technique.[23] After completing the osteotomy on both sides, set screws at the caudal part of the osteotomy are fixed on a prebent rod at the desired angle for the osteotomy. The operator holds the tong while an assistant removes the temporary rod on the other side. Next, the operator gradually reduces the sagittal and/or coronal deformity with his or her right hand

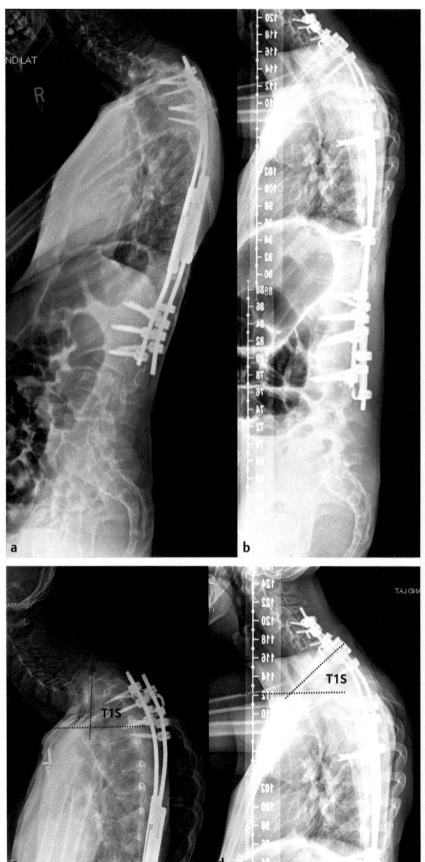

Fig. 14.7 **(a)** Radiographs of a 15-year-old boy who had undergone scoliosis surgery 7 years earlier. He shows cervical spine deformity with proximal junctional kyphosis. **(b)** After multilevel Smith-Petersen osteotomy (at T1–T2, T2–T3, and T5–T6), T1 slope improved from 90 to 40 degrees. Cervical deformity and horizontal gaze corrections were possible after surgical correction of his upper thoracic spine.

to place the prebent lordotic rod within the screw heads, while the assistant fixes the set screws on the cranial part of the osteotomy. Additional reduction or correction of asymmetric reduction is obtained, as needed, using gentle compression across the osteotomy over the rods with screw loosening and retightening.

The laminectomy defect after closing the osteotomy should be reconstructed by allograft or local bone to prevent nonunion of the osteotomy and/or rod fracture. Bisected C7 or T1 spinous processes obtained during the laminectomy are a good source of graft for laminectomy defect reconstruction.

14.5.2 Three-Column Osteotomy below T2–T4: PSO or VCR

PSO and VCR are options for cervical deformity combined with high upper TK or severe PJK after thoracolumbar spinal deformity surgery (▶ Fig. 14.6a,b). The mean correction angle with PSO is 35 to 40 degrees.[18,19,23] VCR is indicated for cases with sharp angular kyphosis, combined sagittal and coronal deformity, and/or those requiring more correction angle than can be achieved with PSO. Some authors believe VCR is safer than PSO at this level because anterior column support can avoid or minimize posterior column shortening and protect the spinal cord. For PSO, rib resections such as in T1 PSO are not always required. Instead, bilateral disarticulations of costovertebral joints are sufficient in many cases for PSO at T2–T4.

For VCR, laminectomies that include the upper and lower 50% of laminae, and bilateral superior and inferior facetectomies are performed, as well as removal of bilateral transverse processes and corresponding ribs. A sufficient amount of rib resection provides room for safe graft or cage insertion. Thoracic nerve root(s) below T2 can be severed proximal to the dorsal root ganglion without causing neurological deficit. Nonabsorbable suture ties are most commonly used to cut thoracic nerve roots. This provides space and decreases tension on the dura during graft insertion.

Bilateral discectomy at the intervertebral disc spaces cephalad and caudal to the osteotomy is the next step to define the resection margin of VCR. The discectomy starts from the posterolateral corner of the disc and extends toward the midline and anterior annulus as much as possible. In cases of rigid deformity, the anterior longitudinal ligament should be released from the posterior side. Endplate preparation requires complete removal of the cartilaginous endplate using ring curettes and/or curved curettes. Preservation of the bony endplate cephalad and caudad is important to prevent graft/cage subsidence.

Resections of pedicles, cancellous bone, and the posterior and lateral wall of the vertebral body are performed in a similar manner to PSO. After finishing one side, temporary rod fixation is required to avoid translation of the unstable spinal column, as in PSO. Most commonly, a titanium mesh cage is filled with local bone and/or allograft. An expandable cage or strut allograft is another option for the interbody graft.

After placement of the cage, a contoured rod with the desired alignment is applied from the cage insertion side. Slight loosening of the temporary rod is helpful for the reduction. After the permanent contoured rod is secured, the temporary rod is replaced with another permanent rod with the same alignment. As in PSO, additional reduction or correction of asymmetric reduction can be obtained, as needed, using gentle compression across the osteotomy over the rods with screw loosening and retightening. Careful attention to neuromonitoring signals is critical throughout the procedure.

14.5.3 Posterior Column Osteotomy (Smith-Petersen Osteotomy) of the Upper Thoracic Spine

SPO is indicated for less severe, nonrigid deformities. Children with PJK after undergoing thoracolumbar deformity correction may be good candidates for this type of osteotomy (▶ Fig. 14.7a, b). However, fixed deformities and those with completely ankylosed segments are not indicated.

After all pedicle screws and lateral mass screws are placed, the osteotomy starts with a V-shaped laminectomy and bilateral symmetric total facet joint resections. The laminectomies consist of the inferior lamina of the cranial vertebra and superior lamina of the caudal vertebra using osteotomes, Kerrison rongeur, or bone scalpels. Corresponding ligamentum flavum and facet joint capsules should be removed completely before closing to avoid spinal cord and nerve root impingement. If the deformity is too rigid or additional correction is needed, transverse process and rib disarticulations are helpful to achieve more correction.

Typically, SPO involves three to four segments, depending on the angle and rigidity of the deformity. Reduction of the osteotomy consists of two steps. The first step is gentle and gradual assembly of a prebent rod with a desired correction angle using reduction clamps connecting to the pedicle screws. Second, intersegmental compression between the pedicle screws over the rods can close the gaps between the laminae. Compression of the heads of the pedicle screws without rod assembly may cause uncontrolled reduction, which may lead to pedicle fracture, anterior column fracture, or segmental translation. Although the reported incidence of neurological complication after SPO is lower than that after three-column osteotomy,[24,25] careful monitoring of possible dural impingement between the laminae and any changes in neuromonitoring signals is critical during the reduction procedure.

14.6 Conclusion

Upper thoracic osteotomy can be a more effective treatment than cervical osteotomies for the surgical correction of cervicothoracic kyphosis in some patients, including those with cervicothoracic or upper TK with high T1 slope and/or high TIA and those with cervical deformity combined with upper thoracic PJK after thoracolumbar fusion. Although upper thoracic osteotomy is a technically demanding procedure, it provides more efficient restoration of C2–C7 SVA and horizontal gaze compared with cervical osteotomy in such patients. Various surgical techniques, including multilevel SPO, PSO, and VCR, can be applied according to deformity characteristics.

References

[1] Deviren V, Scheer JK, Ames CP. Technique of cervicothoracic junction pedicle subtraction osteotomy for cervical sagittal imbalance: report of 11 cases. J Neurosurg Spine. 2011; 15(2):174–181

[2] McClendon J, Jr, O'Shaughnessy BA, Sugrue PA, et al. Techniques for operative correction of proximal junctional kyphosis of the upper thoracic spine. Spine. 2012; 37(4):292–303

[3] Samudrala S, Vaynman S, Thiayananthan T, et al. Cervicothoracic junction kyphosis: surgical reconstruction with pedicle subtraction osteotomy and Smith-Petersen osteotomy. Presented at the 2009 Joint Spine Section Meeting. Clinical article. J Neurosurg Spine. 2010; 13(6):695–706

[4] Theologis AA, Tabaraee E, Funao H, et al. Three-column osteotomies of the lower cervical and upper thoracic spine: comparison of early outcomes, radiographic parameters, and peri-operative complications in 48 patients. Eur Spine J. 2015; 24 Suppl 1:S23–S30

[5] Bailey AS, Stanescu S, Yeasting RA, Ebraheim NA, Jackson WT. Anatomic relationships of the cervicothoracic junction. Spine. 1995; 20(13):1431–1439

[6] Boockvar JA, Philips MF, Telfeian AE, O'Rourke DM, Marcotte PJ. Results and risk factors for anterior cervicothoracic junction surgery. J Neurosurg. 2001; 94(1) Suppl:12–17

[7] Boyle JJ, Milne N, Singer KP. Influence of age on cervicothoracic spinal curvature: an ex vivo radiographic survey. Clin Biomech (Bristol, Avon). 2002; 17(5):361–367

[8] Iyer S, Lenke LG, Nemani VM, et al. Variations in occipitocervical and cervicothoracic alignment parameters based on age: a prospective study of asymptomatic volunteers using full-body radiographs. Spine. 2016; 41(23):1837–1844

[9] Suk KS, Kim KT, Lee SH, Kim JM. Significance of chin-brow vertical angle in correction of kyphotic deformity of ankylosing spondylitis patients. Spine. 2003; 28(17):2001–2005

[10] Bernhardt M, Bridwell KH. Segmental analysis of the sagittal plane alignment of the normal thoracic and lumbar spines and thoracolumbar junction. Spine. 1989; 14(7):717–721

[11] Jackson RP, McManus AC. Radiographic analysis of sagittal plane alignment and balance in standing volunteers and patients with low back pain matched for age, sex, and size. A prospective controlled clinical study. Spine. 1994; 19(14):1611–1618

[12] Ames CP, Smith JS, Eastlack R, et al. International Spine Study Group. Reliability assessment of a novel cervical spine deformity classification system. J Neurosurg Spine. 2015; 23(6):673–683

[13] Lee SH, Kim KT, Seo EM, Suk KS, Kwack YH, Son ES. The influence of thoracic inlet alignment on the craniocervical sagittal balance in asymptomatic adults. J Spinal Disord Tech. 2012; 25(2):E41–E47

[14] Hyun SJ, Kim KJ, Jahng TA, Kim HJ. Clinical impact of T1 slope minus cervical lordosis following multilevel posterior cervical fusion surgery: A minimum 2-year follow-up data. Spine. 2017; 42(24):1859–1864

[15] Tang JA, Scheer JK, Smith JS, et al. ISSG. The impact of standing regional cervical sagittal alignment on outcomes in posterior cervical fusion surgery. Neurosurgery. 2012; 71(3):662–669, discussion 669

[16] Lee SH, Son ES, Seo EM, Suk KS, Kim KT. Factors determining cervical spine sagittal balance in asymptomatic adults: correlation with spinopelvic balance and thoracic inlet alignment. Spine J. 2015; 15(4):705–712

[17] Simmons ED, DiStefano RJ, Zheng Y, Simmons EH. Thirty-six years experience of cervical extension osteotomy in ankylosing spondylitis: techniques and outcomes. Spine. 2006; 31(26):3006–3012

[18] Tokala DP, Lam KS, Freeman BJ, Webb JK. C7 decancellisation closing wedge osteotomy for the correction of fixed cervico-thoracic kyphosis. Eur Spine J. 2007; 16(9):1471–1478

[19] Wang MY, Berven SH. Lumbar pedicle subtraction osteotomy. Neurosurgery. 2007; 60(2) Suppl 1:ONS140–ONS146, discussion ONS146

[20] Chin KR, Ahn J. Controlled cervical extension osteotomy for ankylosing spondylitis utilizing the Jackson operating table: technical note. Spine. 2007; 32(17):1926–1929

[21] Khoueir P, Hoh DJ, Wang MY. Use of hinged rods for controlled osteoclastic correction of a fixed cervical kyphotic deformity in ankylosing spondylitis. J Neurosurg Spine. 2008; 8(6):579–583

[22] Mehdian S, Arun R. A safe controlled instrumented reduction technique for cervical osteotomy in ankylosing spondylitis. Spine. 2011; 36(9):715–720

[23] Lee SH, Kim KT, Suk KS, Kim MH, Park DH, Kim KJ. A sterile-freehand reduction technique for corrective osteotomy of fixed cervical kyphosis. Spine. 2012; 37(26):2145–2150

[24] La Maida GA, Luceri F, Gallozzi F, Ferraro M, Bernardo M. Complication rate in adult deformity surgical treatment: safety of the posterior osteotomies. Eur Spine J. 2015; 24 Suppl 7:879–886

[25] La Marca F, Brumblay H. Smith-Petersen osteotomy in thoracolumbar deformity surgery. Neurosurgery. 2008; 63(3) Suppl:163–170

15 Osteotomy in the Thoracolumbar Spine for Cervical Deformity

Sang Hun Lee, Ki-Tack Kim, Yong-Chan Kim, Cheung Kue Kim, Hyung Suk Juh, and Khaled M. Kebaish

Abstract

Osteotomy in the thoracolumbar spine can correct cervical deformity through a secondary effect on spinopelvic alignment. Compensatory postures to achieve spinopelvic balance in response to thoracolumbar deformity have been described in many studies. In a typical primary thoracolumbar deformity, loss of lumbar lordosis and/or increased thoracic kyphosis are accompanied by increased pelvic tilt. This increase in pelvic tilt is a compensation mechanism of the lower back and hip extensor musculature that shifts the sagittal vertical axis posteriorly, creating cervical hyperlordosis to obtain a horizontal gaze. In patients with thoracolumbar deformity, osteotomy can decrease thoracic kyphosis and increase lumbar lordosis, improving cervical alignment to achieve a more natural lordotic curve. Thoracolumbar osteotomy can correct cervical spine deformity by improving T1 slope and C2–C7 sagittal vertical axis, restoring horizontal gaze without direct correction of cervical alignment. Thoracolumbar osteotomy is performed primarily to address thoracolumbar deformities; the corrective effects on cervical deformity are secondary. However, thoracolumbar osteotomy may be indicated for cervical deformity and thoracolumbar deformity with global sagittal imbalance, especially for fixed cervical deformity such as ankylosing spondylitis, diffuse idiopathic skeletal hyperostosis, or a surgically fused cervical spine with global spinopelvic decompensation. Flexible cervical deformities are treated with corrective surgeries within the cervical spine and are not indications for thoracolumbar osteotomy. Various osteotomy techniques, including the Smith-Petersen osteotomy, pedicle subtraction osteotomy, and vertebral column resection, may be performed, depending on the required degree of correction and location of the deformity.

Keywords: cervical deformity, lumbar osteotomy, osteotomy, pedicle subtraction osteotomy, Smith-Petersen osteotomy, thoracolumbar spine, vertebral column resection

15.1 Thoracolumbar Osteotomy for Cervical Deformity

It is well known that corrective surgeries for thoracolumbar deformity influence cervical spine alignment.[1,2,3,4] In response to spinal malalignment, the human body uses compensatory mechanisms to achieve an upright posture and maintain the head over the pelvis for a horizontal gaze. In primary thoracolumbar deformity, loss of lumbar lordosis (LL) and increased thoracic kyphosis (TK) are accompanied by increased pelvic tilt caused by the compensation mechanisms of the lower back, hip extensor musculature, and cervical hyperlordosis to obtain a horizontal gaze. Pre- and postoperative reciprocal changes in these adjacent regions have been described in many studies of thoracolumbar osteotomy (▶ Fig. 15.1).[5,6,7]

Surgical correction of thoracolumbar kyphosis by osteotomy improves cervical spine alignment from hyperlordosis to a more natural lordotic curve because decreased TK and increased LL do not require compensation to preserve sagittal balance and horizontal gaze. Cervical spine deformity correction without direct correction of cervical alignment but rather through thoracolumbar osteotomy is achieved by the improvement of T1 slope and C2–C7 sagittal vertical axis (SVA), which restore the horizontal gaze (▶ Fig. 15.2).

Thoracolumbar osteotomy is performed primarily to address thoracolumbar deformities, and the corrective effects on cervical deformity are secondary. Thoracolumbar osteotomy may be indicated for cervical deformity in patients with the following conditions:

- Cervical deformity combined with thoracolumbar deformity with global sagittal imbalance. Cervical deformity without thoracolumbar deformity is not an indication for thoracolumbar osteotomy. In patients with cervical and thoracolumbar deformities, corrective surgery should always begin in the thoracolumbar spine because correction of thoracolumbar spine deformity improves global SVA, as well as horizontal gaze. In many cases, residual cervical deformity is tolerable after successful correction of the thoracolumbar deformity. Also, correction of thoracolumbar deformity provides balanced spinopelvic alignment, which is the foundation for evaluating and planning additional correction of cervical deformity. If thoracolumbar deformity correction does not restore horizontal gaze and SVA, additional cervical osteotomies may be required.

- Fixed cervical deformity, such as ankylosing spondylitis (AS), diffuse idiopathic skeletal hyperostosis, or a surgically fused cervical spine with global spinopelvic decompensation. In patients with mobile cervical spine segments, correction of thoracolumbar deformity changes cervical spine alignment. It is difficult to predict the amount of correction in cervical alignment in patients with an "unfused" cervical spine. Flexible deformity (visible on flexion–extension radiographs) or "unfused" deformity (correctable by skeletal traction) is treated with corrective surgery of the cervical spine and is not an indication for thoracolumbar osteotomy. However, the correction of cervical deformity (not a correction of cervical lordosis but a correction of chin–brow vertical angle [CBVA] and SVA in the strict sense) can be expected after thoracolumbar deformity correction with osteotomy because the fused cervical spine does not compensate for changes in the thoracolumbar spine.

15.2 Evaluation of Spinopelvic Alignment in the Ankylosed Spine

15.2.1 Global Spinal Alignment on Radiographs

SVA from the C7 plumb line and CBVA are two of the most important parameters for evaluating global sagittal balance. All patients should undergo detailed preoperative radiographic imaging studies, including standing 36-inch anteroposterior and lateral radiographs, as well as routine cervical, thoracic, and lumbar spine radiographs. The lateral radiograph should include facial bones to enable measurement of CBVA. An additional lateral radiograph with the chin–brow line is needed for patients with severe sagittal imbalance. Standard lateral radiographs do not show the cervical spine and facial bones. Computed tomography (CT) and magnetic resonance imaging (MRI) are necessary to evaluate ossification, fusion, and spinal stenosis. The following basic sagittal alignment parameters should be measured: cervical lordosis (C2 lower endplate [LEP] to C7 LEP), T1 slope, thoracic inlet angle, neck tilt, cervicothoracic angle (C6 upper endplate [UEP] to T4 LEP), TK (T4 UEP to T12 LEP), thoracolumbar angle (T10 UEP to L2 LEP), LL (L1 UEP to L5 LEP), sacral slope, pelvic tilt, and pelvic incidence (PI) (▶ Fig. 15.3).

15.2.2 Fusion Status of Spinal Segments

Patients with AS or diffuse idiopathic skeletal hyperostosis have a variable degree of ossification or pseudarthrosis in the spine, even in the middle of ankylosed segments. Terminating fusion at the junction of incomplete ossification or pseudarthrosis

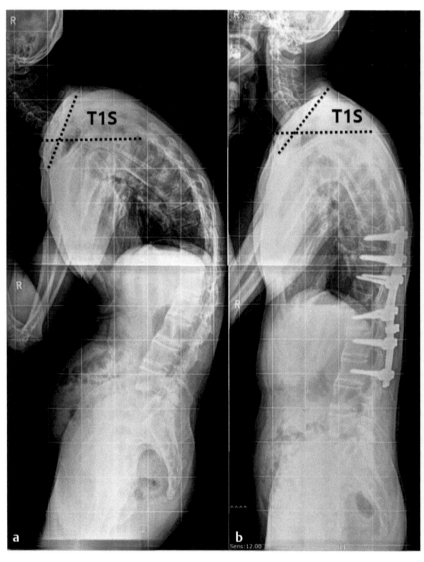

Fig. 15.1 Preoperative **(a)** and postoperative **(b)** whole-spine standing radiographs of a 35-year-old man with ankylosing spondylitis. He had a fused thoracolumbar spine with kyphotic deformity but mobile cervical spine segments. After a T12 pedicle subtraction osteotomy, thoracolumbar kyphosis and C7 sagittal vertical axis were improved significantly. According to the decrease in T1 slope (T1S), his preoperative cervical hyperlordosis changed to a natural lordotic curve without any surgical correction of the cervical spine.

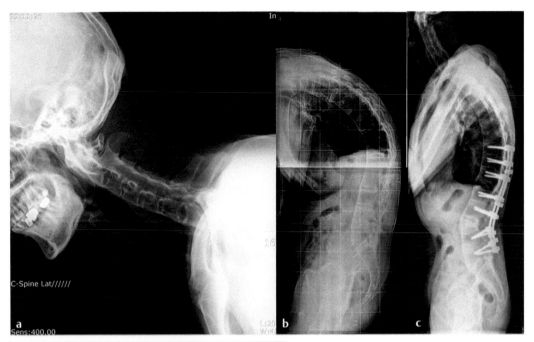

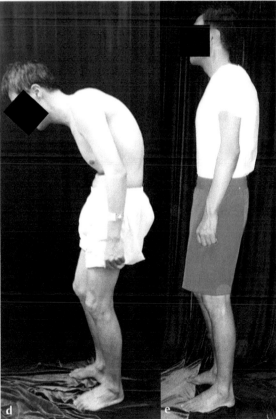

Fig. 15.2 Preoperative cervical spine standing lateral **(a)** and whole-spine **(b)** radiographs of a 53-year-old man with ankylosing spondylitis. Preoperatively, the cervical to the thoracolumbar spine was autofused. Normal cervicothoracic angle (C6–T4) is noted. After L3 pedicle subtraction osteotomy **(c)**, his lumbar lordosis improved from 5 to 35 degrees and C7 sagittal vertical axis improved from 23 to 8 cm. The gross cervical deformity was also corrected according to improvement in thoracolumbar kyphosis. Preoperative **(d)** and postoperative **(e)** photographs of the patient show major correction of global sagittal imbalance. Improvement of the chin–brow vertical angle and restoration of the horizontal gaze were possible through the secondary effects of lumbar osteotomy. No other procedure was performed for the cervical deformity.

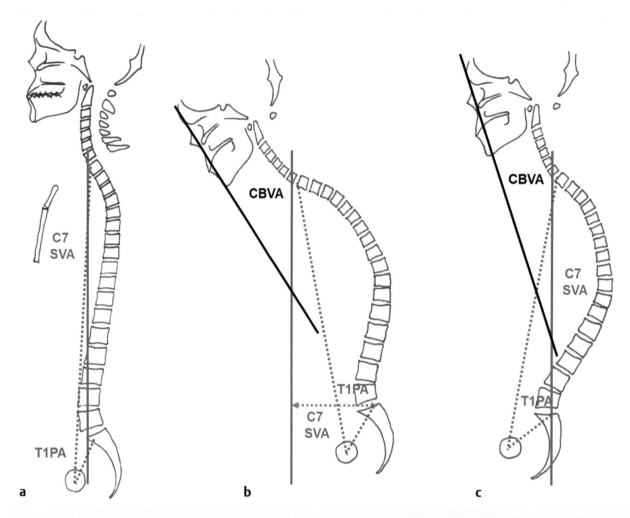

Fig. 15.3 Schematic drawings of **(a)** normal sagittal spinopelvic balance showing normal C7 sagittal vertical axis (SVA; *blue line*) (within 5 cm of the posterosuperior corner of the sacrum) and normal T1 pelvic angle (PA; *red dotted lines*) (< 14 degrees). **(b)** Spinopelvic alignment with global sagittal imbalance. C7 SVA and T1 PA increased. Chin–brow vertical angle (CBVA; *black and blue lines*) increases if the patient has a fused cervical spine. **(c)** Compensated spinopelvic imbalance with the same thoracolumbar kyphosis as shown in **(b)**. The compensation mechanism consists of pelvic retroversion. As a result of pelvic retroversion, C7 SVA is normalized and CBVA decreases but T1 PA does not change.

may cause early junctional failure. Extension of instrumentation within the ankylosed segments can provide more rigid fixation without further loss of motion segments. Cervical, thoracic, and lumbosacral spine flexion–extension radiographs and whole-spine CT scans are required to evaluate fusion.

15.3 Surgical Planning for Thoracolumbar Osteotomy

15.3.1 The Apex of Thoracolumbar Deformity

The ideal level of osteotomy is at the apex of the deformity. However, there are several limitations to performing an osteotomy at the apex. First, if the deformity is diffuse, it can be difficult to locate the apex of the deformity. Second, the apex may be at a challenging level, such as the midthoracic spine, or at a level with epidural scarring from previous laminectomy or transforaminal interbody fusion. Third, an osteotomy at the apex may be less

efficient at restoring SVA compared with an osteotomy at a lower level with the same degree of correction. In such cases, osteotomy at a nonapex level may be a better option.

15.3.2 The Level of the Osteotomy

When patients have diffuse TK or when the apex of the deformity is at the midthoracic spine, the surgeon may consider thoracic multilevel Smith-Petersen osteotomy (SPO) or three-column osteotomy, including pedicle subtraction osteotomy (PSO) or vertebral column resection (VCR), depending on rigidity of the deformity and degree of correction angle required. Multiple SPOs are not indicated in a completely ankylosed or fused spine. PSO and VCR are options for rigid, severe deformity.

When a patient's thoracolumbar junction angle kyphosis is more prominent than TK, and LL is not kyphotic, an osteotomy at the lower thoracic spine (T11 or T12) or the upper lumbar spine (L1 or L2) is an efficient way to correct TK and LL. If the TK and thoracolumbar kyphosis are not severe and the more dominant kyphosis is in the lumbar spine, PSO at L3 or lower may be a good option for correction of the global deformity. A lower lumbar PSO (at L4 or L5) can provide more SVA realignment than upper lumbar PSO with the same degree of correction because of the longer lever arm. However, lower lumbar PSO may be more technically difficult because the anatomical dimensions of pedicles, transverse processes, and vertebral bodies are bigger than in the upper lumbar spine and, in most cases, require pelvic fixation to stabilize distal segments of the spinal column.

15.3.3 Estimation of the Required Degree of Correction

C7 SVA is one of the most important indicators of global spinal alignment. Correction of C7 SVA to within 5 cm of the postero-superior corner of S1 is a good target. However, C7 SVA may not reflect local deformities within the thoracic and/or lumbar spine with compensation through pelvic retroversion. Recently, a novel parameter, T1 pelvic angle (the angle between the line from the axis of the femoral head to the center of the T1 vertebra and the line from the axis of the femoral head to the middle of the S1 UEP) has been proposed to measure true thoracolumbar deformity considering pelvic retroversion and pelvic tilt in patients with sagittal compensation, and it has been shown to correlate with health-related quality-of-life outcomes (▶ Fig. 15.3).[8] T1 pelvic angle of less than 14 degrees is ideal. It is important to preserve 10 to 15 degrees of undercorrection of CBVA in patients with an ankylosed spine from the cervical to thoracolumbar regions. Overcorrection of CBVA may worsen preoperative impairments in horizontal gaze and activities of daily living, such as reading, eating, and walking down stairs.

The degree of correction after spinal osteotomy varies depending on surgical technique, the amount of bone resection, intervertebral disc removal, the required degree of correction, and surgeon experience. Reportedly, the mean degree of correction for SPO is approximately 10 degrees per spinal segment.[9,10] Usually, SPO is performed on three to four segments, depending on the required degree of correction. A conventional PSO can correct from 30 to 40 degrees in the sagittal plane per segment; however, an extensive osteotomy involving the adjacent disc space and vertebral body can increase the degree of correction. When patients need correction in the coronal plane, asymmetric PSO can correct the coronal plane deformity at the same time.[11,12,13,14] VCR provides the largest degree of correction in the sagittal and coronal planes. The reported degree of correction ranges from 37 to 104 degrees in the sagittal plane and as high as 100 degrees in the coronal plane.[15,16,17]

Determining the amount of correction needed is the first step in surgical planning for corrective osteotomy. However, the optimal degree of correction is highly controversial. The oldest and simplest method is to consider only the local area of the deformity, such as LL or thoracolumbar angle. It involves correction of LL to achieve the desired lordotic angle using any osteotomy technique, including SPO, PSO, or VCR. However, the optimal LL is not easy to determine because the reported normal value of LL ranges from 30 to 89 degrees.[18,19,20] LL for a given patient should be proportional to the observed PI. Because of the strong correlation between PI and LL, it is an acceptable goal to reconstruct LL to reach a PI minus LL of less than 10

degrees. Ondra et al[21] proposed a trigonometric calculation of the required degree of correction at the PSO level based on C7 SVA. Although these methods make it easy to predict the degree of correction, they can lead to undercorrection because they do not account for pelvic compensation.

Initial attempts to predict the degree of correction, including pelvic parameters, were performed by van Royen et al.[22] They presented a planning method to predict degree of correction after osteotomy in patients with AS based on CBVA and sacral slope. Le Huec et al[23] proposed a more complicated "full balance integrated" method, including hip flexion and pelvic tilt angles for the calculation of the required degree of correction. Simulation software was later developed. The first software was ASKyphoplan, used by van Royen et al[22] to assist in planning corrective osteotomy for patients with AS. Most recently, the reliability of a free computer program, Surgimap Spine (Nemaris Inc, New York, NY), has been validated.[24,25,26] In a simulation using Surgimap, the level and amount of correction are based on corrected pelvic tilt, which may prevent undercorrection of SVA.[24,25,26] However, the simulation does not account for compensatory changes in the unfused segments of the spine. In addition, the ideal pelvic tilt and actual restoration of pelvic tilt are unpredictable.

Intraoperative radiography is necessary to check whether the planned degree of correction has been achieved. Additional bone resection within the osteotomized segment or additional osteotomy may be required depending on intraoperative radiographic findings.

15.3.4 Thoracolumbar Osteotomy Complications

Although PSO and VCR are useful techniques to correct fixed or rigid thoracolumbar deformity, they are also associated with serious complications. Neurological complications, including spinal cord injury, nerve root injury, and cauda equina, are the primary concern after spinal osteotomy. Clinical studies have reported neurological complication rates after PSO of 4.2 to 11%, with 2.8 to 5.7% of patients experiencing permanent neurological deficit.[27,28,29] Neurological complications after VCR have also been reported. Suk et al[16,17]reported a 6 to 8% rate of transient neurological deficit and a 3 to 6% rate of permanent complete spinal cord injury after posterior VCR in their clinical series. Transient neurological complication rates of 2.7 to 14% and permanent injury rates of 2.8 to 6.3% have also been reported.[27,28,29] In addition to neurological complications, various surgical and medical complications are associated with spinal osteotomy. Surgical complications include surgical site infection, dural tear, cerebrospinal fluid leak, screw malposition, rod fracture, adjacent level fracture, and proximal junctional kyphosis. Medical complications include cardiopulmonary events after anesthesia, blood loss, deep vein thrombosis, pulmonary embolism, and cerebrovascular accident. Clinical series have reported a wide range of overall complication rates, from 25 to 69%.[13,14,15,16,17,18,27] Some studies have reported a higher complication rate for VCR compared with PSO. The greater blood loss and longer operative time associated with VCR compared with PSO may account for this difference.[13,15,16,17,27,28,29] However, several studies have reported no significant difference in complication rates. Lower complication rates, ranging from 17 to 45%, were reported in patients who underwent posterior column osteotomy, including SPO or Ponte osteotomy.[30,31] However, the reported neurological complication rate ranged from 0 to 1.4%, which is much lower than that of three-column osteotomy.[30,31]

15.4 Outcomes of Thoracolumbar Osteotomy for Cervical Sagittal Balance in the Ankylosed Spine

Changes in CBVA, T1 slope, neck tilt, C0–C2 angle (if mobile), and C2–C7 SVA occur after thoracolumbar osteotomy (combined with changes in C7 SVA and global spinal alignment).[32]

15.5 Surgical Techniques

15.5.1 Posterior Column Osteotomy (Smith-Petersen Osteotomy) of the Thoracolumbar Spine

Spinal cord monitoring with somatosensory-evoked potentials and transcranial motor-evoked potentials is used routinely during thoracic SPOs. In lumbar SPOs, free-running electromyography can help prevent nerve root injury. After patient positioning, an intraoperative lateral radiograph is necessary to confirm thoracolumbar spine alignment and locate the level of approach.

A midline skin incision is followed by subperiosteal dissection of the paraspinal muscles to expose the spinous processes, laminae, facet joints, and transverse processes. Exposure typically extends three levels above and below the intended osteotomy level but may be expanded according to instrumentation fixation strength and osteoporosis. Pedicle screws are inserted before performing osteotomy procedures.

The osteotomy starts with a V-shaped laminectomy and bilateral symmetric total facet joint resections. Laminectomy consists of removal of the inferior lamina of the cranial vertebra and superior lamina of the caudal vertebra using osteotomes, Kerrison rongeurs, or bone scalpels. Corresponding ligamentum flavum and facet joint capsules should be removed completely before closing to avoid dural sac and nerve root impingement. Complete facetectomy is important, especially for lumbar SPOs, to prevent postoperative radiculopathy and to achieve optimum degree of correction. If the deformity is too rigid or additional correction is needed, transverse process and rib disarticulation are helpful to obtain more correction in the thoracic spine. SPO is performed in three to four segments, depending on the angle and rigidity of the deformity.

Reduction of the osteotomy starts from gentle and gradual assembly of a prebent rod with a desired correction angle using various reduction clamps connecting to the pedicle screws. After rod assembly, intersegmental compression between the pedicle screws over the rods can close the gaps between the laminae. Compression of the head of pedicle screws without rod assembly may cause uncontrolled reduction, which may be complicated by pedicle fracture, anterior column fracture, or segmental translation. Although the reported incidence of neurological complications after SPO is lower than that after three-column osteotomies, careful monitoring of possible dura impingement between the laminae and any changes in neuromonitoring signals is critical during the reduction procedure. Decortication and bone graft for successful fusion are the final steps for multilevel SPO.

15.5.2 Pedicle Subtraction Osteotomy at the Lumbar Spine

The patient is positioned prone on a surgical table with chest and pelvis pads. Some surgeons prefer a foldable surgical table to close the osteotomy gap, but many surgeons close the osteotomy gap successfully with compression of the pedicle screws on the rod without a folding surgical table. Instrumentation of three segments above and below the osteotomy is typically required, although the length of fixation depends on bone strength and presence of bony ankyloses at the adjacent segments (▶ Fig. 15.4).

Laminectomy and Facet Resection

The first step in PSO is laminectomy at the level of osteotomy with resection of the inferior half of the lamina and inferior articular processes of the upper vertebra using osteotomes and/or bone scalpels. Wide laminectomy helps prevent dural sac buckling and spinal cord/cauda equina impingement; however, a laminectomy defect that is too wide may leave a bone defect that can cause nonunion of the PSO, rod fracture, and instrumentation failure. Laminectomy at the PSO level should be on the bilateral pars and should include all circumferential bony overhangs outside the pedicle border using a Leksell rongeur or variable-sized Kerrison rongeurs. The superior articular processes should be removed close to the superior border of the pedicle, and all circumferential borders of the pedicles should be exposed. The superior articular processes of the lower vertebra need to be removed to avoid nerve root impingement below the osteotomy level.

Transverse Process and Pedicle Removal

The next step is transverse process removal. Muscle attachments, intertransversarii muscles, and psoas muscle to the transverse process should be released with electrocautery and/or a curved curette. After complete isolation of the pedicle borders, the pedicle can be resected using osteotomes while protecting the dura medially and the nerve roots above and below. Thinning the pedicle wall by sequential dilation using curettes or high-speed burr makes pedicle removal easier and safer.

Decancellation of the Vertebral Body and Resection of the Posterior and Lateral Wall of the Vertebral Body

Decancellation of the vertebral body is the next step after removal of the pedicles. When decancellation is performed on one side, a short, temporary rod fixation on the other side is required to avoid fracture and translation of the vertebral column. Variable-sized straight and reversed-angle curettes are

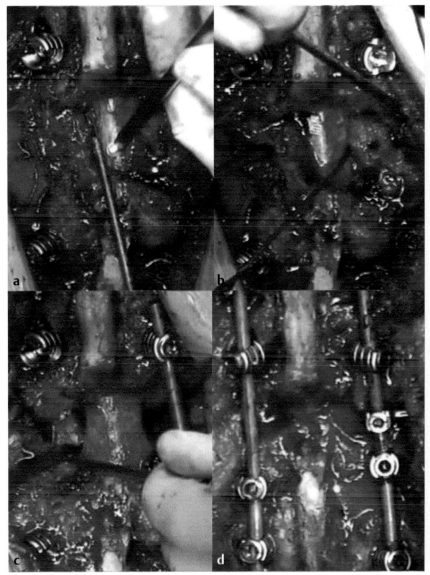

Fig. 15.4 Intraoperative photographs of lumbar pedicle subtraction osteotomy. Sequential steps include **(a)** laminectomy and facet resection, **(b)** transverse process and pedicle removal, **(c)** decancellation of the vertebral body and lateral wall removal, and **(d)** closing of the osteotomy.

used to remove the cancellous bone inside the vertebral body. The posterior wall can be crushed using variable impactors or reversed-angle curettes. The lateral wall of the vertebral body should be removed in a tapered wedge (a blunt osteotome is helpful for gentle closure of the osteotomy). At this stage, segmental arteries on the side of the vertebral body are vulnerable to injury by the osteotomes; subperiosteal dissection of the lateral wall of the vertebral body and protection of the soft tissue with a Cobb elevator are required. To limit cancellous bleeding, homeostatic agents such as thrombin with a collagen sponge are useful. The anterior wall may be left intact to create a greenstick fracture. In a vertebra with a thick, strong anterior wall, the surgeon may need to make a fracture using a blunt osteotome or Cobb elevator. The amount of laminectomy and removal of the posterior wall of vertebral body vary according to the required degree of correction.

Closing the Osteotomy

Partial closure of the osteotomy gap occurs spontaneously after the temporary rod is released. Gentle, gradual compression between the pedicle screws on the rod is the safest way to reduce the osteotomy gap. If the gap does not close easily, more decancellation and vertebral body wall resection are needed rather than forceful reduction. Several methods are recommended to avoid nonunion of the PSO. First, precise laminectomy to minimize or eliminate the gap between the ends of the cephalad and caudad laminae after closing the osteotomy is important. Second, if the laminectomy defect persists after closing the gap, covering the defect with a structural bone graft is helpful. Bisected spinous processes in the midline are good sources for the graft. Third, interbody fusion can be performed at the adjacent segment to stop segmental motion.

15.5.3 Three-Column Osteotomy at the Lower and Midthoracic Spine: T5–T12

Conventional Pedicle Subtraction Osteotomy

For PSO at the level of the thoracic spine, laminectomy, facet, and transverse process resection are similar to the methods described for lumbar PSO. A unique step in thoracic PSO is bilateral rib head disarticulation from the costovertebral junction. A Cobb elevator or blunt osteotome is useful to avoid injury to pleura or segmental vessels. After disarticulating the rib head–vertebral body junction, pedicle resection, decancellation, and closing osteotomy are similar to those of lumbar PSO. Unlike lumbar PSO below L2, too much correction at a single level (more than 35–40 degrees) may cause dural sac infolding and spinal cord impingement. In these cases, a modified PSO preserving the inferior wall of the pedicle at multiple levels is a safer option.

Modified Partial PSO for the Midthoracic Spine

This procedure preserves the inferior wall of the pedicle to avoid overcorrection at any level but provides more correction per segment than does SPO, especially in the midthoracic spine. This osteotomy is appropriate for the completely ossified spinal column, in which case SPO is unfeasible. Partial PSO can be performed with lumbar PSO, as well as combined with conventional SPO, PSO, or VCR to obtain a harmonious correction of the thoracolumbar spine. Kim et al[33] reported a mean correction angle of 18.8 degrees with partial PSO. They recommended partial PSO as an alternative option for deformities that require an intermediate degree of correction between that achievable with SPO and that achievable with conventional PSO (▶ Fig. 15.5 and ▶ Fig. 15.6).

Posterior Vertebral Column Resection

Given that posterior VCR is capable of achieving the largest degree of correction, this technique is indicated for the most severe, rigid deformities. Posterior VCR is effective when it is performed at the apex of the deformity but is technically demanding. Basic procedures are similar to those for PSO. The laminectomies typically need to be wider than those for PSO to expose the upper and lower disc space. Insufficient laminectomy is a common technical pitfall and may cause incomplete removal of intervertebral discs and endplates adjacent to the cage or graft. After transverse process resection, bilateral rib resections are necessary to obtain correction and place a graft.

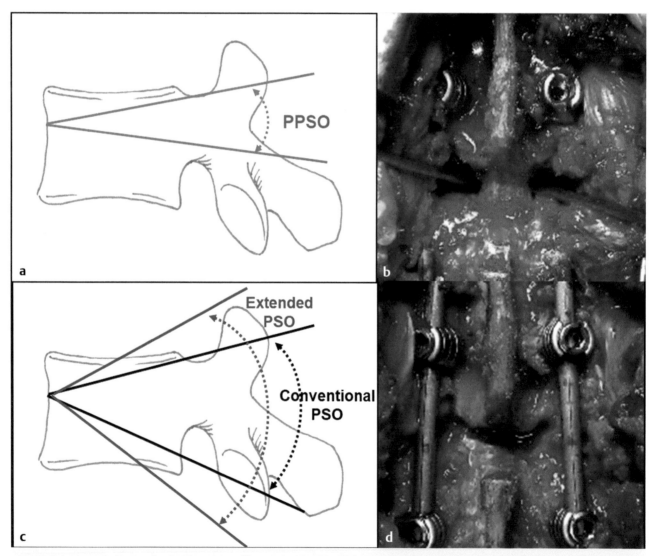

Fig. 15.5 A schematic drawing showing the amount of bone resection achieved through a partial pedicle subtraction osteotomy (PPSO) **(a)** compared with that achieved through a conventional pedicle subtraction osteotomy (PSO) and an extended PSO including the adjacent intervertebral disc space **(b)**. Intraoperative photographs of PPSO, before **(c)** and after **(d)** closing the osteotomy gap.

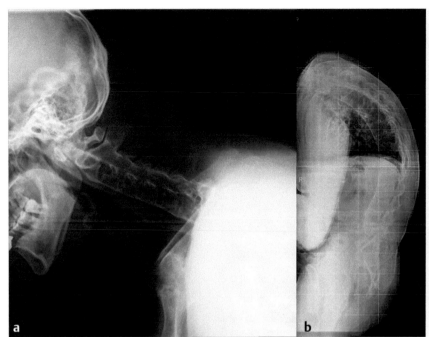

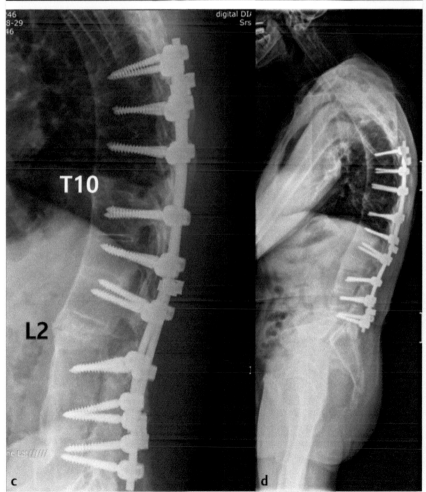

Fig. 15.6 Preoperative cervical spine standing lateral **(a)** and whole-spine **(b)** radiographs of a 48-year-old man with ankylosing spondylitis and thoracolumbar kyphotic deformity. A horizontal gaze was impossible because of his fused kyphotic spine. However, his cervicothoracic angle (C6–T4) was not kyphotic. Upper lumbar pedicle subtraction osteotomy and lower thoracic partial pedicle subtraction osteotomy were planned to correct the thoracolumbar global kyphosis. **(c)** After L2 pedicle subtraction osteotomy and T10 partial pedicle subtraction osteotomy, global and local sagittal imbalance improved significantly. **(d)** Postoperative standing whole-spine radiograph shows major improvement in sagittal balance and chin–brow vertical angle, which improved from 48 to 18 degrees without correction of the cervical spine deformity.

A rib resection point is approximately 1.5 to 2 inches lateral to the costovertebral junction, depending on the size of the interbody graft. Rib resection starts from the distal point after dissection of the intercostal muscles attaching the cranial and caudal ends using a Bovie and/or Cobb elevator. The proximal costochondral junction can be detached with a Cobb elevator or a blunt osteotome to avoid pleura or segmental vessel injuries. Bilateral and posterior wall removal procedures are similar to those of PSO. Before pedicle and vertebral body removal, cutting the unilateral intercostal nerve is helpful to provide a wide working space. Using 1–0 silk or nonabsorbable suture, the intercostal nerve should be tied at a proximal point of the dorsal root ganglion before cutting the nerve root. The tied end is helpful for gentle retraction and protection of the dural sac during graft insertion. For the next step, bilateral posterolateral corner discectomies at the upper and lower intervertebral discs help to locate the portion of vertebral body to be removed. If the posterior VCR is not being used for spinal tumor resection, complete removal of the vertebral body is unnecessary. However, a sufficient amount of vertebral body and both endplates should be removed to place a graft properly.

15.6 Conclusion

Thoracolumbar osteotomy is performed primarily to address thoracolumbar deformities; the corrective effects on cervical deformity are secondary by improving T1 slope and C2–C7 SVA. Thoracolumbar osteotomy may be indicated for cervical deformity for fixed cervical deformity such as AS, diffuse idiopathic skeletal hyperostosis, or a surgically fused cervical spine with global spinopelvic decompensation. Although the ideal level of osteotomy is at the apex of the deformity, osteotomy at a nonapex level may be a better option when (1) the deformity is diffuse; (2) the apex is at a challenging level; or (3) an osteotomy at the apex would be less efficient at restoring SVA compared with an osteotomy at a lower level with the same degree of correction. Estimation of the optimal degree of correction is controversial. Reconstruction of LL to reach a PI minus LL of approximately 10 degrees is the simplest local method. Recently developed computer programs simulate the results of correction, including not only local angle correction but also restoration of pelvic tilt. However, CBVA and T1 slope are the two most important parameters when the purpose of thoracolumbar osteotomy is to correct cervical deformity.

References

[1] Barrey C, Roussouly P, Perrin G, Le Huec JC. Sagittal balance disorders in severe degenerative spine. Can we identify the compensatory mechanisms? Eur Spine J. 2011; 20 Suppl 5:626–633

[2] Diebo BG, Ferrero E, Lafage R, et al. Recruitment of compensatory mechanisms in sagittal spinal malalignment is age and regional deformity dependent: a full-standing axis analysis of key radiographical parameters. Spine. 2015; 40(9):642–649

[3] Ha Y, Schwab F, Lafage V, et al. Reciprocal changes in cervical spine alignment after corrective thoracolumbar deformity surgery. Eur Spine J. 2014; 23 (3):552–559

[4] Ferrero E, Liabaud B, Challier V, et al. Role of pelvic translation and lower-extremity compensation to maintain gravity line position in spinal deformity. J Neurosurg Spine. 2016; 24(3):436–446

[5] Day LM, Ramchandran S, Jalai CM, et al. Thoracolumbar realignment surgery results in simultaneous reciprocal changes in lower extremities and cervical spine. Spine. 2017; 42(11):799–807

[6] Hwang SW, Samdani AF, Tantorski M, et al. Cervical sagittal plane decompensation after surgery for adolescent idiopathic scoliosis: an effect imparted by postoperative thoracic hypokyphosis. J Neurosurg Spine. 2011; 15(5):491–496

[7] Passias PG, Soroceanu A, Scheer J, et al. International Spine Study Group. Magnitude of preoperative cervical lordotic compensation and C2-T3 angle are correlated to increased risk of postoperative sagittal spinal pelvic malalignment in adult thoracolumbar deformity patients at 2-year follow-up. Spine J. 2015; 15(8):1756–1763

[8] Protopsaltis T, Schwab F, Bronsard N, et al. International Spine Study Group. The T1 pelvic angle, a novel radiographic measure of global sagittal deformity, accounts for both spinal inclination and pelvic tilt and correlates with health-related quality of life. J Bone Joint Surg Am. 2014; 96(19):1631–1640

[9] La Marca F, Brumblay H. Smith-Petersen osteotomy in thoracolumbar deformity surgery. Neurosurgery. 2008; 63(3) Suppl:163–170

[10] Smith-Petersen MN, Larson CB, Aufranc OE. Osteotomy of the spine for correction of flexion deformity in rheumatoid arthritis. J Bone Joint Surg Am. 1945; 27(1):1–11

[11] Boachie-Adjei O, Ferguson JAI, Pigeon RG, Peskin MR. Transpedicular lumbar wedge resection osteotomy for fixed sagittal imbalance: surgical technique and early results. Spine. 2006; 31(4):485–492

[12] Cecchinato R, Berjano P, Aguirre MF, Lamartina C. Asymmetrical pedicle subtraction osteotomy in the lumbar spine in combined coronal and sagittal imbalance. Eur Spine J. 2015; 24 Suppl 1:S66–S71

[13] Kim KT, Park DH, Lee SH, Lee JH. Results of corrective osteotomy and treatment strategy for ankylosing spondylitis with kyphotic deformity. Clin Orthop Surg. 2015; 7(3):330–336

[14] Kim KT, Suk KS, Cho YJ, Hong GP, Park BJ. Clinical outcome results of pedicle subtraction osteotomy in ankylosing spondylitis with kyphotic deformity. Spine. 2002; 27(6):612–618

[15] Dorward IG, Lenke LG, Stoker GE, Cho W, Koester LA, Sides BA. Radiographic and clinical outcomes of posterior column osteotomies in spinal deformity correction. Spine. 2014; 39(11):870–880

[16] Suk SI, Chung ER, Kim JH, Kim SS, Lee JS, Choi WK. Posterior vertebral column resection for severe rigid scoliosis. Spine. 2005; 30(14):1682–1687

[17] Suk SI, Kim JH, Kim WJ, Lee SM, Chung ER, Nah KH. Posterior vertebral column resection for severe spinal deformities. Spine. 2002; 27(21):2374–2382

[18] Bernhardt M, Bridwell KH. Segmental analysis of the sagittal plane alignment of the normal thoracic and lumbar spines and thoracolumbar junction. Spine. 1989; 14(7):717–721

[19] Berthonnaud E, Dimnet J, Roussouly P, Labelle H. Analysis of the sagittal balance of the spine and pelvis using shape and orientation parameters. J Spinal Disord Tech. 2005; 18(1):40–47

[20] Vialle R, Levassor N, Rillardon L, Templier A, Skalli W, Guigui P. Radiographic analysis of the sagittal alignment and balance of the spine in asymptomatic subjects. J Bone Joint Surg Am. 2005; 87(2):260–267

[21] Ondra SL, Marzouk S, Koski T, Silva F, Salehi S. Mathematical calculation of pedicle subtraction osteotomy size to allow precision correction of fixed sagittal deformity. Spine. 2006; 31(25):E973–E979

[22] van Royen BJ, Scheerder FJ, Jansen E, Smit TH. ASKyphoplan: a program for deformity planning in ankylosing spondylitis. Eur Spine J. 2007; 16(9):1445–1449

[23] Le Huec JC, Leijssen P, Duarte M, Aunoble S. Thoracolumbar imbalance analysis for osteotomy planification using a new method: FBI technique. Eur Spine J. 2011; 20 Suppl 5:669–680

[24] Akbar M, Terran J, Ames CP, Lafage V, Schwab F. Use of Surgimap Spine in sagittal plane analysis, osteotomy planning, and correction calculation. Neurosurg Clin N Am. 2013; 24(2):163–172

[25] Langella F, Villafañe JH, Damilano M, et al. Predictive accuracy of SurgimapTM surgical planning for sagittal imbalance: A cohort study. Spine. 2017; 42(22):E1297–E1304

[26] Park YS, Kim HS, Baek SW, Oh JH. Preoperative computer-based simulations for the correction of kyphotic deformities in ankylosing spondylitis patients. Spine J. 2014; 14(10):2420–2424

[27] La Maida GA, Luceri F, Gallozzi F, Ferraro M, Bernardo M. Complication rate in adult deformity surgical treatment: safety of the posterior osteotomies. Eur Spine J. 2015; 24 Suppl 7:879–886

[28] Lenke LG, Newton PO, Sucato DJ, et al. Complications after 147 consecutive vertebral column resections for severe pediatric spinal deformity: a multicenter analysis. Spine. 2013; 38(2):119–132

[29] Sciubba DM, Yurter A, Smith JS, et al. International Spine Study Group (ISSG). A comprehensive review of complication rates after surgery for adult deformity: A reference for informed consent. Spine Deform. 2015; 3(6):575–594

[30] Geck MJ, Macagno A, Ponte A, Shufflebarger HL. The Ponte procedure: posterior only treatment of Scheuermann's kyphosis using segmental posterior shortening and pedicle screw instrumentation. J Spinal Disord Tech. 2007; 20 (8):586–593

[31] Pizones J, Sánchez-Mariscal F, Zúñiga L, Izquierdo E. Ponte osteotomies to treat major thoracic adolescent idiopathic scoliosis curves allow more effective corrective maneuvers. Eur Spine J. 2015; 24(7):1540–1546

[32] Smith JS, Shaffrey CI, Lafage V, et al. International Spine Study Group. Spontaneous improvement of cervical alignment after correction of global sagittal balance following pedicle subtraction osteotomy. J Neurosurg Spine. 2012; 17 (4):300–307

[33] Kim KT, Park DH, Lee SH, Suk KS, Lee JH, Park KJ. Partial pedicle subtraction osteotomy as an alternative option for spinal sagittal deformity correction. Spine. 2013; 38(14):1238–1243

16 Congenital Cervical Deformity and Hemivertebra

Joshua M. Pahys and Amer F. Samdani

Abstract

Congenital cervical scoliosis presents a wide range of challenges for the clinician, from simple to complex. The potential for associated anomalies needs to be evaluated early, including formal renal and cardiac assessments. A preoperative MRI is also necessary to screen for intraspinal anomalies that may also need to be addressed. Failure of formation produces either a wedge vertebra or a hemivertebra. Failure of segmentation produces partial to complete fusion from one vertebra to another. Congenital spinal deformities can present with an isolated anomaly up to a multilevel combination of failure of formation and/or segmentation. Fully segmented hemivertebrae have the highest chance for progression compared to a fully incarcerated hemivertebra. Congenital cervical deformity presents a unique challenge in that there is less possibility for compensation above the anomaly. This can result in significant torticollis and/or progressive compensatory deformities in the thoracolumbar spine. Bracing is not an effective treatment for congenital cervical deformity but has been used to prevent soft-tissue contractures prior to surgical intervention. Preoperative halo traction can be utilized to reduce the magnitude of some deformities prior to surgery, most notably in cases of severe cervical kyphosis. Hemivertebra resection has been described in several case reports. This typically requires a combined anterior-posterior approach to accommodate the course of the vertebral artery. The future of treatment for congenital scoliosis is certainly encouraging. With the continued improvement in modern instrumentation, intraoperative navigation, and intraoperative neuromonitoring, the safety and efficacy of treatment for congenital scoliosis continues to move in a positive direction.

Keywords: congenital scoliosis, cervical deformity, torticollis, hemivertebra, Klippel–Feil syndrome

16.1 Introduction

Congenital anomalies of the spine result from abnormal vertebral development during weeks 4 to 6 of gestation that results in asymmetric growth of the spine. The overall incidence of congenital scoliosis is approximately 1 in every 1,000 live births.[1] Isolated anomalies are likely sporadic with little genetic tendency. However, a 5 to 10% risk of congenital scoliosis for future siblings of patients with multiple vertebral anomalies has been reported.[2]

16.2 Classification

Congenital scoliosis is classically described as a failure of segmentation, formation, or a mixed form.[3] Approximately 80% of anomalies may be classified as either failures of segmentation or formation, with 20% being a mixed form. Segmentation defects involve bony bars between adjacent segments.[4] A block vertebra results from bilateral segmentation defects with fusion of the disc spaces between the involved vertebrae. A unilateral

bar typically occurs on the concave side of a curve. A unilateral unsegmented bar is a bony bar fusing both the disc spaces and/or facets on one side of the spine. The unsegmented bar does not contain growth plates and therefore does not grow.

Failure of formation produces either a wedge vertebra or a hemivertebra. A wedge vertebra represents partial failure of vertebral body formation on one side but maintains two pedicles. In contrast, a hemivertebra represents complete failure of formation of half the vertebra. There are three main types of hemivertebrae: fully segmented (65%), partially segmented (22%), and nonsegmented/incarcerated (12%).[2,4] A fully segmented hemivertebra possesses a normal disc both above and below the anomaly. A partially segmented hemivertebra is fused to the neighboring vertebra on one side with an open disc space on the opposite side. An incarcerated hemivertebra has no intervening disc space between the adjacent vertebrae.[3] An excellent illustration of these anomalies can be viewed in a previous congenital scoliosis review by Hedequist and Emans.[5]

Kawakami et al[6] proposed a three-dimensional (3D) classification for congenital scoliosis utilizing 3D computed tomography (CT) reconstructions. This 3D imaging allows for the evaluation of several types of laminae that were consistently found, as well as provide a more detailed appreciation of severe deformities not possible with biplanar radiographs alone. The authors described four types of congenital vertebral anomalies: type 1: solitary simple; type 2: multiple simple; type 3: complex; type 4: segmentation failure. More recently, Williams et al[7] reported on the initial validation of a new Classification of Early-Onset Scoliosis (C-EOS). C-EOS encompasses patient age, etiology (including congenital), major Cobb angle, kyphosis, and annual progression ratio (APR). Excellent interobserver reliability was reported. However, neither of the two studies specifies any correlations with these new classification schemes and the risk of progression and/or patient outcomes.

16.3 Natural History

Determining which congenital curves will progress rapidly is difficult. In general terms, 25% of curves do not progress, 25% progress slowly, and 50% display rapid progression.[8] The determinants of curve progression depend on the type of anomaly, its location, and the age of the patient. Normal longitudinal growth of the spine is a summation of the growth occurring at the superior and inferior endplates of the vertebral bodies. The presence and quality of the disc spaces surrounding an anomalous vertebral segment will predict the potential for asymmetric growth, as healthy discs typically portend curve progression. Fully segmented hemivertebrae have a higher potential for progression, as definable intervertebral discs signify the presence of growth potential.[3]

McMaster and Ohtsuka[3] reported on the rate of worsening in patients with various types of congenital spine anomalies. The anomaly that is the most at risk for progression is the unilateral bar with contralateral hemivertebra, followed by a unilateral bar, a hemivertebra, a wedge vertebra, and a block vertebra, which is the least likely to cause any significant deformity. A "hemimetameric shift" occurs when a hemivertebra on one side is balanced by another on the opposite side of the spine, separated by one normal vertebra. This is most commonly found in the thoracic spine. Intuitively, it would appear that the asymmetric growth potential should balance in this circumstance. However, these deformities still progress in up to 30% of patients.[9] With regard to patient age, curve progression is typically most rapid before age 5 and during the adolescent growth spurt.[10] Curves in the thoracolumbar spine appear to progress more rapidly than those in the upper thoracic and cervical spine.[5]

16.3.1 Compensatory Deformity

Unlike in the thoracolumbar spine, there is less possibility for compensation above a cervical deformity. Furthermore, a cervical hemivertebra is often associated with other malformations such as Klippel–Feil syndrome, which further reduces the number of flexible segments available to allow for any significant compensation.[11] This often results in an increasing head tilt. This resultant torticollis and shoulder imbalance are two particular cosmetic abnormalities of congenital cervical anomalies.[12] If the deformity is significant enough, the head tilt can lead to soft-tissue contractures of the neck musculature and outward facial asymmetry.[13] In an attempt to achieve a more horizontal gaze, the patient may develop a compensatory curve in the upper thoracic spine, or a considerable trunk shift to the side of the cervical convexity if additional congenital anomalies are present in the thoracic spine.[11,14] At times, a child will compensate for a primary cervical deformity with a long thoracolumbar deformity. If treatment of the cervical deformity is not undertaken in a timely manner, then the thoracolumbar deformity may become fixed (▶ Fig. 16.1a, c, d).

16.4 Associated Anomalies

The spine develops between 4 and 6 weeks of gestation along with the genitourinary, musculoskeletal, and cardiovascular systems. Therefore, many patients with congenital scoliosis also manifest abnormalities in other organ systems. These anomalies may be isolated or in association with the VACTERL syndrome (vertebral anomalies, anorectal atresia, cardiac anomalies, tracheoesophageal fistula, renal and limb anomalies).[15] The musculoskeletal system should be examined closely for other anomalies in the cervical spine (Klippel–Feil syndrome), upper extremity (Sprengel's deformity or radial deficiency), and/or lower extremity (developmental dysplasia of the hip).

Genitourinary abnormalities are observed in 20 to 40% of these children. These are usually anatomic abnormalities with normal renal function. However, a renal ultrasound or evaluation of the kidneys on the spine MRI is recommended for all of these patients.[16] Cardiac abnormalities occurred in 18 to 26% of patients in one series of congenital scoliosis.[17] Ventricular septal defects tend to be the most common finding. Prior to any surgical intervention, an echocardiogram with an evaluation should be performed by a cardiologist if indicated.[5] Neural axis abnormalities occur in up to 40% of patients with congenital scoliosis.[15]

A wide variety of abnormalities are observed including diastematomyelia, intradural lipoma, syringomyelia, Chiari malformation, and tethered cord. Shen et al[17] recently reported a 43%

incidence of intraspinal anomalies in 226 patients with congenital scoliosis, with diastematomyelia being the most common condition. In this study, intraspinal anomalies were identified more frequently in patients with a thoracic hemivertebra and/or failure of segmentation and mixed diagnosis. Two recent reports demonstrated a significantly higher incidence of intraspinal anomalies in patients with congenital scoliosis and rib abnormalities than in those without.[18]

Clinical indicators of intraspinal anomalies can include skin stigmata such as hairy patch or skin dimple[19] or asymmetric abdominal reflexes. Neurosurgical intervention is recommended for any anomaly which tethers the cord prior to attempting surgical correction of the deformity. An MRI examination of the entire spine from occiput to sacrum is recommended prior to any surgical intervention.[17]

16.5 Commonly Associated Conditions

16.5.1 Klippel–Feil Syndrome

Klippel–Feil syndrome is described as a triad of congenital fusion of two or more cervical vertebrae, a short neck, and low hairline. The presence of Klippel-Feil syndrome is unknown, as the majority of individuals who have this condition are typically asymptomatic. Brown et al[20] reported an overall prevalence of 0.71% of congenital cervical fusions present in a study of 1,400 skeletal cervical spine specimens. Of these specimens, approximately 75% of the congenital fusions were noted in the first three cervical vertebrae (fusion of C2–C3 was the most common). The majority of these patients had three or fewer cervical segments fused overall. Hensinger et al[21] developed a classification system to describe the location and extent of cervical fusions in this patient population. Type I demonstrates a fusion of the second and third cervical vertebrae with occipitalization of the atlas; type II is a long fusion with an abnormal occipitocervical junction; and type III demonstrates two block fusion segments with a single open interspace. Type III was postulated to have the worst prognosis, given the potential for overuse of a single mobile disc space between two long lever arms. However, long-term data from other studies have not shown an increase in neurologic problems in these patients.[22] Pizzutillo et al[23] reported that patients with hypermobility of the upper cervical spine were at an increased risk for neurologic problems, whereas those with involvement of the lower cervical spine were at an increased risk for early degenerative disease.

16.5.2 Larsen Syndrome

Larsen syndrome is a connective tissue disorder caused by mutations of the Filamin B gene. Clinical presentations typically include multiple joint dislocations, clubfoot, heart defects, and neonatal tracheomalacia.[24] Patients with Larsen syndrome commonly demonstrate cervical spine deformities, most notably progressive kyphosis, that has been reported to cause paralysis and death.[25] Cervical spine imaging is mandatory after diagnosis of Larsen syndrome to evaluate for any abnormalities and/or instability (▶ Fig. 16.2a–c).[26] Circumferential decompression and fusion is required in the presence of myelopathy with cord compression.[27]

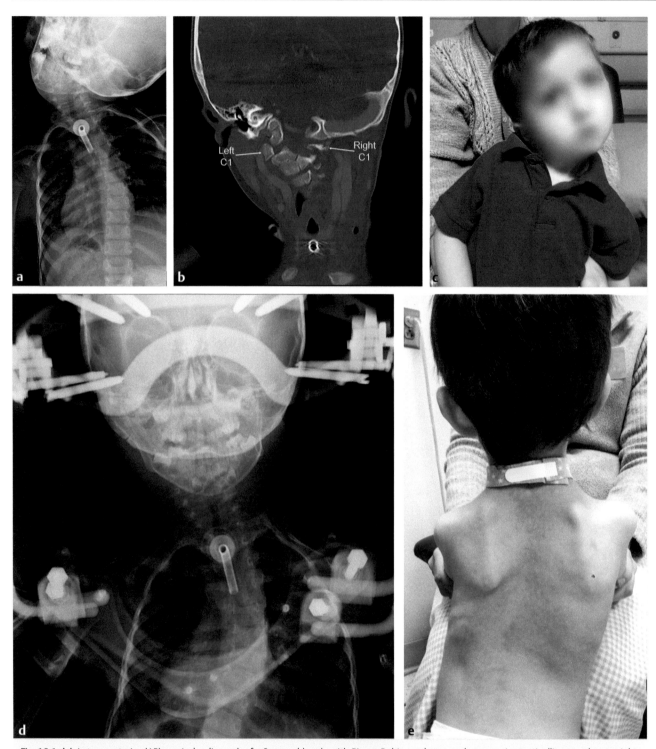

Fig. 16.1 **(a)** Anteroposterior (AP) cervical radiograph of a 3-year-old male with Pierre–Robin syndrome and progressive torticollis secondary to right-side C1 hypoplasia. **(b)** Coronal CT scan demonstrating hypoplasia of the right C1 lateral mass relative to the left lateral mass. **(c)** Clinical photograph of the patient with notable torticollis and right shoulder elevation. **(d)** Perioperative AP radiograph after sternocleidomastoid release and placement of a halo vest to achieve passive correction of the torticollis. Note the presence of a right thoracic compensatory scoliosis. **(e)** One year postoperative clinical photo after occiput to C3 posterior spinal fusion. *(Continued)*

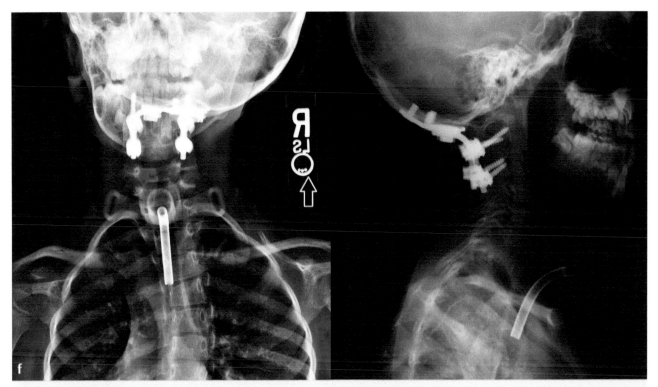

Fig 16.1 (*Continued*) **(f)** Three year postoperative AP/lateral radiographs after occiput to C3 posterior spinal fusion. Compensatory right thoracic scoliosis has nearly completely resolved.

16.5.3 Goldenhar Syndrome

Goldenhar syndrome is a congenital disorder from the abnormal development of the first and second branchial arches. Clinical manifestations include craniofacial macrosomia, vertebral anomalies, and cardiac and renal defects.[28] Cervical spine fusions/hemivertebrae have been reported in 8 to 61% of cases and occipitalization of the atlas in 5 to 30%, as well as odontoid hypoplasia and basilar invagination.[29] Cervical spine instability can result from these anomalies requiring craniocervical fusion.

16.5.4 Mucopolysaccharidosis

Mucopolysaccharidosis (MPS) disorders (Morquio disease and Hurler syndrome) result from an autosomal recessive defect resulting in the accumulation of keratin sulfate and chondroitin-6 sulfate.[30] The glycosaminoglycan accumulation results in odontoid hypoplasia leading to atlantoaxial instability and canal compromise, which are virtually universal in this condition. This has led to the recommendation by some authors for prophylactic occipitocervical fusion in selected cases.[31]

16.6 Treatment

16.6.1 Bracing

Brace treatment for congenital scoliosis has been historically ineffective and therefore not recommended for thoracolumbar congenital deformities.[32] Similarly, brace treatment for congenital cervical deformities has also been shown to be ineffective at correcting the curve or slowing/arresting progression of the deformity.[11,12] Ruf et al[11] reported that bracing was unable to influence the unbalanced spinal growth in their series of patients with cervical hemivertebra. Dubousset[12] reported on seven patients with an isolated hemi-atlas. The deformity was progressive despite efforts at conservative management with brace wear, and all required a fusion. Dr. Dubousset states, "bracing will not correct the deformity or help avoid surgery." However, the author goes on to report that "...bracing in these patients [with congenital cervical deformity] may prevent contractures of soft tissues and may retain the possibility of passive correction." Thus, in some patients, the authors of this chapter prefer to place patients in a cervical collar and perform regular stretching exercises at home in an effort to maintain flexibility of the soft tissues prior to surgical intervention. This passive stretch may allow a reasonable correction of the deformity without the need for a significant vertebral resection at the time of fusion.

16.6.2 Casting

Demirkiran et al[33] reported that serial derotational body casts can be effective as a delay tactic for significant thoracolumbar congenital deformities. The authors demonstrated a modest reduction in the deformity with serial body castings and were able to delay invasive surgical intervention for an average of 26 months, with the argument that older, larger patients are better able to tolerate surgery. As stated earlier with regard to bracing, this has not been shown to be applicable to congenital cervical deformities.

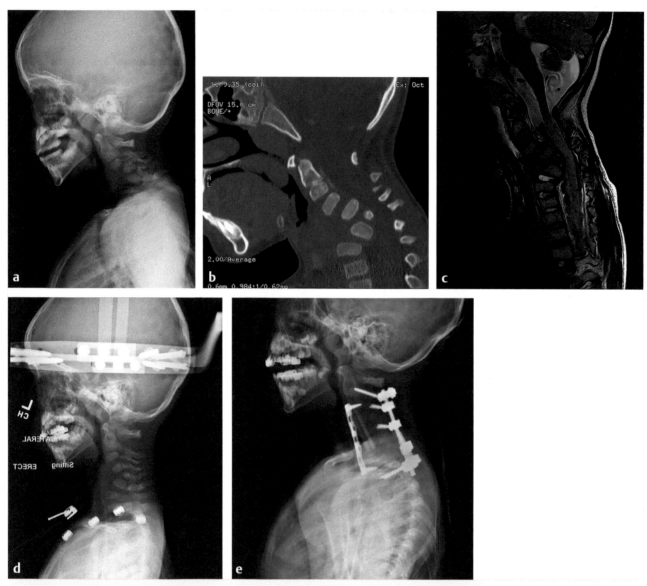

Fig. 16.2 (a) Lateral radiograph of a 4-year-old male with Larsen syndrome and progressive myelopathy and ataxia secondary to progressive cervical kyphosis. (b) Sagittal CT scan demonstrates a wedge vertebra at C5. Complete anteroposterior dissociation from C2 to C7 was also noted, which is a reported phenomenon in the cervical spine of patients with Larsen syndrome. (c) Sagittal T2-weighted MRI demonstrates cord compression and cord signal change. (d) Lateral erect radiograph in preoperative halo gravity traction. (e) Lateral radiograph 2 years status post C3–C5 corpectomy and C2–T2 anteroposterior spinal fusion. Fusion was required from C2 to T2 in order to safely span the area of complete anteroposterior dissociation from C2 to C7.

16.6.3 Preoperative Halo Vest/Halo Gravity Traction

Dubousset[12] described gradual correction of congenital torticollis with a halo cast in an effort to stretch the soft tissues and achieve a passive correction prior to occipitocervical fusion. The authors of this chapter have used this technique with a halo vest prior to definitive treatment, most commonly in cases of torticollis due to an isolated hemi-atlas. The patient is placed in a halo vest and gradually stretched over 3 to 7 days to achieve a horizontal gaze, thus achieving a slight diastasis on the concavity of the craniocervical deformity. A posterior spinal fusion is then performed from the occiput to C2 or C3 without the need for resection of the C1 hemivertebra (▶ Fig. 16.1a–f).[12,34]

Preoperative halo gravity traction can also be performed in an effort to reduce the magnitude of the deformity prior to surgery. This is generally effective only if there is an isolated congenital anomaly and less so if there is an extensive, immobile congenital fusion mass. Preoperative halo gravity traction has been safely performed by the authors for cases of severe congenital cervical kyphosis in an effort to reduce the severity of the angulation prior to anterior decompression/resection. This can only be performed in a cognitively intact patient who is able to follow commands and verbalize any neurologic complaints. Additional traction weight is applied gradually over a 5- to 14-day period with frequent around-the-clock neurologic assessments (▶ Fig. 16.2a–e). Extreme caution must be exercised, especially in patients who present with existing myelopathy due to anterior cord compression from the angular kyphosis. Cases of quadriplegia and death have been reported as a result of progressive kyphosis in this patient population.[26,35,36]

16.6.4 In Situ Fusion and Hemiepiphysiodesis

Surgical treatment should be considered in patients with congenital cervical deformity with resultant severe disfigurement or in patients with proven or expected deterioration.[11] Given the rarity of these conditions, the literature on its surgical treatment is limited. Several authors have advocated for in situ bilateral fusion or unilateral fusion of the convexity (hemiepiphysiodesis) to avoid the complexity and potential morbidity of a cervical vertebral resection. As stated earlier, a certain amount of passive correction can be achieved with preoperative halo vest and/or halo gravity traction for isolated anomalies/ hemivertebra spanning one to two segments and less so for multilevel rigid deformities, or if a congenital bar is present.

Obeid et al[37] described the successful hemiepiphysiodesis of a cervicothoracic scoliosis due to a C7 hemivertebra. A unilateral fusion was performed on the convexity from C6 to T1 using intraoperative navigation for pedicle screw placement. However, long-term results were not reported.

Winter et al[38] reported on the outcomes of 290 patients who underwent posterior fusion for congenital scoliosis. A modest correction of 28% was obtained with posterior fusion alone which increased to 36% correction with the use of Harrington instrumentation. Curve progression after fusion greater than 10 degrees ("bending of the fusion mass") was seen in 26% of patients. The authors recommended a concomitant anterior convex fusion in the setting of a unilateral bar to prevent progression of the curve after posterior fusion, especially if a contralateral hemivertebra is also present. The study did not specifically evaluate each region of the spine but did report that some of the cases were in the cervicothoracic region.

16.6.5 Hemivertebra Resection

Hemivertebra excision/resection has been reported as an effective means of definitive treatment for progressive congenital scoliosis. It is most often described in the thoracolumbar spine and has even been reported to be successful in patients as young as 1 year of age.[39] However, there are only a few reports of hemivertebra resection in the cervical spine, given the rarity of the deformity as well as the challenges of the local anatomy and vasculature.[11,14,40] A posterior-only approach is typically sufficient and comparatively less invasive in achieving satisfactory correction of congenital deformities in the thoracolumbar spine.[39] The cervical spine is complicated by the anatomic course of the vertebral arteries, which most commonly requires a combined anteroposterior approach.

Proponents of hemivertebra excision for congenital cervical deformities argue that there is little possibility for compensation above the hemivertebra, and further they are often associated with other malformations such as Klippel–Feil syndrome. Thus, there is typically little flexibility for compensation below the deformity as well. Furthermore, the patient's attempt to achieve a horizontal gaze in the setting of a congenital torticollis will often result in a compensatory trunk shift to the side of the cervical convexity.[11,12]

Deburge and Briard[14] presented a case report of a 14-year-old patient with Klippel–Feil syndrome and a C7 hemivertebra causing progressive torticollis. The patient underwent a four-stage procedure: (1) anterior C7 hemivertebra resection; (2) removal of C7 posterior elements creating a 30-degree wedge; (3) awake closed manual reduction of the osteotomy site with a halo cast; and (4) anterior fusion with instrumentation from C6 to T1. The patient was maintained in a halo cast for 3 months and was stable with neutral alignment at 2 years postoperatively. The authors stressed that the surgeon must perform a meticulous resection of the uncus anteriorly, the posterolateral corner of the pedicle, and the transverse process in order to minimize the potential for vertebral artery injury.

More recently, Ruf et al[11] reported on three patients with mean age of 9 years who underwent combined anteroposterior cervical hemivertebra resection. The hemivertebrae were located at C2–CC3, C3–CC4, and C3–C5, respectively. This procedure, as described by the authors, was completed in a two-stage process beginning with a complete laminectomy of the involved vertebra (e). This was followed by removal of the entire posterior facet and posterior wall of the foramen transversarium to expose the nerve root and vertebral artery. The vertebral artery was then protected and gently retracted laterally with a vessel loop to allow for posterior removal of the pedicle. An anterior cervical approach then followed, either on the same day or in a staged fashion. The anterior wall of the foramen transversarium was then removed, followed by the hemivertebra in its entirety along with the adjacent intervertebral discs. If there was a congenital fusion present, an appropriate wedge (30 degrees) was resected in the fusion mass to achieve an adequate correction. The anterior gap was then closed by bending the head to the convex side. Instrumented anterior fusion was then performed. The authors report this can be supplemented with an additional posterior instrumentation, compression, and fusion if necessary for stability, or if there is any residual kyphosis after the anterior procedure. In this study, the authors report appropriate correction of the deformity without any neurovascular injuries at an average follow-up of over 4 years.

16.7 Conclusion

Congenital cervical deformity with or without a hemivertebra is a relatively rare phenomenon that is typically associated with other anomalies both orthopaedic and systemic. There is a high prevalence of cardiac or renal anomalies, which require assessment at the time of diagnosis. Other diagnoses such as Klippel–Feil, Larsen, or Goldenhar syndromes often accompany congenital cervical deformities. Conservative treatment with brace wear is classically ineffective for progressive disfiguring deformities. However, resection of cervical hemivertebra requires a complex combined anteroposterior resection and fusion due to the presence of the vertebral artery. When clear progression is observed in these patients, treatment should be undertaken to minimize the complexity of the required surgical intervention and to prevent compensatory curves from becoming structural. While technically demanding, this procedure has demonstrated encouraging results in several case reports.

References

[1] Giampietro PF, Blank RD, Raggio CL, et al. Congenital and idiopathic scoliosis: clinical and genetic aspects. Clin Med Res. 2003; 1(2):125–136

[2] Wynne-Davies R. Congenital vertebral anomalies: aetiology and relationship to spina bifida cystica. J Med Genet. 1975; 12(3):280–288

[3] McMaster MJ, Ohtsuka K. The natural history of congenital scoliosis. A study of two hundred and fifty-one patients. J Bone Joint Surg Am. 1982; 64 (8):1128–1147

[4] Hedequist D, Emans J. Congenital scoliosis. J Am Acad Orthop Surg. 2004; 12 (4):266–275

[5] Hedequist D, Emans J. Congenital scoliosis: a review and update. J Pediatr Orthop. 2007; 27(1):106–116

[6] Kawakami N, Tsuji T, Imagama S, Lenke LG, Puno RM, Kuklo TR, Spinal Deformity Study Group. Classification of congenital scoliosis and kyphosis: a new approach to the three-dimensional classification for progressive vertebral anomalies requiring operative treatment. Spine. 2009; 34(17):1756–1765

[7] Williams BA, Matsumoto H, McCalla DJ, et al. Development and initial validation of the Classification of Early-Onset Scoliosis (C-EOS). J Bone Joint Surg Am. 2014; 96(16):1359–1367

[8] McMaster MJ. Congenital scoliosis. In: Weinstein SL, ed. The Pediatric Spine: Principles and Practice. 2 ed. Philadelphia, PA: Lippincott Williams & Wilkins; 2001:161–178

[9] Shawen SB, Belmont PJ, Jr, Kuklo TR, et al. Hemimetameric segmental shift: a case series and review. Spine. 2002; 27(24):E539–E544

[10] Dimeglio A. Growth in pediatric orthopaedics. J Pediatr Orthop. 2001; 21 (4):549–555

[11] Ruf M, Jensen R, Harms J. Hemivertebra resection in the cervical spine. Spine. 2005; 30(4):380–385

[12] Dubousset J. Torticollis in children caused by congenital anomalies of the atlas. J Bone Joint Surg Am. 1986; 68(2):178–188

[13] Manaligod JM, Bauman NM, Menezes AH, Smith RJ. Cervical vertebral anomalies in patients with anomalies of the head and neck. Ann Otol Rhinol Laryngol. 1999; 108(10):925–933

[14] Deburge A, Briard JL. Cervical hemivertebra excision. J Bone Joint Surg Am. 1981; 63(8):1335–1339

[15] Basu PS, Elsebaie H, Noordeen MH. Congenital spinal deformity: a comprehensive assessment at presentation. Spine. 2002; 27(20):2255–2259

[16] Buckley PS, Guille JT. Evaluation of the patient with a congenital spinal deformity. Semin Spine Surg. 2010; 22(3):110–112

[17] Shen J, Wang Z, Liu J, Xue X, Qiu G. Abnormalities associated with congenital scoliosis: a retrospective study of 226 Chinese surgical cases. Spine. 2013; 38 (10):814–818

[18] Ghandhari H, Tari HV, Ameri E, Safari MB, Fouladi DF. Vertebral, rib, and intraspinal anomalies in congenital scoliosis: a study on 202 Caucasians. Eur Spine J. 2015; 24(7):1510–1521

[19] McMaster MJ. Occult intraspinal anomalies and congenital scoliosis. J Bone Joint Surg Am. 1984; 66(4):588–601

[20] Brown MW, Templeton AW, Hodges FJ, III. The incidence of acquired and congenital fusions in the cervical spine. Am J Roentgenol Radium Ther Nucl Med. 1964; 92:1255–1259

[21] Hensinger RN, Lang JE, MacEwen GD. Klippel-Feil syndrome; a constellation of associated anomalies. J Bone Joint Surg Am. 1974; 56(6):1246–1253

[22] Guille JT, Miller A, Bowen JR, Forlin E, Caro PA. The natural history of Klippel-Feil syndrome: clinical, roentgenographic, and magnetic resonance imaging findings at adulthood. J Pediatr Orthop. 1995; 15(5):617–626

[23] Pizzutillo PD, Woods M, Nicholson L, MacEwen GD. Risk factors in Klippel-Feil syndrome. Spine. 1994; 19(18):2110–2116

[24] McKay SD, Al-Omari A, Tomlinson LA, Dormans JP. Review of cervical spine anomalies in genetic syndromes. Spine. 2012; 37(5):E269–E277

[25] Campbell RM, Jr. Spine deformities in rare congenital syndromes: clinical issues. Spine. 2009; 34(17):1815–1827

[26] Johnston CE, II, Birch JG, Daniels JL. Cervical kyphosis in patients who have Larsen syndrome. J Bone Joint Surg Am. 1996; 78(4):538–545

[27] Sakaura H, Matsuoka T, Iwasaki M, Yonenobu K, Yoshikawa H. Surgical treatment of cervical kyphosis in Larsen syndrome: report of 3 cases and review of the literature. Spine. 2007; 32(1):E39–E44

[28] Feingold M, Baum J. Goldenhar's syndrome. Am J Dis Child. 1978; 132 (2):136–138

[29] Healey D, Letts M, Jarvis JG. Cervical spine instability in children with Goldenhar's syndrome. Can J Surg. 2002; 45(5):341–344

[30] Montaño AM, Tomatsu S, Gottesman GS, Smith M, Orii T. International Morquio A Registry: clinical manifestation and natural course of Morquio A disease. J Inherit Metab Dis. 2007; 30(2):165–174

[31] White KK, Steinman S, Mubarak SJ. Cervical stenosis and spastic quadriparesis in Morquio disease (MPS IV). A case report with twenty-six-year follow-up. J Bone Joint Surg Am. 2009; 91(2):438–442

[32] Winter RB, Moe JH, MacEwen GD, Peon-Vidales H. The Milwaukee brace in the nonoperative treatment of congenital scoliosis. Spine. 1976; 1(2):85–96

[33] Demirkiran HG, Bekmez S, Celilov R, Ayvaz M, Dede O, Yazici M. Serial derotational casting in congenital scoliosis as a time-buying strategy. J Pediatr Orthop. 2015; 35(1):43–49

[34] Hensinger RN. Congenital anomalies of the cervical spine. Clin Orthop Relat Res. 1991(264):16–38

[35] Madera M, Crawford A, Mangano FT. Management of severe cervical kyphosis in a patient with Larsen syndrome. Case report. J Neurosurg Pediatr. 2008; 1 (4):320–324

[36] Muzumdar AS, Lowry RB, Robinson CE. Quadriplegia in Larsen syndrome. Birth Defects Orig Artic Ser. 1977; 13 3C:202–211

[37] Obeid I, Taieb A, Vital JM. Circumferential convex growth arrest by posterior approach for double cervicothoracic curves in congenital scoliosis. Eur Spine J. 2013; 22(9):2126–2129

[38] Winter RB, Moe JH, Lonstein JE. Posterior spinal arthrodesis for congenital scoliosis. An analysis of the cases of two hundred and ninety patients, five to nineteen years old. J Bone Joint Surg Am. 1984; 66(8):1188–1197

[39] Ruf M, Harms J. Posterior hemivertebra resection with transpedicular instrumentation: early correction in children aged 1 to 6 years. Spine. 2003; 28 (18):2132–2138

[40] Chen Z, Qiu Y, Zhu Z, et al. Posterior-only hemivertebra resection for congenital cervicothoracic scoliosis: correcting neck tilt and balancing the shoulders. Spine. 2018; 43(6):394–401

17 Risk Stratification and Frailty in Complex Cervical Surgery

Emily K. Miller and Christopher I. Shaffrey

Abstract

Accurate risk stratification is essential for preoperative patient counseling, surgical planning, comparing intersurgeon outcomes, and prediction of anticipated complication rates for the development of quality metric ranges. Traditional statistical methods have identified many patient, surgical, and systems factors that associate with increased risk of complications or other adverse outcomes. Current research focuses on taking these factors and generating clinically useful tools to estimate individual risk. The American Society of Anesthesiologists has been used to classify patients and predict surgical risk for years; however, it only assesses medical comorbidities and does not account for other patient factors that may affect outcome. Frailty indices provide a comprehensive assessment of all patient factors to generate more individualized patient risk scores. Invasiveness indices provide a quantitative method to compare risk of various surgical procedures and will likely be a useful tool for individualized surgical planning. Advanced predictive modeling uses complex algorithms to identify patterns in large datasets to combine assessments of patient and surgical factors to provide an individualized risk score for each patient. Multidisciplinary team conferences are also used as a method of risk stratification. Though less quantitative and more subject to bias, this does provide an opportunity to coordinate care efforts to improve preoperative patient optimization, investigate eligibility for other treatment options, optimize planned surgical procedure, and ensure that all perioperative providers know specific risks for individual patients. This chapter provides an overview of the currently available tools and the future areas of investigation in this field.

Keywords: risk stratification, frailty, invasiveness, predictive modeling, multidisciplinary

17.1 Introduction

The practice of individualized medicine is on the rise in all fields of medicine. When discussing risks and benefits of a particular procedure with patients, surgeons often rely on average values and use gestalt to estimate whether a given patient has higher or lower than average risk. Risk stratification research focuses on factors that are associated with severe complications and/or poor outcomes in order to improve preoperative predictions of risk. As risk stratification tools grow progressively more reliable and comprehensive, it becomes possible to give patients a more accurate assessment of their personal risk undergoing a given procedure.

Spine surgery, including complex cervical surgery, has a very high rate of complications. In a prospective database of 78 cervical deformity patients, 44% had at least one complication and 24% had at least one major complication.[1] Among those patients who underwent three-column osteotomy procedures in the cervical spine, the complication rate was 60% and the reoperation rate was 33%.[2] Advances in surgery and anesthesia have made surgery available to older patients with more comorbidities by reducing the physiologic impact.[3] Given this degree of risk associated with cervical spine operations, improved preoperative risk stratification is essential to identify those patients at highest risk of severe complication. It is important that those patients who are at highest risk may also be those who have the greatest potential benefit. In adult spinal deformity, despite the higher rate of complications in older patients (62% in those older than 75 years[4]), these patients also tend to experience greater improvement in pain and disability with surgical treatment.[5] Given the large discrepancy between potential benefit and potential harm, adequate preoperative risk stratification strategies are essential, particularly for elderly patients undergoing high-risk procedures, to minimize morbidity and mortality.

Risk stratification is also an important tool in cost-effectiveness strategies,[6,7,8] development of quality metric ranges in health policy, and accurate comparisons of intersurgeon complication rates. Minimization of complication incidence, identification of patients most likely to benefit from postoperative intensive care, and preoperative discharge planning are all potential cost-effectiveness methods that rely on adequate risk stratification. Additionally, when analyzing interventions and changes in surgical technique for efficacy, accurate risk stratification of patients is essential to control for patient factors. Health policy interventions are already comparing hospital outcomes to impact payments. As comparing interfacility and intersurgeon complication rates becomes standard practice, accurate risk stratification analysis of patients is essential to weight complication rates by patient population risk. If the current system continues to move toward bundled payments, it is important to quantify risk of complications depending on specific procedure and patient factors since payments need to be adjusted accordingly. All of these upcoming challenges in health policy rely on accurate patient and procedure risk stratification.

Given the importance of accurate risk stratification, this chapter investigates the current status of risk stratification tools, how these tools can be applied specifically to complex cervical deformity, and where further efforts are needed. Fortunately, risk stratification has become increasingly present in recent research, with many new tools and strategies being developed. As these methods become more quantitative and prognostic, avoiding inappropriately restrictive health policy regulations is essential to prevent some patients from receiving necessary care.

17.2 Retrospective Regression Models

By using regression models, researchers have identified many factors associated with worse outcomes based on complication incidence, reoperation rate, quality of life, length of hospital stay, readmission rate, and discharge to facility.[9] These factors can be divided into patient factors (▶ Table 17.1) and surgical factors (▶ Table 17.2).[9,10,11,12] However, given the number of identified contributors to preoperative risk, it is impossible to accurately assess and weigh each of these measurements in a routine office visit. In order to remedy this issue, risk tools were developed.

17.3 Risk Stratification Tools

The American Society of Anesthesiologists (ASA) classification scheme, first introduced in 1941 to evaluate overall health status of patients prior to surgery (▶ Table 17.3),[13,14] has long been used as a risk stratification tool to identify those patients at the highest risk. Key advantages of the ASA classification are ease of use and prevalence, but the main disadvantage is that it focuses only on comorbidities and does not take into account other patient or surgical factors. The ASA has been shown to have a strong correlation with major complication incidence and increased length of stay.[15] The Charlson Comorbidity Index is a similar tool that estimates a patient's 10-year mortality, is associated with complication incidence, and is occasionally used for risk stratification (▶ Table 17.4).[16]

Table 17.1 Patient factors

Diagnosed medical comorbidities	Overall preoperative functional status	Psychological factors	Other
Heart disease Bleeding/Clotting Disorder Peripheral vascular disease Prior CVA Lung disease Kidney disease Osteoporosis Diabetes Hypertension Neurological comorbidity Cancer BMI	Totally dependent Partially dependent Independent Difficulty with specific ADLs, iADLs, mobility	Preoperative pain catastrophizing Kinesophobia Confidence Optimism Motivation Self-efficacy Stress Depression Social support Dementia Poor cognition	Substance use/abuse (especially smoking) Chronological age Gender Race Coagulation profile (low platelets, high PTT, high INR) Prealbumin Preoperative education classes Peer support

Abbreviations: BMI, body mass index; CVA, cerebrovascular accident; iADLs, instrumental activities of daily living; INR, international normalized ratio; PTT, partial thromboplastin time.

Table 17.2 Surgical factors

Invasiveness of the procedure	Level of surgical skill	Systems factors
Operative time Osteotomy Pelvic fixation Fusion length Blood loss	Years of practice Volume of complex procedures	Facility volume Designated spine team (anesthesia/nursing) Preoperative steroid use Hospital size

Table 17.3 American Society of Anesthesiologists

Class	Definition
1	No comorbidities (healthy, non-smoking, minimal substance use)
2	Mild systemic disease (well-controlled hypertension or diabetes, current smoker)
3	Severe systemic disease (poorly controlled hypertension/diabetes/COPD, mild congestive heart failure)
4	Severe systemic disease that is a constant threat to life (recent [<3 mo] myocardial infarction, cerebrovascular accident, transient ischemic event, sepsis)
5	Moribund patient not expected to survive without the surgery (ruptured aortic aneurysm, massive trauma)
6	Brain-dead patient undergoing organ removal for donation

Abbreviation: COPD, chronic obstructive pulmonary disease.

Table 17.4 Charlson Comorbidity Index

Points given	Comorbidity
1	Myocardial infarct, congestive cardiac insufficiency, peripheral vascular disease, dementia, cerebrovascular disease, chronic pulmonary disease, connective tissue disease, diabetes without complications, ulcers, chronic disease of the liver or cirrhosis
2	Lymphoma, leukemia, benign tumors, diabetes with complications, moderate or severe renal disease, hemiplegia
3	Moderate or severe liver disease
6	Malignant tumor, metastatic cancer, AIDS

17.4 Frailty

In the last 5 years, research has focused on frailty as a potential predictor of poor outcomes following surgery. As a measure of physiologic rather than chronologic age,[17] frailty has been shown to be a better predictor of increased complication rate, longer length of hospital stay, and worse postoperative health-related quality-of-life (HRQoL) scores than chronologic age alone in general surgery.[18,19,20,21] Frailty is a comprehensive overview of patient factors which could potentially contribute to increased surgical risk including comorbidities, mental health, physical health, social support, and functional status. Given the aging population in the United States and worldwide,[22] and the fact that surgeries are now being made available to older patients with more comorbidities,[3] accurate risk stratification including all patient factors is especially critical.

Three recent studies in spine surgery have published an association between frailty and complications; however, most of these studies have utilized the modified frailty index. Frailty indices are based on the concept that frailty can be measured as an accumulation of deficits in all areas of health. The modified frailty index was developed by analyzing the National Surgical Quality Improvement Program (NSQIP) database and identifying 11 recorded variables that corresponded to 16 of the 70 variables in the Canadian Study of Health and Aging Frailty Index.[23,24,25,26] However, when Searle et al tested precision and accuracy of frailty indices created following the recommended rubric, a frailty index was found to be precise and accurate as long as enough (30–40) variables were included in the model, but frailty measurements were unstable and imprecise at lower numbers, especially below 10 variables.[27] In other words, the precise variable composition of the frailty index was found to not impact the calculation of frailty as long as enough variables were included in the model. There is no study comparing accuracy of frailty measurements using the modified frailty index to full frailty indices (those including at least 30–40 variables) or to other frailty calculators such as the frailty phenotype. While the modified frailty index has been shown to be another useful risk stratification tool similar to the ASA, it is not yet established whether this is an accurate measure of frailty. Additionally, these studies were all performed using the NSQIP database. Large national databases rely on current procedural terminology[28] to identify patients by diagnosis which leads to inclusion discrepancies, they only record complications for 30 days postoperatively, and they have been shown to underreport complications compared to surgeon-maintained databases. This leads to significant discrepancies in reporting.[29]

The Cervical Deformity Frailty Index (CD-FI), developed by the International Spine Study Group, includes 40 variables and was developed utilizing the validated methodology mentioned earlier. It has been shown to be associated with major complication (▶ Fig. 17.1).[30] The Adult Spinal Deformity Frailty Index (ASD-FI), on which the CD-FI was based, has been more extensively studied and validated in multiple databases with strong associations with both major complication incidence and hospital length of stay. Based on these data, it has been established that frailty is a good risk stratification tool for spine surgery. The main advantage of developing a frailty-based risk stratification tool is that it is a comprehensive evaluation of all preoperative patient factors that affect individual risk of complications, increased length of hospital stay, and other adverse events.

17.5 Invasiveness

While patient factors can increase individual risk of complication with a given procedure, the invasiveness of the specific procedure performed can significantly alter the anticipated risk. Surgical factors such as performance of three-column osteotomies and pelvic fixation have a substantial impact on the risk of a given procedure regardless of patient physiologic status. The Spine Surgery Invasiveness Index (SSII), developed by Mirza et al, generates an invasiveness score based only on number of levels fused, instrumented, and decompressed (▶ Table 17.5).[31] This tool was validated through association with blood loss and operative time and has been shown to have a significant correlation with surgical-site infection.[32,33] However, this tool is not useful for differentiating between similar procedures (such as anterior cervical discectomy and fusion

Fig. 17.1 Incidence of major complications.

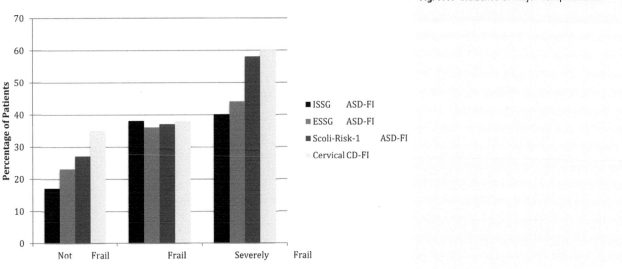

Table 17.5 Surgical factors included in invasiveness indices

Spine Surgery Invasiveness Index	Adult Deformity Surgery Complexity Index (ADSCI)	Adult Spinal Deformity Surgical Invasiveness Score
Number of levels fused	Number of levels fused	Number of levels fused
Number of levels decompressed	Number of levels decompressed	Number of levels decompressed
Number of levels instrumented	Number of levels instrumented	Number of levels instrumented
	Number of cemented levels	Number of anterior lumbar interbody fusions
	Number of interbody fusions	Number of transforaminal/posterior lumbar interbody fusions
	Number of Smith–Petersen osteotomies	
	Number of pedicle subtraction osteotomies	Number of Smith–Peterson osteotomies
	Number of posterior vertebral column resections	Number of three-column osteotomies
	Pelvic fixation	Pelvic fixation
	Revision vs. primary	Revision vs. primary

with and without anterior plating) and is, therefore, less helpful for assessing specific procedure risk for a given patient. The Adult Deformity Surgery Complexity Index (ADSCI) and the Adult Spinal Deformity Surgical Invasiveness Score (ASDSIS), developed by Pellisé et al and Neuman et al in 2017, focus on comparing invasiveness of ASD surgeries (▶ Table 17.5). Both models had improved correlation with blood loss and surgery duration compared to the SSII in ASD surgery.[34,35] No results have been published yet looking at associations with complication rate and outcome; however, research is currently ongoing. Further research will be needed to determine whether variations in invasiveness can mediate the increased risk of complications and adverse events for frail patients.

17.6 Predictive Modeling

Advanced predictive modeling, a new and exciting approach to Big Data, has allowed for significant advances in outcomes research. Over the last decade, predictive modeling has led to the development of very accurate models for surgical outcomes analyses. Unlike predictive modeling, traditional statistical methods are designed to test specific hypotheses, rely on many required assumptions, and produce odds/hazard ratios for each variable. While traditional statistical methods, like regressions, are based on averages of large groups, predictive analytics identifies patterns in large datasets in order to create accurate, patient-specific predictive models. Complex computer algorithms and even artificial intelligence analyze hundreds to thousands of patients with hundreds of variables to build models to predict a specific outcome of interest without any control group or hypothesis. Those variables found in frailty or invasiveness indices can easily be incorporated into a large predictive model.

Assuming that the dataset is complete and accurate, multiple types of models can be developed for a single outcome of interest within a given dataset to identify which has the greatest utility for the aims of the model. These models can be combined to improve the overall accuracy of the model. However, accuracy, generalizability, and transparency of models must be balanced in order to ensure utility of the model. A very accurate model for a specific population may not be generalizable to other datasets or it may be so complicated that the maker does not know exactly how the model is making its predictions.

In ASD, advanced predictive modeling has been used to examine risk of proximal junctional kyphosis, risk of major complications, and likelihood of reaching Oswestry Disability Index (ODI) minimal clinically important difference (MCID) at 2

years following surgery. For proximal junctional kyphosis/proximal junctional failure, the model accuracy was 87.6% with an area under the receiver operating characteristics (AUROC) of 0.89.[36] For major complications, the model accuracy was 86.3% with an AUROC of 0.89.[37] For ODI MCID, the model accuracy was 86% with an AUROC of 0.96. Patients predicted to meet MCID had significantly greater mean quality-adjusted life-years (QALYs) at 2 years postsurgery than those patients not predicted to meet MCID. Using predictive modeling, authors were able to predict 2-year QALYs gained in ASD patients.[38] With the addition of artificial intelligence, accurate predictive models can be used as a point-of-care decision tool to aid in surgical decision making and preoperative patient counseling.

17.7 Multidisciplinary Teams

Another new risk stratification technique is to assess each individual patient in a multidisciplinary preoperative evaluation conference to assess patient risk of surgery, whether that risk can be minimized, and alternative treatments to surgery. At the Virginia Mason Medical Center (VMMC), patients are presented at monthly multidisciplinary conferences including an internist, a physiatrist, physical therapists, two designated complex spine anesthesiologists, the nurses who coordinate the complex spine cases, and the operating neurosurgeon and orthopaedic surgeon. All participants in the conference have an equal voice in deciding who might benefit from further nonoperative management, who requires further medical optimization prior to operative treatment, and who can proceed directly to operative management.[39,40] Unlike the tools mentioned previously, multidisciplinary conferences are more subject to personal bias, knowledge, and expertise of the conference participants. At VMMC, out of 100 patients who were reviewed by the multidisciplinary team who had previously been recommended for lumbar spine fusion by an outside surgeon, the team recommended nonoperative management for 58. In the 42 operative patients, there were no 30-day complications.[10] Through this protocol, they limited surgical care to only lower-risk patients. While this significantly decreased the number of complications, it may have excluded some patients who might have substantially benefited.

Additionally, VMMC also started several new systems interventions aimed at minimizing risk with surgery concurrently with the study on multidisciplinary conferences. Potential systems interventions to minimize risk include offering a preoperative course for patients; having a designated spine surgery team including nurses, operating room technicians, and anesthesiologists; having two surgeons performing the procedure bilaterally simultaneously to minimize operative times; maintaining easily visible tracking boards for laboratory parameters and blood product availability; and staging the operation to promote patient physiologic stability, standardized sign-out protocols, observation in the ICU postoperatively, and early mobilization with physical therapy.[39,40] These interventions are likely confounding variables in assessing the impact of multidisciplinary risk stratification.

17.8 Key Points/Summary/Clinical Application

1. Accurate, comprehensive risk stratification is essential:
   - As insurance reimbursements and health policies are increasingly dependent on outcomes, individual patients must be risk stratified in order to determine anticipated outcomes, hospital length of stay, and complication rate.
   - Risk stratification is necessary to accurately compare inter-surgeon and interfacility outcomes.
   - Individualized risk assessment allows for more personalized surgical planning. Surgical invasiveness could be tailored to accommodate higher risk patients to decrease their individual risk of complication or poor outcome.
   - Patient–surgeon decision-making discussions would have more personalized estimations of risk and expectations for recovery so that patients can make better informed decisions. This may lead to increased patient satisfaction following surgical intervention.
2. Currently utilized tools such as the ASA and CCI focus only on comorbidities. While they are useful estimates for anesthesiologists predicting medical complications perioperatively (ASA) or for predicting 10-year mortality (CCI), their value for predicting surgical complications and length of stay is limited by only focusing on a single-patient factor (comorbidities).
3. Preoperative frailty assessment is a much more comprehensive score incorporating all patient factors contributing to increased risk of surgical intervention.
   - The CD-FI is strongly associated with increased risk of major complications and can be used as a preclinical review of systems survey to provide patients with a personalized risk estimate.
   - There are numerous other frailty assessment tools that are well studied and validated that could be included in primary care preoperative patient clearance for surgery. These scales have been shown to correlate well with frailty indices like the CD-FI.
   - The modified frailty index, though potentially a good risk stratification tool, is not a measurement of frailty and is not a comprehensive assessment of patient factors.
4. Invasiveness scores, including the SSII, the ADSCI, and the ASDSIS, require further investigation prior to implementation in clinical practice.
   - The SSII is the only one of the three indices that has been shown to correlate with a complication (surgical-site infection). The others have only been validated as measures of invasiveness looking at estimated blood loss and operative time.
   - The SSII, while useful for distinguishing between major and minor procedures, is not detailed enough to differentiate between comparable procedures with minor changes in surgical strategy. More detailed indices need to be developed for specific surgical procedures.
   - The ADSCI and ASDSIS are very detailed and are good for determining invasiveness for ASD surgery; however, they have not yet published results demonstrating correlation with complication incidence or other outcomes of interest. This research is ongoing.
5. Advanced predictive modeling is the future of risk stratification. Eventually, predictive models will be able to assess individual risk of a given procedure, incorporating all pertinent factors that might impact a specific outcome like complication incidence. However, these tools are not currently available for use in a clinical setting.
6. Multidisciplinary conferences, as a risk stratification tool, are subject to bias of the providers involved, but could also lead to improved preoperative patient optimization and improved coordination for the surgical team during surgery.
   - Including primary care physicians and other providers in preoperative planning can improve preoperative patient optimization through interventions like smoking cessation counseling and osteoporosis treatment.
   - Including other spine specialists, such as interventional spine physicians and physical therapists, could improve risk–benefit discussions with patients by providing a more thorough discussion of potential alternatives to surgery or lack thereof.
   - Including anesthesiologists, operating room nurses, and internists in the conferences ensures that on the day of the surgery, everyone on the surgical team knows the patient and potential risks for that patient.

References

[1] Smith JS, Ramchandran S, Lafage V, et al. International Spine Study Group. Prospective multicenter assessment of early complication rates associated with adult cervical deformity surgery in 78 patients. Neurosurgery. 2016; 79 (3):378–388

[2] Theologis AA, Tabaraee E, Funao H, et al. Three-column osteotomies of the lower cervical and upper thoracic spine: comparison of early outcomes, radiographic parameters, and peri-operative complications in 48 patients. Eur Spine J. 2015; 24 Suppl 1:S23–S30

[3] Ambler GK, Brooks DE, Al Zuhir N, et al. Effect of frailty on short- and mid-term outcomes in vascular surgical patients. Br J Surg. 2015; 102(6):638–645

[4] Acosta FL, Jr, McClendon J, Jr, O'Shaughnessy BA, et al. Morbidity and mortality after spinal deformity surgery in patients 75 years and older: complications and predictive factors. J Neurosurg Spine. 2011; 15(6):667–674

[5] Smith JS, Shaffrey CI, Glassman SD, et al. Spinal Deformity Study Group. Risk-benefit assessment of surgery for adult scoliosis: an analysis based on patient age. Spine. 2011; 36(10):817–824

[6] Hughes M, Lip GY, Guideline Development Group, National Clinical Guideline for Management of Atrial Fibrillation in Primary and Secondary Care, National Institute for Health and Clinical Excellence. Stroke and thromboembolism in atrial fibrillation: a systematic review of stroke risk factors, risk stratification schema and cost effectiveness data. Thromb Haemost. 2008; 99:295–304

[7] Kanis JA, Borgstrom F, De Laet C, et al. Assessment of fracture risk. Osteoporos Int. 2005; 16(6):581–589

[8] Sheldon R, O'Brien BJ, Blackhouse G, et al. for the Canadian Implantable Defibrillator Study (CIDS) Investigators. Effect of clinical risk stratification on cost-effectiveness of the implantable cardioverter-defibrillator: the Canadian implantable defibrillator study. Circulation. 2001; 104(14):1622–1626

[9] Ames CP, Scheer JK, Lafage V, et al. Adult spinal deformity: epidemiology, health impact, evaluation, and management. Spine Deform. 2016; 4(4): 310–322

[10] Buchlak QD, Yanamadala V, Leveque JC, Sethi R. Complication avoidance with pre-operative screening: insights from the Seattle spine team. Curr Rev Musculoskelet Med. 2016; 9(3):316–326

[11] Flanigan DC, Everhart JS, Glassman AH. Psychological factors affecting rehabilitation and outcomes following elective orthopaedic surgery. J Am Acad Orthop Surg. 2015; 23(9):563–570

[12] Wang K, Vitale M. Risk stratification: perspectives of the patient, surgeon, and health system. Spine Deform. 2016; 4(1):1–2

[13] Wolters U, Wolf T, Stützer H, Schröder T. ASA classification and perioperative variables as predictors of postoperative outcome. Br J Anaesth. 1996; 77 (2):217–222

[14] Keats AS. The ASA classification of physical status–a recapitulation. Anesthesiology. 1978; 49(4):233–236

[15] Phan K, Kim JS, Lee NJ, Kothari P, Cho SK. Relationship between ASA scores and 30-day readmissions in patients undergoing anterior cervical discectomy and fusion. Spine. 2017; 42(2):85–91

[16] Whitmore RG, Stephen JH, Vernick C, et al. ASA grade and Charlson Comorbidity Index of spinal surgery patients: correlation with complications and societal costs. Spine J. 2014; 14(1):31–38

[17] Rockwood K, Song X, MacKnight C, et al. A global clinical measure of fitness and frailty in elderly people. CMAJ. 2005; 173(5):489–495

[18] Farhat JS, Velanovich V, Falvo AJ, et al. Are the frail destined to fail? Frailty index as predictor of surgical morbidity and mortality in the elderly. J Trauma Acute Care Surg. 2012; 72(6):1526–1530, discussion 1530–1531

[19] Joseph B, Pandit V, Sadoun M, et al. Frailty in surgery. J Trauma Acute Care Surg. 2014; 76(4):1151–1156

[20] Kim SW, Han HS, Jung HW, et al. Multidimensional frailty score for the prediction of postoperative mortality risk. JAMA Surg. 2014; 149(7):633–640

[21] Schuurmans H, Steverink N, Lindenberg S, Frieswijk N, Slaets JP. Old or frail: what tells us more? J Gerontol A Biol Sci Med Sci. 2004; 59(9):M962–M965

[22] Yancik R. Population aging and cancer: a cross-national concern. Cancer J. 2005; 11(6):437–441

[23] Phan K, Kim JS, Lee NJ, et al. Frailty is associated with morbidity in adults undergoing elective anterior lumbar interbody fusion (ALIF) surgery. Spine J. 2017; 17(4):538–544

[24] Ali R, Schwalb JM, Nerenz DR, Antoine HJ, Rubinfeld I. Use of the modified frailty index to predict 30-day morbidity and mortality from spine surgery. J Neurosurg Spine. 2016; 25(4):537–541

[25] Leven DM, Lee NJ, Kothari P, et al. Frailty index is a significant predictor of complications and mortality after surgery for adult spinal deformity. Spine. 2016; 41(23):E1394–E1401

[26] Flexman AM, Charest-Morin R, Stobart L, Street J, Ryerson CJ. Frailty and postoperative outcomes in patients undergoing surgery for degenerative spine disease. Spine J. 2016; 16(11):1315–1323

[27] Searle SD, Mitnitski A, Gahbauer EA, Gill TM, Rockwood K. A standard procedure for creating a frailty index. BMC Geriatr. 2008; 8(24):24

[28] American Medical Association. Current Procedural Terminology: CPT 2016. Chicago, IL: American Medical Association; 2016

[29] Poorman GW, Passias PG, Buckland AJ, et al. International Spine Study Group (ISSG). Comparative analysis of perioperative outcomes using nationally derived hospital discharge data relative to a prospective multicenter surgical database of adult spinal deformity surgery. Spine. 2017; 42(15):1165–1171

[30] Miller EK, Ailon T, Neuman BJ, et al. International Spine Study Group. Assessment of a novel adult cervical deformity frailty index as a component of preoperative risk stratification. World Neurosurg. 2018; 109:e800–e806

[31] Mirza SK, Deyo RA, Heagerty PJ, Turner JA, Lee LA, Goodkin R. Towards standardized measurement of adverse events in spine surgery: conceptual model and pilot evaluation. BMC Musculoskelet Disord. 2006; 7:53

[32] Mirza SK, Deyo RA, Heagerty PJ, et al. Development of an index to characterize the "invasiveness" of spine surgery: validation by comparison to blood loss and operative time. Spine. 2008; 33(24):2651–2661, discussion 2662

[33] Cizik AM, Lee MJ, Martin BI, et al. Using the spine surgical invasiveness index to identify risk of surgical site infection: a multivariate analysis. J Bone Joint Surg Am. 2012; 94(4):335–342

[34] Pellisé F, Vila-Casademunt A, Núñez-Pereira S, et al. The Adult Deformity Surgery Complexity Index (ADSCI): a valid tool to quantify the complexity of posterior adult spinal deformity surgery and predict postoperative complications. Spine J. 2018; 18(2):216–225

[35] Neuman BJ, Ailon T, Klineberg E, et al. Development and validation of a novel adult spinal deformity surgical invasiveness score: analysis of 464 patients. Neurosurgery. 2018; 82(6):847–853

[36] Scheer JK, Osorio JA, Smith JS, et al. International Spine Study Group. Development of validated computer-based preoperative predictive model for proximal junction failure (PJF) or clinically significant PJK with 86% accuracy based on 510 ASD patients with 2-year follow-up. Spine. 2016; 41(22):E1328–E1335

[37] Scheer JK, Smith JS, Schwab F, et al. International Spine Study Group. Development of a preoperative predictive model for major complications following adult spinal deformity surgery. J Neurosurg Spine. 2017; 26(6):736–743

[38] Scheer JK, Oh T, Smith JS, Shaffrey CI, Daniels AH, Sciubba DM, Hamilton DK, Protopsaltis TS, Passias PG, Hart RA, Burton DC, Bess S, Lafage R, Lafage V, Schwab F, Klineberg EO, Ames CP, International Spine Study Group. Development of a validated computer-based preoperative predictive model for pseudarthrosis with 91% accuracy in 336 adult spinal deformity patients. Neurosurg Focus. 2018 Nov 1; 45(5):E11

[39] Sethi RK, Pong RP, Leveque JC, Dean TC, Olivar SJ, Rupp SM. The Seattle Spine Team Approach to adult deformity surgery: a systems-based approach to perioperative care and subsequent reduction in perioperative complication rates. Spine Deform. 2014; 2(2):95–103

[40] Yanamadala V, Kim Y, Buchlak QD, et al. Multidisciplinary evaluation leads to the decreased utilization of lumbar spine fusion: an observational cohort pilot study. Spine. 2017; 42(17):E1016–E1023

18 Surgical and Neurological Complications

Brandon B. Carlson, Han Jo Kim, and Justin S. Smith

Abstract

Cervical deformity surgeries tend to be high-risk procedures, and recent prospective reports have demonstrated complication rates as high as 43.6% in this patient population. These patients are exposed to multiple medical and surgical risks, including development of new neurological deficits, associated with their surgeries. This chapter summarizes general surgical and neurologic risks associated with cervical spine surgery and presents the limited literature currently available that is specific to cervical deformity surgery. In the preoperative setting, this may help surgeons with surgical planning and may also serve as a valuable resource for the appropriate preoperative counseling of patients. Additionally, if complications are encountered, surgeons will be better equipped to recognize, handle, and mange patients appropriately and judiciously in order to optimize patient outcomes.

Keywords: pseudarthrosis, dysphagia, C5 palsy, infection, instrumentation failure

18.1 Introduction

Cervical deformity surgery typically involves technically demanding and high-risk procedures with specific surgical goals. These procedures can have substantial impact for improving quality of life; however, many techniques used to correct deformities can increase complication risks. Surgeons treating cervical deformity patients should clearly understand the risks and counsel their patients extensively prior to surgery regarding possible complications. A recent prospective study of cervical deformity patients demonstrated an overall early (within 30 days of surgery) complication rate of 43.6%[1] and another study of patients undergoing three-column osteotomies reported a complication rate of 56.5% within 90 days of surgery.[2] Complications may have transient or lasting effects and may alter functional status and/or quality of life permanently. The incidence of complications may vary based on diagnosis, surgical factors, and confounding patient factors. Some complications may be realized during surgery, while others may not be readily appreciated until postoperatively. Treating complications may range from observation to acute surgical intervention. Surgeons treating cervical deformity should understand the possible adverse events related to cervical surgery in general, the surgical approaches, and the complications specifically associated with deformity surgery. This chapter discusses surgical and neurological complications associated with cervical deformity surgery and presents the supporting literature and suggested management strategies.

18.2 Surgical Complications

Surgical complications during cervical spinal procedures may be directly related to the region and type of surgery, surgical approaches, underlying pathology, or patient factors. Cervical deformity surgery has higher reported complication rates compared to other cervical procedures, based on recent prospective reports.[1,2] Awareness of these potential complications allows surgeons to accurately counsel their patients, identify problems earlier, and implement appropriate treatments as necessary. This section discusses surgical complications associated with the anterior cervical approach, vascular injuries, dural tears and cerebrospinal leaks, wound complications and infections, pseudarthrosis, and instrumentation-associated complications. Surgical complications are summarized in ▶ Table 18.1.

18.2.1 Anterior Cervical Approach Complications

The anterior cervical spine approach described by Smith and Robinson provides a generally safe and reproducible surgical dissection.[3] Compared to the posterior cervical approach, the anterior approach has unique risks and complications including vascular, neurologic, tracheal, and esophageal injuries. These complications can vary in severity depending on structures involved and extent of injury.

Several nerves are at risk during anterior cervical surgery. Surgical level determines the risk for different nerves. The hypoglossal nerve is at highest risk during anterior exposures from C1 through C3. These injuries are extremely rare with a reported incidence of 0.01%.[4] Palsy of the hypoglossal nerve results in ipsilateral tongue deviation and difficulty swallowing due to impairment of food transport toward the back of the mouth. The superior laryngeal nerve is typically at highest risk at C3–C4 and has a reported injury incidence of 0 to 1.25%.[5] This nerve has two branches: internal (sensory) and external (motor). Injury to the internal branch may result in aspiration difficulties, while injuries to the external branch may result in a monotone voice due to loss of cricothyroid muscle function. The recurrent laryngeal nerve (RLN) is vulnerable at multiple levels and usually injured via a traction-type injury as it sits in the tracheoesophageal groove. Damage to this nerve may result in hoarseness or loss of voice due to partial or complete paralysis of the posterior cricoarytenoid muscle in the larynx. The sympathetic chain is also at risk during the anterior exposure as it lies on the lateral margins of the longus colli. Careful medial to lateral elevation of the longus colli muscles while exposing the vertebral bodies reduces the risk to these structures. Injury to the sympathetic chain can result in a Horner syndrome (ptosis, miosis, and anhydrosis). The incidence of Horner syndrome has been reported to be 0.06 to 1%.[6,7]

Airway compromise or respiratory failure is an important and life-threatening complication associated with anterior cervical surgery. Causes of airway compromise can be soft-tissue swelling, hematoma, instrumentation failure, or graft dislodgement. The overall risk for reintubation after anterior cervical surgery is low with a reported rate of 0.5% in a large retrospective database study.[8] They found this rate increased to 1.6% in procedures involving 3 + levels; however, they were unable to specifically stratify cervical deformity procedures. Other factors

Table 18.1 Summary of complications, rates, and risk factors associated with cervical spine surgery

	Rates	Risk factors
Cervical deformity surgery	43.6–56.5%	
Surgical complications		
Airway compromise	0.6–1.6%	Male, older age, operative time, hematoma, 3 + levels
Esophageal perforation	0–3.4%	Retractors, instruments, implant erosion
Dysphagia	47–50%	Operative time, increased operative levels, C2–C4 segments, rhBMP use, smoking, endocrine disorder
Vascular injuries	0.7–1.4%	Anomalous vertebral artery, wide corpectomy, malpositioned hardware, Grade 4 osteotomies, tumor/infection procedures
Dural tears and CSF leaks	0–18%	OPLL, revision procedures
Infection	0.2–1.6% (anterior) 0.7–4.7% (posterior)	Combined surgical approaches, tobacco use, IV drug abuse, malnutrition, obesity
Epidural hematoma	0.09%	
Pseudarthrosis	0–54%	Number of levels fused, graft material, surgical technique, tobacco use
Implant malposition or pullout	0.085–7%	Surgical level (axial > subaxial), pseudarthrosis, corpectomy
Neurological complications		
Hypoglossal nerve	0.01%	C1–C3 exposure
Superior laryngeal nerve	0–1.25%	C3–C4 exposure
Sympathetic chain and Horner syndrome	0.06–1%	Anterior exposure lateral to longus colli
Recurrent laryngeal nerve palsy	1.8–2.8% (primary) 14.1 (revision)	Traction, retractors, post-op swelling, cervicothoracic junction surgery, revision procedures
Spinal cord injury	0.0–1%	Stenosis/spondylosis, intubation, positioning, instrumentation, technical mistakes, deformity correction
C5 palsy	0–12.1% (anterior) 0–30% (posterior)	Pathogenesis not fully understood
C8 nerve injury	14%	Three-column osteotomy

Abbreviations: CSF, cerebrospinal fluid; OPLL, ossification of the posterior longitudinal ligament; rhBMP, recombinant human bone morphogenetic protein.

reported as associated with postoperative airway compromise are male gender, older age, increased number of comorbidities, hematoma, and prolonged operations.[8,9] In patients with acute airway decompensation, etiologies such as hematoma, cerebrospinal fluid (CSF) leak, or plate/graft dislodgement should be considered and may require emergent intervention. Based on a recent prospective report of cervical deformity procedures, respiratory failure occurred in 5.1% of patients.[1] This higher rate may be explained by more levels fused, marked changes in cervical alignment, or longer procedures due to the complexity associated with deformity correction procedures.

Several methods for managing airway edema or postoperative airway protection in higher-risk patients have been described. A randomized controlled trial using perioperative steroids to reduce prevertebral soft-tissue swelling demonstrated decreased airway edema, improved swallowing, and shortened hospital stay.[10] Utilization of steroids both topically and systemically has been described; however, proper dosing, method of application, and duration of use have not been fully studied. Topical retropharyngeal steroids should be used with caution in patients with known chronic corticosteroid use. A case report by Lee et al of two patients suggested this application can lead to increased

esophageal perforation risk.[11] For high-risk patients, surgeries with combined approaches, or prolonged procedures, surgeons may also consider continuing postoperative intubation in a monitored intensive care unit for airway protection. Type of surgery and patient factors need to be carefully considered and discussed with patients when planning extensive deformity procedures that may utilize an anterior or combined approach.

Esophageal perforation injuries are rare and have reported rates of 0 to 3.4%.[12,13] Mortality has been reported as 20% if missed within 24 hours and up to 50% if treatment is delayed for more than 24 hours.[14] Perforation injuries may occur during retractor placement, instrumentation, or from dislodged screws, plates, or grafts. Esophageal damage may be noticed at the time of surgery or be discovered in a delayed fashion due to implant/graft erosion over time. Patients present with dysphagia, odynophagia, infection, aspiration, or airway compromise. Diagnosis can be made with endoscopy, contrast-enhanced computed tomography (CT) scans, and/or barium-enhanced esophagrams. Treatment can be complex and may require percutaneous endoscopic gastrostomy tube placement for nutrition, intravenous antibiotics to prevent infection, and possible repair or reconstruction with the assistance of otolaryngology and thoracic surgeons. These can be devastating and potentially life-threatening injuries.

Like esophageal injuries, tracheal injuries are extremely rare during anterior cervical surgery and are usually associated with retractor placement, perforation by a sharp instrument, or erosion by an implant or graft. These injuries can be complex to treat and often require the expertise of a head and neck surgeon. There are no specific reports of tracheal injuries during cervical deformity surgery.

Dysphagia and dysphonia are well-known associated adverse events following anterior cervical surgery and occur far more commonly than esophageal or tracheal perforation injuries. The true incidence of dysphagia has been difficult to define in the literature; however, three prospective studies have reported rates of 48%,[15] 50%,[16] and 47%[17] in the early postoperative periods. Patients should be counseled about the risks of dysphagia after anterior surgery. Factors reported to be associated with the occurrence of dysphagia include increased operative time, greater number of surgical levels, angle from C2 to C7, use of self-retaining retractors, elevated endotracheal cuff pressure, ventral instrumentation size and placement, procedures including more proximal cervical exposure (C2–C4), use of recombinant human bone morphogenetic protein-2 (rhBMP-2), staged surgery, presence of an endocrine disorder, and smoking.[15,16,18,19,20,21,22] Although most cases of dysphagia resolve without intervention, resolution can take several months or longer and may impart significant morbidity on patient recovery. Patients with refractory symptoms after 6 to 9 months may require further evaluation and referral to an otolaryngologist. Surgeons should be vigilant in evaluating a patient with new-onset or worsening dysphagia in the late postoperative period and should consider the possibility of implant or graft erosion causing esophageal perforation. Early postoperative dysphagia was reported at 11.5% overall after cervical deformity procedures; however, this rate increased to 24.1% in the subset of patients with combined anterior-posterior procedures.[1]

Dysphonia rates have also been difficult to define in the literature. One reason is poor standardization defining the condition. Another reason is there is wide variation in reported incidence between studies that relied on patients to self-report this complication and those that utilized laryngoscopy. The most common cause of dysphonia after anterior cervical surgery is RLN injury or palsy. RLN injury has been associated with traction injury, postoperative soft-tissue swelling, surgery at the cervicothoracic junction, and revision surgery. Incidence of RLN injury has been reported from 1.8 to 2.8% for primary surgeries and up to 14.1% for revision procedures.[23,24,25] Cadaveric studies demonstrated the RLN has a more predictable course on the patient's left side and historically it was believed that approaching this side may lower injury rates; however, recent studies have shown similar injury rates when approaching from the right or left sides.[23,25] Recent cervical deformity literature has not reported high rates of dysphonia; however, surgeons should be aware of this risk if utilizing an anterior or combined approach for deformity surgery, especially in revision cases.

18.2.2 Vascular Injuries

Vascular injuries can occur during anterior or posterior cervical surgery. Vertebral artery injuries are uncommon during cervical spine surgery with reported rates from 0.07 to 1.4%.[1,26,27,28,29] The vertebral arteries have variable locations based on cervical level; however, they tend to be less commonly encountered during a typical anterior exposure. Anomalous vertebral artery anatomy in the subaxial spine has been reported in up to 20% of the population.[30] Tortuous and/or ectopic arteries may be encountered during ventral or dorsal exposure, corpectomy procedures, or during instrumentation placement. With normal vascular anatomy, factors such as performing a wide corpectomy, Grade 4 osteotomy (complete uncovertebral joint resection to the transverse foramen),[31] or treating tumor and infection-related conditions can increase the risks of vertebral artery injuries as well. Careful evaluation of preoperative MRI or contrast-enhanced CT scans allows surgeons to identify abnormal anatomy and plan appropriately.[32] In a large, multicenter AO Spine database review of 16,582 cervical spine cases, 14 vertebral artery injuries were identified and of these, 50% had anomalous vessel anatomy on preoperative imaging identified during postoperative review.[29]

The anatomy of the vertebral arteries is classically described as four segments, V1–V4. V1 runs from the subclavian artery to the C6 transversarium and ventral to the C7 transverse process. V2 describes the segment within the transversarium from C6 to C1. The third segment (V3) extends from the atlas to the foramen magnum, and V4 is intradural from the foramen magnum to the posterior inferior cerebellar artery and joins the contralateral vertebral artery to become the basilar artery. Vascular injuries may occur at any of the four segments. In the subaxial spine, the vertebral arteries take a more predictable pathway than the atlantoaxial regions. Arterial injury rates are low for the subaxial spine for both lateral mass and pedicle screw instrumentation. Abumi et al reported 1 arterial injury among 712 cervical pedicle screws placed (0.6%).[33] Despite the theoretical risk to surrounding structures during subaxial lateral mass instrumentation, there are no specific reports of arterial injury in the modern literature. Nevertheless, undoubtedly this complication does occur at some low rate. In contrast, instrumentation of the atlantoaxial spine has higher reported rates of arterial injury from 4.1 to 8.2%, particularly with transarticular screws.[30] Given that some patients with cervical deformity may require instrumentation of these segments, surgeons should carefully examine preoperative imaging and should consider preoperative CT or magnetic resonance angiography to clearly define the vascular anatomy. If surgeons are planning a three-column osteotomy at C7, preoperative CT with angiography is required to carefully assess the vertebral arteries and their course at the cervicothoracic junction. This is critical for safely performing this procedure at the cervicothoracic junction. Reported vascular injuries during deformity corrective procedures are low, ranging from 0 to 1.3%[1,2,34,35]; however, injury to these structures can be catastrophic and life-threatening.

In the event of an injury, tamponade, embolization, surgical repair, and ligation are all considerations for treatment. Direct ligation should be the last treatment option with reported mortality rates of up to 12%.[30] Prompt consultation with a vascular surgeon should be considered if a vertebral artery injury is suspected. If local bleeding control is obtained, immediate postoperative angiography is recommended. Patients should be monitored in intensive care units for changes in neurologic function. Treatment goals should be focused on preventing vertebrobasilar ischemia and cerebrovascular events.

18.2.3 Dural Tears and Cerebrospinal Fluid Leaks

Dural tears or cerebral spinal leaks are uncommon during cervical spine surgery. Reported incidence in anterior cervical surgery is 0 to 8.3%.[36,37] CSF leaks are more common during revision surgery and procedures involving ossification of the posterior longitudinal ligament, with rates reported as high as 32% for the latter.[38] Incidental durotomies may also be encountered during posterior procedures and rates between 0.3 and 13% have been reported, with rates as high as 18% for revision procedures. CSF leaks can cause delayed physical therapy initiation, prolonged hospital stays, increased healthcare costs, wound complications, and need for additional surgeries. Among 78 cervical deformity cases, two (2.6%) dural tears were reported.[1] If encountered, treatments may include direct repair with or without a synthetic sealant adjunct. Proper multilayer wound closure is critical and many authors recommend subfascial drains (with careful monitoring of drain output) or lumbar drains. Pseudomeningocele formation is rare with reported incidence of 0.08%.[39] For refractory symptomatic cases, a peritoneal shunt or revision surgery may be considered. Patients with dural tears are at risk for other complications including delayed wound healing, prolonged recovery, pulmonary complications, meningitis, or even death.[40]

18.2.4 Wound Complications and Infections

Surgical-site wound complications and infections are rare occurrences in spinal surgery. Reported rates of deep infection after anterior surgery range from 0.2 to 1.6% and for posterior surgery range from 0.7 to 4.7%.[41] Recent reports have illustrated slightly higher infection rates in patients undergoing cervical deformity surgery with infection rates of 0% for anterior-only, 7.9% for posterior-only, and 6.8% for combined approaches.[1] Of these, 6.4% were deep infections. These rates did not have significant associations with demographic factors; however, other studies have shown alcohol consumption, tobacco use, intravenous drug abuse, malnutrition, and obesity to predispose spinal patients to surgical-site infections.[42,43] These modifiable risk factors should be considered during preoperative optimization. Surgical-site infections can range from superficial to deep and have a wide range of necessary treatments. Patients may require surgical debridement, instrumentation removal or exchange, and possibly complex wound closure or flap reconstruction. Organism-specific antibiosis is often required and long-term suppression may be necessary.

Another wound-related complication that can have devastating effects is symptomatic epidural hematoma. If an epidural hematoma is suspected, early identification and surgical evacuation is key for neurological recovery. A report by Schroeder et al in 2017 demonstrated a 0.09% incidence of symptomatic epidural hematomas among 16,582 cervical spine surgeries.[44] Among patients with known hematomas, those with delayed diagnosis had higher rates of residual neurological deficits and showed no improvement in health-related quality of life metrics at final follow-up. Surgeons should be aware of this complication, make prompt diagnosis, and institute immediate treatment to help achieve optimal neurologic recovery.

18.2.5 Pseudarthrosis

Pseudarthrosis is the failure of bony fusion after a spinal arthrodesis procedure. This is a known complication with surgery of any spinal region. In the cervical spine, pseudarthrosis can occur after anterior or posterior procedures. Nonunions may be asymptomatic; however, they may result in pain, recurrence of radicular or myelopathic symptoms, deformity, graft dislodgement, or instrumentation failure. Development of pseudarthrosis is multifactorial and may be associated with the number of surgical levels, graft type, biomechanical stability, and host factors. Reports over the last three decades have attempted to elucidate the factors associated with pseudarthrosis and guide surgeons toward optimal treatment.

Reported pseudarthrosis rates range from 0 to 11% for single-level surgery,[45,46,47,48] 0 to 63% for two levels,[45,48,49,50] and 0 to 54% for three or more levels.[49,51,52,53,54] These studies include other confounding variables such as use of autograft versus allograft, variable use of ventral instrumentation, and variations in endplate preparation. Despite these differences, it is described and accepted that nonunion rates increase as more levels are fused in the anterior cervical spine. For patients undergoing deformity correction surgery, multiple levels may need to be approached and these patients should be counseled regarding the nonunion risks associated with multilevel surgery.

In addition to the number of fusion levels, interbody graft material has been associated with different pseudarthrosis rates. Interbody grafts can be made of autograft, allograft, or synthetic materials such as PEEK, titanium, or carbon fiber. There are conflicting reports regarding potential differences in radiographic pseudarthrosis rates between autograft and allograft materials, especially with multilevel surgery.[48,49,53,55] Additional factors, such as packing material and surgical technique, may help explain these differing results. In addition, similar fusion rates have been reported between structural autograft and synthetic cage materials in anterior cervical procedures.[49,56,57] Standalone interbody devices are also used for cervical fusion; however, the literature related to their efficacy and associated pseudarthrosis rates, especially in multilevel constructs, has yet to be fully reported.

Ventral fixation is also a variable that may impact pseudarthrosis rates. While some reports suggest similar fusion rates with and without anterior plating, a recent meta-analysis suggests that anterior instrumentation improves pseudarthrosis rates, even in single-level surgery.[58] Modern instrumentation includes locking screw technology to increase the fixation rigidity and to help prevent toggling or pullout. Recently, dynamic plate designs have been introduced with the theoretical advantage of maintaining graft and implant load-sharing and possibly increasing fusion rates; however, further studies are needed to determine their clinical impact.

Patient host factors can substantially impact bony fusion rates. The most relevant factor identified in the literature is smoking or tobacco exposure.[59] Other factors such as comorbidities, presence of metabolic bone disorders, or malnutrition should always be considered during preoperative optimization and counseling and may impact surgical outcomes.

Close patient follow-up is necessary to monitor patients for pseudarthrosis. Measuring the interspinous distance on dynamic cervical radiographs is one method for detecting motion after cervical fusion surgery with 2 mm or less of motion being highly associated with solid arthrodesis.[60] Fine-cut CT scanning is the radiographic study of choice for evaluating cervical fusions; however, all radiographic methods have limitations and surgical exploration remains the gold standard for assessing complete arthrodesis.[61]

18.2.6 Implant-Associated Complications

Cervical spine deformity surgery usually involves applying instrumentation to the spinal segments. Instrumentation can be inserted into the ventral and/or dorsal spine through various methods. In the anterior spine, ventrally placed plates and screws can be applied to bridge across fusion segments. Alternatively, interbody devices with integrated fixation screws have also been developed. In the posterior cervical spine, wiring techniques, lateral mass screws, pedicle screws, translaminar screws, and transarticular screws have all been utilized. Regardless of technique, implant placement always poses risks during and after surgery.

Screw malposition in the cervical spine can be a detrimental complication. In the anterior spine, improper screw length can lead to iatrogenic spinal cord injury (SCI) and paralysis. This complication was more prevalent when nonlocking bicortical screws were used. With the evolution of locking cancellous screw and plate technology, this complication is now uncommon. Alternatively, depending on plate placement and screw angle, screws may violate adjacent disc spaces, neuroforamina, or vertebral arteries. With posterior fixation, spinal cord, nerve root, facet joint, or arterial injuries can occur, particularly in the atlantoaxial segments. Harms and Melcher reported the incidence of malpositioned screws as 0 to 4% in the atlas and 0 to 7% in the axis.[62] In the subaxial spine, pedicle breaches are less common and insertion techniques using anatomic landmarks[63] or by direct pedicle palpation after laminoforaminotomy[64] have both been shown to be safe and effective.

Screw pullout, breakage, and fixation failure are rare but do occur. A recently published review of 12,903 patients identified 11 cases (0.085%) that required reoperation for malpositioning or screw pullout.[65] In the cervical spine, this may be associated with distal junctional kyphosis and this topic is covered in subsequent chapters. Instrumentation can fatigue and fail in the presence of pseudarthrosis. In addition, several reports have demonstrated high failure rates and graft dislodgement after multilevel anterior corpectomy procedures.[66,67,68,69] Despite reports with low fixation failure rates in cervical deformity cohorts, surgeons should be aware of these risks if corpectomy or osteotomies are necessary for deformity correction. We present a case of hardware failure and screw pullout in ▶ Fig. 18.1.

18.3 Neurological Complications

Neurologic injuries associated with cervical deformity surgery are not uncommon and may have transient or permanent effects. Injuries may occur at the spinal cord and/or nerve root levels. Which nerves can be affected differs based on anterior versus posterior surgical approaches. Additionally, injuries to peripheral nerves may be encountered as a result of positioning during surgery. Factors contributing to potential injury should be identified and considered at all phases of treatment. This section will review potential neurological complications including spinal cord injuries and nerve root injuries associated with cervical deformity surgery. Neurological complications are summarized in ▶ Table 18.1.

18.3.1 Spinal Cord Injury

Iatrogenic SCI is uncommon during cervical spine surgery with reported rates from 0.0 to 1%.[70,71,72,73] These injuries may occur during multiple steps of the surgery including intubation, positioning, instrumentation, decompression, technical mistakes, and/or deformity correction. Intraoperative hypotension can also cause SCI, especially in patients with preexisting spinal cord compression due to underlying cervical pathology.

Intubation-associated or positioning SCI has been reported with neck extension.[74] Multiple conditions such as Down syndrome, rheumatoid arthritis, ankylosing spondylitis, infection, tumor, or other inflammatory arthropathies may predispose patients to instability; however, SCI after intubation was found to be more likely associated with stenosis and spondylosis rather than instability.[74] Surgeons should collaborate closely with anesthesiologists and neurologists and consideration should be given to utilizing fiberoptic intubation to minimize SCI risk during the presurgical phases.

Intraoperative SCI may result from multiple etiologies. Neuromonitoring can help alert a surgeon of neurological changes during decompression, instrumentation, or corrective maneuvers. Neuromonitoring may include motor evoked potentials (MEPs), somatosensory evoked potentials (SSEPs), and electromyography (EMGs). Based on spinal cord anatomy, trauma to the anterior cord motor tracts may be best identified by MEPs, while dorsal injuries to the sensory tracts may first be identified by changes in SSEPs. Surgeons should utilize neuromonitoring during cervical deformity surgery and incorporate this information intraoperatively to help ensure spinal cord safety. Once neuromonitoring changes are identified, a prompt evaluation of all possible contributing factors should be performed by treatment team members and swift interventions should be performed as indicated. If changes occurred after a surgical step, this step should be assessed and reversed if possible. Hemoglobin level, mean arterial pressure, and the technical aspects of neuromonitoring should always be checked.

Cervical deformity corrective maneuvers can be high risk. SCI has been reported during cervical extension osteotomies in both seated and prone positions; however, most neurologic injuries are transient and permanent deficits are not common.[1,75,76,77,78] Delayed presentation of SCI in the postoperative period can be caused by acute fixation failure or epidural hematoma. Prompt identification, emergency MRI, and possible emergent surgical intervention may be required for treatment.

After SCI has been identified, treatment algorithms often depend on the underlying etiology or surgeon's preference. There is controversial data supporting the use of steroids after SCI. Some centers routinely use steroids, while others may not. Maintenance of spinal cord perfusion is critical and patients with SCI should be in monitored settings with consideration of maintaining an elevated mean arterial pressure for the early postoperative period (e.g., 85 mm Hg for 3–5 days). Ensuring cord decompression and stabilization will provide an environment for maximal recovery; however, prognosis after SCI is difficult to determine acutely and continued slow recovery may continue for several months or longer after surgery.

18.3.2 Nerve Root Complications

New cervical nerve root deficits are possible during both anterior and posterior procedures. The most commonly reported deficits involve the C5 nerve root. This may manifest as isolated deltoid weakness and/or sensory deficits with or without pain in the C5 dermatome. It is unilateral in the majority of patients and bilateral in 8% of cases.[79] Reported incidence of C5 nerve root palsy associated with anterior procedures ranges from 0 to 12.1%[80,81,82] and 0 to 30% for posterior procedures, with an average incidence of 4.6%.[79,83,84,85,86,87] In a study of 78 cervical deformity cases, C5 palsy occurred in 6.4% of patients.[1] The pathogenesis of this complication after cervical spine surgery is not fully understood. Sakaura et al have suggested five possible pathways that operate independently or together. Elements of intraoperative trauma, traction or tethering of the C5 root following cord shift after decompression, spinal cord ischemia, segmental spinal cord dysfunction, and possible reperfusion injury may all contribute to this complication.[79] Once identified, treatment algorithms are not clearly defined. Surgeons should first review imaging studies for any cause of nerve root com-

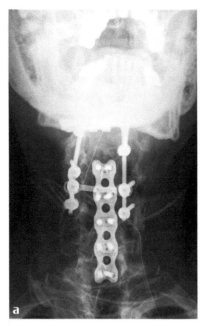
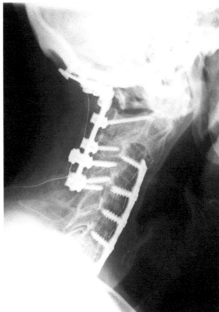
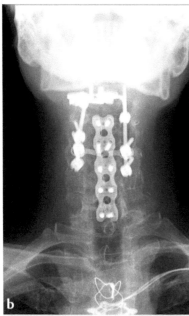
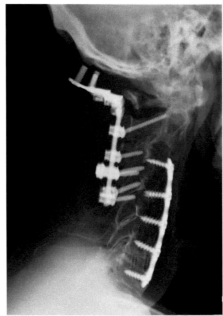

Fig. 18.1 Case example: This 62-year old male had a previous C3–C7 anterior cervical discectomy performed several years prior. He had been recently treated by another surgeon and underwent a posterior procedure occiput to C5 for cervical spondylosis and myelopathy (a). He presented 10 days after surgery with complaints that he could feel that his plate was loose and he had an inability to maintain a horizontal gaze (b). He underwent a revision procedure and was found to have a failed fixation proximally as well as a pseudarthrosis at C6–C7. Revision included occiput to C7 instrumentation, structural allograft augmentation from occiput to C2, along with off-label use of recombinant human bone morphogenetic protein-2 and iliac crest autograft.

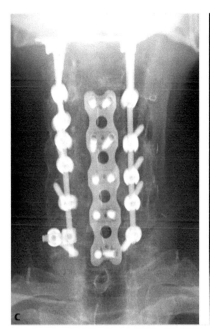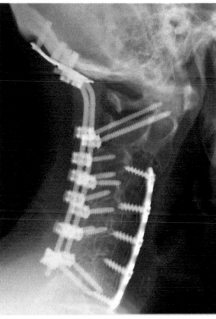

Fig 18.1 (*Continued*) **(c)** This case demonstrates acute instrumentation failure with screw pullout as well as an unrecognized C6–C7 pseudarthrosis at the lowest level of a previous multilevel anterior cervical fusion.

pression. Electromyogram may also be obtained to rule out brachial plexopathy if suspected. In the absence of etiology requiring intervention, treatment is supportive with physical therapy to prevent shoulder stiffness or sequelae due to immobility. With incomplete motor weakness, conservative and supportive treatment has led to complete resolution within 2 years.[79,81,85] In the largest reported series of C5 palsies, 54.2% had complete resolution of symptoms, 25.4% had residual deficits, and 17.0% had no recovery (3.4% lost to follow-up).[82] Patients should be counseled carefully if this complication is identified in the postoperative period.

Injury to the C2 nerve root is a known complication associated with C1 fixation. Protection of the nerve may prevent injury and some authors advocate intentional sacrifice due to the proximity of instrumentation for atlantoaxial fixation. Postoperative neuralgia may result from either distraction injury, severing the nerve or from hardware irritation. Treatment is typically symptomatic supportive care.

C8 nerve root injuries are most commonly associated with extension-type osteotomies in the low cervical spine with a reported incidence of 14%.[88] Other studies on three-column osteotomies in the cervical spine report non-C5 motor deficits from 0 to 8.7%.[2,35] Advances in neuromonitoring may have positively impacted and lowered these rates by giving surgeons direct feedback during the procedure. Surgeons performing three-column osteotomies in the lower cervical spine should ensure adequate decompression of the C8 nerve roots and analyze neuromonitoring data closely during corrective maneuvers. C8–T1 palsies manifest in specific intrinsic hand muscles and sensory distributions. Surgeons should be familiar with these myotome and dermatome patterns. C8–T1 motor innervation is specific for the abductor and flexor pollicis brevis, opponens pollicis, and the lateral two lumbricals via their contributions to the median nerve. The sensory dermatome specific to C8–T1 includes the medial antebrachial cutaneous nerve which provides sensation to the medial volar and dorsal forearm.[89] If a C8 nerve palsy is identified postoperatively,

obtaining a CT scan should be considered in order to assess the foramen. If the nerves are adequately decompressed, surgeons should consider implementing physical therapy and observing for recovery.

18.4 Conclusion

Cervical deformity surgery has procedure-related risks that are similar to other cervical procedures; however, recently reported complication rates are higher in cervical deformity than in other cervical pathology cohorts. Knowledge of the potential surgical and neurological complications allows surgeons to perform comprehensive preoperative counseling with patients and manage postoperative expectations appropriately. Even with meticulous surgical technique, treating cervical deformities may result in complications. These complications should be identified and managed appropriately to help ensure optimal patient outcomes.

References

[1] Smith JS, Ramchandran S, Lafage V, et al. International Spine Study Group. Prospective multicenter assessment of early complication rates associated with adult cervical deformity surgery in 78 patients. Neurosurgery. 2016; 79 (3):378–388

[2] Smith JS, Shaffrey CI, Lafage R, et al. ISSG. Three-column osteotomy for correction of cervical and cervicothoracic deformities: alignment changes and early complications in a multicenter prospective series of 23 patients. Eur Spine J. 2017; 26(8):2128–2137

[3] Smith GW, Robinson RA. The treatment of certain cervical-spine disorders by anterior removal of the intervertebral disc and interbody fusion. J Bone Joint Surg Am. 1958; 40-A(3):607–624

[4] Ames CP, Clark AJ, Kanter AS, et al. Hypoglossal nerve palsy after cervical spine surgery. Global Spine J. 2017; 7(1) Suppl:37S–39S

[5] Tempel ZJ, Smith JS, Shaffrey C, et al. A multicenter review of superior laryngeal nerve injury following anterior cervical spine surgery. Global Spine J. 2017; 7(1) Suppl:7S–11S

[6] Bertalanffy H, Eggert HR. Complications of anterior cervical discectomy without fusion in 450 consecutive patients. Acta Neurochir (Wien). 1989; 99 (1–2):41–50

[7] Traynelis VC, Malone HR, Smith ZA, et al. Rare complications of cervical spine surgery: Horner's syndrome. Global Spine J. 2017; 7(1) Suppl:103S–108S

[8] Marquez-Lara A, Nandyala SV, Fineberg SJ, Singh K. Incidence, outcomes, and mortality of reintubation after anterior cervical fusion. Spine. 2014; 39 (2):134–139

[9] Lim S, Kesavabhotla K, Cybulski GR, Dahdaleh NS, Smith ZA. Predictors for airway complications following single- and multilevel anterior cervical discectomy and fusion. Spine. 2017; 42(6):379–384

[10] Jeyamohan SB, Kenning TJ, Petronis KA, Feustel PJ, Drazin D, DiRisio DJ. Effect of steroid use in anterior cervical discectomy and fusion: a randomized controlled trial. J Neurosurg Spine. 2015; 23(2):137–143

[11] Lee SH, Mesfin A, Riew KD. Delayed esophageal perforation after anterior cervical fusion and retropharyngeal steroid use: a report of two cases. Spine J. 2015; 15(10):e75–e80

[12] Fountas KN, Kapsalaki EZ, Machinis T, Robinson JS. Extrusion of a screw into the gastrointestinal tract after anterior cervical spine plating. J Spinal Disord Tech. 2006; 19(3):199–203

[13] Hershman SH, Kunkle WA, Kelly MP, et al. Esophageal perforation following anterior cervical spine surgery: case report and review of the literature. Global Spine J. 2017; 7(1) Suppl:28S–36S

[14] Orlando ER, Caroli E, Ferrante L. Management of the cervical esophagus and hypofarinx perforations complicating anterior cervical spine surgery. Spine. 2003; 28(15):E290–E295

[15] Frempong-Boadu A, Houten JK, Osborn B, et al. Swallowing and speech dysfunction in patients undergoing anterior cervical discectomy and fusion: a prospective, objective preoperative and postoperative assessment. J Spinal Disord Tech. 2002; 15(5):362–368

[16] Bazaz R, Lee MJ, Yoo JU. Incidence of dysphagia after anterior cervical spine surgery: a prospective study. Spine. 2002; 27(22):2453–2458

[17] Smith-Hammond CA, New KC, Pietrobon R, Curtis DJ, Scharver CH, Turner DA. Prospective analysis of incidence and risk factors of dysphagia in spine surgery patients: comparison of anterior cervical, posterior cervical, and lumbar procedures. Spine. 2004; 29(13):1441–1446

[18] Finn MA, MacDonald JD. C2-C3 anterior cervical fusion: technical report. Clin Spine Surg. 2016; 29(10):E536–E541

[19] Kang SH, Kim DK, Seo KM, Lee SY, Park SW, Kim YB. Swallowing function defined by videofluoroscopic swallowing studies after anterior cervical discectomy and fusion: a prospective study. J Korean Med Sci. 2016; 31(12):2020–2025

[20] Liu J, Hai Y, Kang N, Chen X, Zhang Y. Risk factors and preventative measures of early and persistent dysphagia after anterior cervical spine surgery: a systematic review. Eur Spine J. 2018; 27(6):1209–1218

[21] Nagoshi N, Tetreault L, Nakashima H, et al. Risk factors for and clinical outcomes of dysphagia after anterior cervical surgery for degenerative cervical myelopathy: results from the AOSpine International and North America Studies. J Bone Joint Surg Am. 2017; 99(13):1069–1077

[22] Wang T, Ma L, Yang DL, et al. Factors predicting dysphagia after anterior cervical surgery: a multicenter retrospective study for 2 years of follow-up. Medicine (Baltimore). 2017; 96(34):e7916

[23] Beutler WJ, Sweeney CA, Connolly PJ. Recurrent laryngeal nerve injury with anterior cervical spine surgery risk with laterality of surgical approach. Spine. 2001; 26(12):1337–1342

[24] Erwood MS, Hadley MN, Gordon AS, Carroll WR, Agee BS, Walters BC. Recurrent laryngeal nerve injury following reoperative anterior cervical discectomy and fusion: a meta-analysis. J Neurosurg Spine. 2016; 25(2):198–204

[25] Kilburg C, Sullivan HG, Mathiason MA. Effect of approach side during anterior cervical discectomy and fusion on the incidence of recurrent laryngeal nerve injury. J Neurosurg Spine. 2006; 4(4):273–277

[26] Burke JP, Gerszten PC, Welch WC. Iatrogenic vertebral artery injury during anterior cervical spine surgery. Spine J. 2005; 5(5):508–514, discussion 514

[27] Rampersaud YR, Moro ER, Neary MA, et al. Intraoperative adverse events and related postoperative complications in spine surgery: implications for enhancing patient safety founded on evidence-based protocols. Spine. 2006; 31 (13):1503–1510

[28] Lunardini DJ, Eskander MS, Even JL, et al. Vertebral artery injuries in cervical spine surgery. Spine J. 2014; 14(8):1520–1525

[29] Hsu WK, Kannan A, Mai HT, et al. Epidemiology and outcomes of vertebral artery injury in 16582 cervical spine surgery patients: an AOSpine North America Multicenter Study. Global Spine J. 2017; 7(1) Suppl:21S–27S

[30] Peng CW, Chou BT, Bendo JA, Spivak JM. Vertebral artery injury in cervical spine surgery: anatomical considerations, management, and preventive measures. Spine J. 2009; 9(1):70–76

[31] Ames CP, Smith JS, Scheer JK, et al. International Spine Study Group. A standardized nomenclature for cervical spine soft-tissue release and osteotomy for deformity correction: clinical article. J Neurosurg Spine. 2013; 19(3):269–278

[32] Ebraheim NA, Xu R, Ahmad M, Heck B. The quantitative anatomy of the vertebral artery groove of the atlas and its relation to the posterior atlantoaxial approach. Spine. 1998; 23(3):320–323

[33] Abumi K, Shono Y, Ito M, Taneichi H, Kotani Y, Kaneda K. Complications of pedicle screw fixation in reconstructive surgery of the cervical spine. Spine. 2000; 25(8):962–969

[34] Kim HJ, Piyaskulkaew C, Riew KD. Comparison of Smith-Petersen osteotomy versus pedicle subtraction osteotomy versus anterior-posterior osteotomy types for the correction of cervical spine deformities. Spine. 2015; 40 (3):143–146

[35] Wollowick AL, Kelly MP, Riew KD. Pedicle subtraction osteotomy in the cervical spine. Spine. 2012; 37(5):E342–E348

[36] Edwards CC, II, Heller JG, Murakami H. Corpectomy versus laminoplasty for multilevel cervical myelopathy: an independent matched-cohort analysis. Spine. 2002; 27(11):1168–1175

[37] Hannallah D, Lee J, Khan M, Donaldson WF, Kang JD. Cerebrospinal fluid leaks following cervical spine surgery. J Bone Joint Surg Am. 2008; 90(5):1101–1105

[38] Smith MD, Bolesta MJ, Leventhal M, Bohlman HH. Postoperative cerebrospinal-fluid fistula associated with erosion of the dura. Findings after anterior resection of ossification of the posterior longitudinal ligament in the cervical spine. J Bone Joint Surg Am. 1992; 74(2):270–277

[39] Ailon T, Smith JS, Nassr A, et al. Rare complications of cervical spine surgery: pseudomeningocoele. Global Spine J. 2017; 7(1) Suppl:109S–114S

[40] Eismont FJ, Wiesel SW, Rothman RH. Treatment of dural tears associated with spinal surgery. J Bone Joint Surg Am. 1981; 63(7):1132–1136

[41] Fehlings MG, Smith JS, Kopjar B, et al. Perioperative and delayed complications associated with the surgical treatment of cervical spondylotic myelopathy based on 302 patients from the AOSpine North America Cervical Spondylotic Myelopathy Study. J Neurosurg Spine. 2012; 16(5):425–432

[42] Olsen MA, Nepple JJ, Riew KD, et al. Risk factors for surgical site infection following orthopaedic spinal operations. J Bone Joint Surg Am. 2008; 90(1): 62–69

[43] Pahys JM, Pahys JR, Cho SK, et al. Methods to decrease postoperative infections following posterior cervical spine surgery. J Bone Joint Surg Am. 2013; 95(6):549–554

[44] Schroeder GD, Hilibrand AS, Arnold PM, et al. Epidural hematoma following cervical spine surgery. Global Spine J. 2017; 7(1) Suppl:120S–126S

[45] Bohlman HH, Emery SE, Goodfellow DB, Jones PK. Robinson anterior cervical discectomy and arthrodesis for cervical radiculopathy. Long-term follow-up of one hundred and twenty-two patients. J Bone Joint Surg Am. 1993; 75 (9):1298–1307

[46] Samartzis D, Shen FH, Lyon C, Phillips M, Goldberg EJ, An HS. Does rigid instrumentation increase the fusion rate in one-level anterior cervical discectomy and fusion? Spine J. 2004; 4(6):636–643

[47] Wang JC, McDonough PW, Endow K, Kanim LE, Delamarter RB. The effect of cervical plating on single-level anterior cervical discectomy and fusion. J Spinal Disord. 1999; 12(6):467–471

[48] Zdeblick TA, Ducker TB. The use of freeze-dried allograft bone for anterior cervical fusions. Spine. 1991; 16(7):726–729

[49] Samartzis D, Shen FH, Matthews DK, Yoon ST, Goldberg EJ, An HS. Comparison of allograft to autograft in multilevel anterior cervical discectomy and fusion with rigid plate fixation. Spine J. 2003; 3(6):451–459

[50] Wang JC, McDonough PW, Endow KK, Delamarter RB. Increased fusion rates with cervical plating for two-level anterior cervical discectomy and fusion. Spine. 2000; 25(1):41–45

[51] Bolesta MJ, Rechtine GR, II, Chrin AM. Three- and four-level anterior cervical discectomy and fusion with plate fixation: a prospective study. Spine. 2000; 25(16):2040–2044, discussion 2045–2046

[52] Emery SE, Fisher JR, Bohlman HH. Three-level anterior cervical discectomy and fusion: radiographic and clinical results. Spine. 1997; 22(22):2622–2624, discussion 2625

[53] Papadopoulos EC, Huang RC, Girardi FP, Synnott K, Cammisa FP, Jr. Three-level anterior cervical discectomy and fusion with plate fixation: radiographic and clinical results. Spine. 2006; 31(8):897–902

[54] Wang JC, McDonough PW, Kanim LE, Endow KK, Delamarter RB. Increased fusion rates with cervical plating for three-level anterior cervical discectomy and fusion. Spine. 2001; 26(6):643–646, discussion 646–647

[55] Shriver MF, Lewis DJ, Kshettry VR, Rosenbaum BP, Benzel EC, Mroz TE. Pseudoarthrosis rates in anterior cervical discectomy and fusion: a meta-analysis. Spine J. 2015; 15(9):2016–2027

[56] Hwang SL, Lee KS, Su YF, et al. Anterior corpectomy with iliac bone fusion or discectomy with interbody titanium cage fusion for multilevel cervical degenerated disc disease. J Spinal Disord Tech. 2007; 20(8):565–570

[57] Topuz K, Colak A, Kaya S, et al. Two-level contiguous cervical disc disease treated with peek cages packed with demineralized bone matrix: results of 3-year follow-up. Eur Spine J. 2009; 18(2):238–243

[58] Fraser JF, Härtl R. Anterior approaches to fusion of the cervical spine: a meta-analysis of fusion rates. J Neurosurg Spine. 2007; 6(4):298–303

[59] Hilibrand AS, Fye MA, Emery SE, Palumbo MA, Bohlman HH. Impact of smoking on the outcome of anterior cervical arthrodesis with interbody or strut-grafting. J Bone Joint Surg Am. 2001; 83-A(5):668–673

[60] Cannada LK, Scherping SC, Yoo JU, Jones PK, Emery SE. Pseudoarthrosis of the cervical spine: a comparison of radiographic diagnostic measures. Spine. 2003; 28(1):46–51

[61] Buchowski JM, Liu G, Bunmaprasert T, Rose PS, Riew KD. Anterior cervical fusion assessment: surgical exploration versus radiographic evaluation. Spine. 2008; 33(11):1185–1191

[62] Harms J, Melcher RP. Posterior C1-C2 fusion with polyaxial screw and rod fixation. Spine. 2001; 26(22):2467–2471

[63] Abumi K, Itoh H, Taneichi H, Kaneda K. Transpedicular screw fixation for traumatic lesions of the middle and lower cervical spine: description of the techniques and preliminary report. J Spinal Disord. 1994; 7(1):19–28

[64] Albert TJ, Klein GR, Joffe D, Vaccaro AR. Use of cervicothoracic junction pedicle screws for reconstruction of complex cervical spine pathology. Spine. 1998; 23(14):1596–1599

[65] Peterson JC, Arnold PM, Smith ZA, et al. misplaced cervical screws requiring reoperation. Global Spine J. 2017; 7(1) Suppl:46S–52S

[66] Sasso RC, Ruggiero RA, Jr, Reilly TM, Hall PV. Early reconstruction failures after multilevel cervical corpectomy. Spine. 2003; 28(2):140–142

[67] Vaccaro AR, Falatyn SP, Scuderi GJ, et al. Early failure of long segment anterior cervical plate fixation. J Spinal Disord. 1998; 11(5):410–415

[68] Wang JC, Hart RA, Emery SE, Bohlman HH. Graft migration or displacement after multilevel cervical corpectomy and strut grafting. Spine. 2003; 28 (10):1016–1021, discussion 1021–1022

[69] Zdeblick TA, Bohlman HH. Cervical kyphosis and myelopathy. Treatment by anterior corpectomy and strut-grafting. J Bone Joint Surg Am. 1989; 71 (2):170–182

[70] Cramer DE, Maher PC, Pettigrew DB, Kuntz C, IV. Major neurologic deficit immediately after adult spinal surgery: incidence and etiology over 10 years at a single training institution. J Spinal Disord Tech. 2009; 22(8):565–570

[71] Daniels AH, Riew KD, Yoo JU, et al. Adverse events associated with anterior cervical spine surgery. J Am Acad Orthop Surg. 2008; 16(12):729–738

[72] Emery SE, Bohlman HH, Bolesta MJ, Jones PK. Anterior cervical decompression and arthrodesis for the treatment of cervical spondylotic myelopathy. Two to seventeen-year follow-up. J Bone Joint Surg Am. 1998; 80(7):941–951

[73] Daniels AH, Hart RA, Hilibrand AS, et al. Iatrogenic spinal cord injury resulting from cervical spine surgery. Global Spine J. 2017; 7(1) Suppl:84S–90S

[74] Hindman BJ, Palecek JP, Posner KL, et al. Cervical spinal cord, root, and bony spine injuries: a closed claims analysis. Anesthesiology. 2011; 114(4): 782–795

[75] Etame AB, Than KD, Wang AC, La Marca F, Park P. Surgical management of symptomatic cervical or cervicothoracic kyphosis due to ankylosing spondylitis. Spine. 2008; 33(16):E559–E564

[76] Langeloo DD, Journee HL, Pavlov PW, de Kleuver M. Cervical osteotomy in ankylosing spondylitis: evaluation of new developments. Eur Spine J. 2006; 15 (4):493–500

[77] Simmons EH. The surgical correction of flexion deformity of the cervical spine in ankylosing spondylitis. Clin Orthop Relat Res. 1972; 86(86):132–143

[78] Tokala DP, Lam KS, Freeman BJ, Webb JK. C7 decancellisation closing wedge osteotomy for the correction of fixed cervico-thoracic kyphosis. Eur Spine J. 2007; 16(9):1471–1478

[79] Sakaura H, Hosono N, Mukai Y, Ishii T, Yoshikawa H. C5 palsy after decompression surgery for cervical myelopathy: review of the literature. Spine. 2003; 28(21):2447–2451

[80] Hashimoto M, Mochizuki M, Aiba A, et al. C5 palsy following anterior decompression and spinal fusion for cervical degenerative diseases. Eur Spine J. 2010; 19(10):1702–1710

[81] Ikenaga M, Shikata J, Tanaka C. Radiculopathy of C-5 after anterior decompression for cervical myelopathy. J Neurosurg Spine. 2005; 3(3):210–217

[82] Thompson SE, Smith ZA, Hsu WK, et al. C5 palsy after cervical spine surgery: a multicenter retrospective review of 59 cases. Global Spine J. 2017; 7(1) Suppl:64S–70S

[83] Chen Y, Chen D, Wang X, Guo Y, He Z. C5 palsy after laminectomy and posterior cervical fixation for ossification of posterior longitudinal ligament. J Spinal Disord Tech. 2007; 20(7):533–535

[84] Greiner-Perth R, Elsaghir H, Böhm H, El-Meshtawy M. The incidence of C5-C6 radiculopathy as a complication of extensive cervical decompression: own results and review of literature. Neurosurg Rev. 2005; 28(2):137–142

[85] Imagama S, Matsuyama Y, Yukawa Y, et al. Nagoya Spine Group. C5 palsy after cervical laminoplasty: a multicentre study. J Bone Joint Surg Br. 2010; 92 (3):393–400

[86] Minoda Y, Nakamura H, Konishi S, et al. Palsy of the C5 nerve root after mid-sagittal-splitting laminoplasty of the cervical spine. Spine. 2003; 28 (11):1123–1127

[87] Takemitsu M, Cheung KM, Wong YW, Cheung WY, Luk KD. C5 nerve root palsy after cervical laminoplasty and posterior fusion with instrumentation. J Spinal Disord Tech. 2008; 21(4):267–272

[88] Simmons ED, DiStefano RJ, Zheng Y, Simmons EH. Thirty-six years experience of cervical extension osteotomy in ankylosing spondylitis: techniques and outcomes. Spine. 2006; 31(26):3006–3012

[89] Stoker GE, Kim HJ, Riew KD. Differentiating c8-t1 radiculopathy from ulnar neuropathy: a survey of 24 spine surgeons. Global Spine J. 2014; 4(1):1–6

19 Medical Complications

Flynn Andrew Rowan, Ananth S. Eleswarapu, and Eric Klineberg

Abstract

Medical complications following surgical correction of adult cervical deformity (ACD) are not uncommon. This chapter discusses the medical complications that are commonly encountered following ACD surgery, as well as their risk factors, prevention, and management.

Keywords: dysphagia, dysphonia, infection, pneumonia, respiratory failure

19.1 Introduction

Adult spinal deformity (ASD) surgery has a greater potential for complications than most other spinal surgeries. This is in part due to the patient population, which tends to be older and with greater underlying comorbidities, as well as the increased physiologic demands that such surgeries place on patients. These complications include surgical as well as medical complications, the latter of which is the focus of this chapter. An understanding of these potential pitfalls allows the thoughtful surgeon to prevent, anticipate, recognize, and potentially mitigate their impact.

Though there is ample literature concerning the development of medical complications following ASD surgery in general, there is a relative paucity of literature regarding adult cervical deformity (ACD) surgery, in particular. While there is considerable overlap in the principles that may lead to development of complications between these two groups of patients, there are also considerable differences, as presented in ▶ Table 19.1. This chapter will focus on those complications more closely related to ACD.

19.2 Complications

Many patients undergoing surgery for ACD are elderly, and may have a myriad of underlying medical comorbidities. Because of the extensive physiologic toll that such a surgical intervention has on a patient, it is not surprising that perioperative and postoperative medical complications are common. Overall

Table 19.1 Comparison of complication rates between adult cervical deformity surgery and adult spinal deformity surgery

	Adult cervical deformity surgery	Adult spinal deformity surgery
Dysphagia/dysphonia	11.5%	<2%
Infection	6.4–7.9%	2.4–4%
Pneumonia	5.2%	0.6%
Respiratory failure	5.1%	0.6%
Pulmonary embolus	1.3–3.9%	1–2%
Deep venous thrombosis	10%	0.7%

complication rates (both medical and surgical) have been reported as high as 26.8% in large series of ASD patients, with the majority of these representing cardiac, pulmonary, infectious, or gastrointestinal complications.[1,2,3] Studies addressing ACD specifically have identified overall complication rates as high as 67%.[4,5] ▶ Table 19.1 presents a summary of the most common types of postoperative medical complications following ASD.

19.2.1 Dysphagia/Dysphonia

Dysphagia and dysphonia are perhaps the most common complication following ACD surgery, though this is most often transient. Because of its transient nature, as well as the fact that many patients may not complain about the presence of mild dysphagia, determining the true incidence is difficult. In a multicenter study of 78 patients undergoing ACD surgery, the International Spine Study Group (ISSG) found a dysphagia rate of 11.5%.[5] A single-institution study found that only 2.6% of patients had severe, long-term dysphagia that required use of a feeding tube.[4] There are many reasons for this high incidence. First, much like any anterior cervical surgery, retraction of the trachea and esophagus may lead to symptoms of dysphagia and dysphonia. Second, the presence of cervical deformity—kyphosis in particular—may result in an underlying swallowing dysfunction that can be exacerbated following surgery.[6] Anatomic changes in alignment of the trachea and esophagus may play a role, especially with a long-standing fixed deformity. Correction of a significant, long-standing kyphosis can place these structures in tension, resulting in dysphagia and dysphonia.[7] Furthermore, the use of recombinant human bone morphogenetic protein (rhBMP) has been shown to promote dysphagia.[8,9]

With the high incidence, and multiple etiologies of dysphagia and dysphonia, it may be difficult to be completely prevented, particularly with anterior approaches or large deformity corrections. However, surgical technique may be able to mitigate some of the severity. Although many patients with underlying deformity may have intubation difficulty, the use of advanced intubation techniques can be useful to prevent the airway trauma associated with prolonged or multiple intubation attempts. Care should be taken during anterior approaches to avoid excessive or prolonged traction on the esophagus and trachea. While intraoperative steroid application has demonstrated success in reducing the rate of dysphagia, it is the authors' belief that the accompanying risk of infection surpasses any benefit, particularly in the setting of these large complex deformities.[9]

19.2.2 Infection

While infection following anterior cervical surgery is fortunately rare, it is more common following posterior cervical exposures. The increased operative time and blood loss associated with deformity surgery may also contribute to an increased risk compared to other posterior cervical procedures. The ISSG multicenter study found a 6.4% rate of deep surgical-site infection and a superficial infection rate of 3.8%.[5] Grosso et al found a similar rate of 7.9% for deep infections.[4] Interestingly, these rates are substantially higher than the ISSG and other groups have reported for deformity surgery in general, ranging from 2.4 to 4%.[1,2]

As with any other surgery, infection prevention starts with appropriate preparation of the surgical site. In contrast to other areas of spinal surgery, the abundance of hair in the posterior cervical region requires further preparation. Hair should be clipped short to minimize contamination of the surgical site. Ideally, this should be performed in the preoperative holding area to prevent airborne contamination of the operating room. Furthermore, our institution utilizes a standardized protocol involving intraoperative irrigation with dilute Betadine, as well as topical vancomycin powder for the posterior cervical approach.[10]

Wound complications in the posterior cervical spine are common. Wound closure is also critical, and should be performed in a layered fashion. Closing the deep muscle, nuchal fascia, and superficial muscle in separate layers is recommended. The skin is often closed with nonabsorbable suture to allow them to be left in place longer to allow the underlying tissue to heal. Postoperatively, routine wound inspection should be performed to assess for any signs of early infection or dehiscence. Posterior cervical wound healing has been shown to be dependent on nutrition.[11,12] Especially in this patient population, nutritional depletion is common and can be compounded postoperatively by dysphagia. Supplementation with nasogastric feeds, protein shakes, or other modalities is critical to provide the building blocks for successful wound healing.

19.2.3 Respiratory Complications

The most common cause of death following surgery for ASD is respiratory failure.[13] Respiratory complications following ACD surgery are common, and are multifactorial. Because of the intimate anatomic relationship of the trachea with the cervical spine and its alignment, deformity correction may alter the airway dynamics.[6] The presence of dysphonia may be associated with respiratory complications. Dysphagia may predispose patients to silent aspiration events that can contribute to the development of pneumonitis, pneumonia, or respiratory distress. Lastly, the use of an immobilizing collar postoperatively may further depress respiratory function. The ISSG reported respiratory failure in 5.1% of ACD patients.[5] Similarly, Grosso et al identified pneumonia in 5.2% of patients postoperatively.[4] This compares to the ASD cohort, wherein the ISSG reported pneumonia in only 0.6% of patients, and the need for reintubation occurred only 0.3% of the time.[14]

For these reasons, respiratory status should be closely monitored following cervical deformity surgery. Communication with the anesthesia providers is critical. Consideration of postoperative transfer to the intensive care unit (ICU) or other higher-level care units should be considered, particularly in a patient with prolonged operative time or any underlying respiratory difficulties. Furthermore, the use of continuous pulse oximetry should be considered in the acute and subacute postoperative period.

19.2.4 Deep Venous Thrombosis/ Pulmonary Embolism

Surgical procedures involving the cervical spine are historically associated with low rates of deep venous thrombosis (DVT) or pulmonary embolism (PE), with rates of approximately 1 to 2%.[15] However, because of the greater physiologic demands of deformity surgery as well as the frequency of combined anterior-posterior procedures, there may be an increased risk in those undergoing ACD surgery. The existing literature is highly varied, with rates of PE ranging from 1.3 to 3.9%, and DVT as high as 44%.[4,5,15,16] Thus, while there are limited data available, what literature does exist may reflect a legitimate increase in thrombotic complications.

Prevention of thrombotic complications must be tailored to each individual patient. While mechanical devices and early mobilization are relatively benign means to help prevent DVT, the use of pharmaceutical anticoagulants is controversial. The risk of epidural hematoma or wound hematoma/seroma with pharmacologic agents may outweigh their benefit.

19.3 Risk Factors for Complications

As in all surgery, appropriate preoperative planning is instrumental to improve operative outcomes. This is particularly true with regard to the appreciation of patient comorbidities prior to elective deformity surgery. Numerous studies have sought to identify perioperative risk factors that may predict postoperative complications in patients undergoing ASD surgery.[17,18,19,20,21,22,23] However, many of these studies have addressed ASD surgery in general, and thus are not specific to cervical deformity.

Among the risk factors considered for those undergoing deformity surgery, the most common modifiable factors include abuse of drugs or alcohol, tobacco use, and obesity. In all cases, patients should be counseled and encouraged to adjust these modifiable risk factors through diet, exercise, and substance cessation prior to proceeding with ASD surgery. Nonmodifiable factors include patient age as well as underlying medical diagnoses such as cardiac, pulmonary, or renal diseases. These nonmodifiable factors also increase the risk of postoperative complications. These diagnoses should be identified during preoperative assessment, and appropriate clearance and perioperative management should be sought by the patients, cardiologist, internist, as well as surgical anesthesiologist.

Although several conditions can lead to cervical deformity, these conditions should be identified and assessed for expectant management postoperatively. Among these conditions are inflammatory conditions such as rheumatoid arthritis and ankylosing spondylitis, neurologic deterioration such as Parkinson disease, and neuromuscular disorders such as myasthenia gravis.[24] Lastly, deformity may be secondary to other causes including trauma, postradiation, or postoperative.

19.3.1 Age

There are conflicting data in the literature supporting the hypothesis that elderly patients are at greater risk of postoperative medical complications. A recent study by the Spinal Deformity Study Group found a dramatic increase in overall complications with increasing age for patients undergoing deformity surgery in general. They stratified patients into the age groups of 25 to 44, 45 to 64, and 65 to 85 and identified rates of complications of 17, 42, and 71%, respectively.[19] However, these results were not divided into medical versus surgical complications. In contrast, the ISSG did not find age to be a risk factor among those with specific cervical deformity, though their study may be underpowered to detect such a difference.[5]

19.3.2 Medical Comorbidities

The presence of medical comorbidities is not surprising given the advanced age of many patients undergoing ACD surgery. This can make the intraoperative and postoperative care of these patients more challenging. Underlying respiratory illnesses should be considered, considering the elevated risk of

respiratory complications following ACD surgery. Furthermore, the presence of increasing medical comorbidities has been found to be an independent predictor of hospital readmission.[25]

19.4 Effect of Complications on Patient Outcomes

There is insufficient literature available regarding outcomes in those who develop complications following ACD correction, compared to those who do not experience complications. However, the available literature does suggest that most patients can expect overall improvement.[4,5,16] Medical complications following deformity surgery are associated with increased perioperative cost as well as length of stay.[26,27,28] Complications do not, however, appear to have an impact on long-term patient-reported outcomes following ASD surgery, with similar improvements in Oswestry Disability Index (ODI), SF-36, Scoliosis Research Society (SRS), and patient satisfaction scores seen at 2-year follow-up in patients with and without perioperative complications.[29,30,31]

19.5 Case Example

▶ Fig. 19.1 shows the AP and lateral radiographs of a 72-year-old female who presented with disabling neck pain and trouble maintaining a horizontal gaze. In addition to a clear sagittal plane deformity, she also had a profound coronal plane deformity resulting in a "cock-robin" position of her head. In addition,

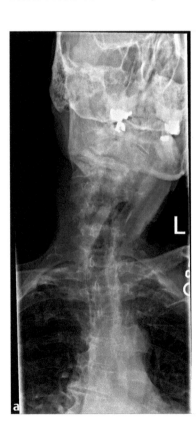
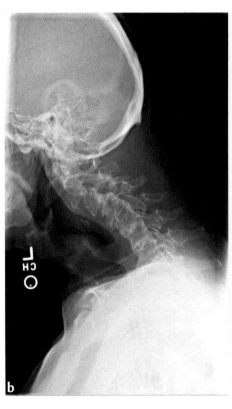

Fig. 19.1 Preoperative radiographs. **(a)** A rigid coronal plane deformity that resulted in a "cock-robin" head position. **(b)** A neutral latera, demonstrating significant loss of normal lordosis.

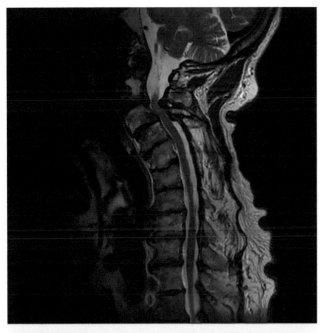

Fig. 19.2 Representative image on sagittal MRI which shows severe upper cervical stenosis, most pronounced at C2/C3.

history and physical exam revealed signs and symptoms consistent with cervical myelopathy, which was confirmed on MRI (▶ Fig. 19.2).

The patient was taken to the operating room where she underwent a combined anterior-posterior decompression, fusion, and deformity correction (▶ Fig. 19.3). Postoperatively, she was admitted to the ICU for ventilatory support due to airway swelling. She was unable to wean from ventilatory support, and on postoperative day 5 the decision was made to undergo tracheotomy, which can be seen in the radiographs of ▶ Fig. 19.3.

One month later, she underwent downsizing and eventual decannulation of the tracheostomy. She was satisfied with her surgical result. She could ambulate without difficulty and noted improvement in her clinical symptoms of myelopathy and her downward gaze.

This scenario highlights several aspects discussed in this chapter. The patient had several risk factors for postoperative airway difficulties, including advanced age, a combined anterior and posterior approach, prolonged surgical time, and correction of a rigid, lordotic deformity. Despite the significant improvement in cervical alignment and head positioning, the correction of such a rigid deformity may have contributed to altered alignment and/or tension of her airway with resultant swelling.

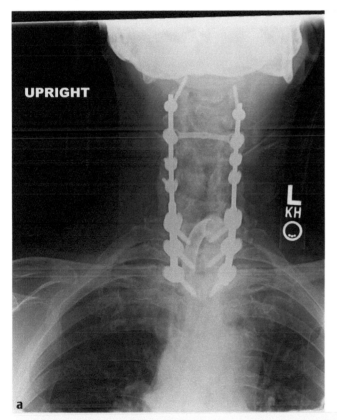
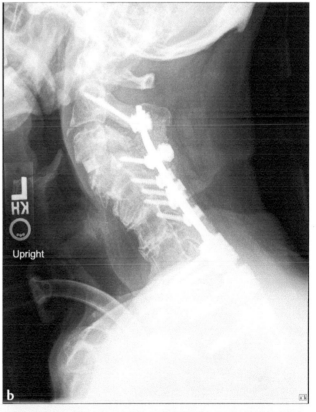

Fig. 19.3 Upright postoperative radiographs. **(a)** Restoration of coronal plane alignment. Lateral radiograph is seen in **(b)**, demonstrating improved alignment, as well as surgical tracheostomy.

References

[1] Sciubba DM, Yurter A, Smith JS, et al. International Spine Study Group (ISSG). A comprehensive review of complication rates after surgery for adult deformity: a reference for informed consent. Spine Deform. 2015; 3(6):575–594

[2] Charosky S, Guigui P, Blamoutier A, Roussouly P, Chopin D, Study Group on Scoliosis. Complications and risk factors of primary adult scoliosis surgery: a multicenter study of 306 patients. Spine. 2012; 37(8):693–700

[3] Blamoutier A, Guigui P, Charosky S, Roussouly P, Chopin D, Study Group on Scoliosis. Surgery of lumbar and thoracolumbar scolioses in adults over 50. Morbidity and survival in a multicenter retrospective cohort of 180 patients with a mean follow-up of 4.5 years. Orthopaedics & Traumatology: Surgery & Research. 2012; 98(5):528–535

[4] Grosso MJ, Hwang R, Krishnaney AA, Mroz TE, Benzel EC, Steinmetz MP. Complications and outcomes for surgical approaches to cervical kyphosis. J Spinal Disord Tech. 2015; 28(7):E385–E393

[5] Smith JS, Ramchandran S, Lafage V, et al. International Spine Study Group. Prospective multicenter assessment of early complication rates associated with adult cervical deformity surgery in 78 patients. Neurosurgery. 2016f; 79 (3):378–388

[6] Randall DR, Strong EB, Belafsky PC. Altered pharyngeal structure and dynamics among patients with cervical kyphosis. Laryngoscope. 2017; 127 (8):1832–1837

[7] Radcliff KE, Bennett J, Stewart RJ, et al. Change in angular alignment is associated with early dysphagia after anterior cervical discectomy and fusion. Clin Spine Surg. 2016; 29(6):248–254

[8] Fineberg SJ, Ahmadinia K, Oglesby M, Patel AA, Singh K. Hospital outcomes and complications of anterior and posterior cervical fusion with bone morphogenetic protein. Spine. 2013; 38(15):1304–1309

[9] Edwards CC, II, Dean C, Edwards CC, Phillips D, Blight A. Can dysphagia following anterior cervical fusions with rhBMP-2 be reduced with local Depomedrol application? A prospective, randomized, placebo-controlled, double-blind trial. Spine. 2016; 41(7):555–562

[10] Tomov M, Mitsunaga L, Durbin-Johnson B, Nallur D, Roberto R. Reducing surgical site infection in spinal surgery with betadine irrigation and intrawound vancomycin powder. Spine. 2015; 40(7):491–499

[11] Sebastian A, Huddleston P, III, Kakar S, Habermann E, Wagie A, Nassr A. Risk factors for surgical site infection after posterior cervical spine surgery: an analysis of 5,441 patients from the ACS NSQIP 2005–2012. Spine J. 2016; 16 (4):504–509

[12] Lee NJ, Kothari P, Kim JS, et al. Nutritional status as an adjunct risk factor for early postoperative complications following posterior cervical fusion. Spine. 2017; 42(18):1367–1374

[13] Hamilton DK, Kong C, Hiratzka J, et al. Patient satisfaction after adult spinal deformity surgery does not strongly correlate with health-related quality of life scores, radiographic parameters, or occurrence of complications. Spine. 2017; 42(10):764–769

[14] Smith JS, Klineberg E, Lafage V, et al. International Spine Study Group. Prospective multicenter assessment of perioperative and minimum 2-year postoperative complication rates associated with adult spinal deformity surgery. J Neurosurg Spine. 2016; 25(1):1–14

[15] Epstein NE. Intermittent pneumatic compression stocking prophylaxis against deep venous thrombosis in anterior cervical spinal surgery: a prospective efficacy study in 200 patients and literature review. Spine. 2005; 30 (22):2538–2543

[16] Etame AB, Wang AC, Than KD, La Marca F, Park P. Outcomes after surgery for cervical spine deformity: review of the literature. Neurosurg Focus. 2010; 28 (3):E14

[17] Sansur CA, Smith JS, Coe JD, et al. Scoliosis research society morbidity and mortality of adult scoliosis surgery. Spine. 2011; 36(9):E593–E597

[18] Schwab FJ, Hawkinson N, Lafage V, et al. International Spine Study Group. Risk factors for major peri-operative complications in adult spinal deformity surgery: a multi-center review of 953 consecutive patients. Eur Spine J. 2012; 21(12):2603–2610

[19] Smith JS, Shaffrey CI, Glassman SD, et al. Spinal Deformity Study Group. Risk-benefit assessment of surgery for adult scoliosis: an analysis based on patient age. Spine. 2011; 36(10):817–824

[20] Daubs MD, Lenke LG, Cheh G, Stobbs G, Bridwell KH. Adult spinal deformity surgery: complications and outcomes in patients over age 60. Spine. 2007; 32 (20):2238–2244

[21] Smith JS, Shaffrey CI, Berven S, et al. Spinal Deformity Study Group. Improvement of back pain with operative and nonoperative treatment in adults with scoliosis. Neurosurgery. 2009; 65(1):86–93, discussion 93–94

[22] Carreon LY, Puno RM, Dimar JR, II, Glassman SD, Johnson JR. Perioperative complications of posterior lumbar decompression and arthrodesis in older adults. J Bone Joint Surg Am. 2003; 85-A(11):2089–2092

[23] Cloyd JM, Acosta FL, Jr, Cloyd C, Ames CP. Effects of age on perioperative complications of extensive multilevel thoracolumbar spinal fusion surgery. J Neurosurg Spine. 2010; 12(4):402–408

[24] Shen FH, Samartzis D, Fessler RG, eds. Textbook of the Cervical Spine. Maryland Heights, MO: Saunders (Elsevier); 2015

[25] Schairer WW, Carrer A, Deviren V, et al. Hospital readmission after spine fusion for adult spinal deformity. Spine. 2013; 38(19):1681–1689

[26] Worley N, Marascalchi B, Jalai CM, et al. Predictors of inpatient morbidity and mortality in adult spinal deformity surgery. Eur Spine J. 2016; 25(3):819–827

[27] Diebo BG, Jalai CM, Challier V, et al. Novel index to quantify the risk of surgery in the setting of adult spinal deformity: a study on 10,912 patients from the Nationwide Inpatient Sample. Clin Spine Surg. 2017; 30(7):E993–E999

[28] Fischer CR, Terran J, Lonner B, et al. Factors predicting cost-effectiveness of adult spinal deformity surgery at 2 years. Spine Deform. 2014; 2(5):415–422

[29] Yeramaneni S, Robinson C, Hostin R. Impact of spine surgery complications on costs associated with management of adult spinal deformity. Curr Rev Musculoskelet Med. 2016; 9(3):327–332

[30] Auerbach JD, Lenke LG, Bridwell KH, et al. Major complications and comparison between 3-column osteotomy techniques in 105 consecutive spinal deformity procedures. Spine. 2012; 37(14):1198–1210

[31] Schwartz DM, Auerbach JD, Dormans JP, et al. Neurophysiological detection of impending spinal cord injury during scoliosis surgery. J Bone Joint Surg Am. 2007; 89(11):2440–2449

20 Relationship of Cervical Spondylotic Myelopathy to Cervical Deformity

Peter G. Passias

Abstract

This chapter delves into the interconnectedness of cervical deformity (CD) and cervical spondylotic myelopathy (CSM). CDs are an increasingly recognized combination of clinical and radiographic entities. While CD can occur in the absence of neurological dysfunction, its presence has been shown to be strongly associated with CSM, as malalignment of the cervical spine itself causes the spinal cord to be compressed or altered in contour in ways to accommodate the deformity, leading to similar neurologic symptoms. This chapter goes through the pathophysiology of CSM, its natural history and clinical presentation, and then delves into other CSM etiologies that are associated with CD, including ossification of the posterior longitudinal ligament, Chiari malformations, and atlantoaxial dislocations. What follows is in-depth understanding of how CD and CSM are related and share many of the same neurologic symptoms and the relevant radiographic parameters and clinical outcome metrics used to assess patients with both CSM and CD. The surgical and technical goals of treatment for patients with both CD and CSM are described, with an emphasis on the fact that both the spinal cord compression and spinal malalignment need to be taken into account when planning the appropriate treatment for these patients.

Keywords: cervical deformity, cervical spondylotic myelopathy, surgical correction, spinal cord compression, spinal malalignment, kyphosis

20.1 Introduction

Cervical spondylotic myelopathy (CSM) is a clinical condition that arises secondary to degenerative changes in the cervical spinal column.[1,2] It is characterized by several clinical symptoms and signs on clinical examination that are consistent with dysfunction of the spinal cord, typically including elements of hand clumsiness and gait impairment. When the spinal cord becomes compressed as degenerative changes occur in the spine, long tract signs arise. CSM is the most common cause of myelopathy in patients older than 55 years.[3,4] Thorough patient history and physical examination can allow for early diagnosis and prevention of further neurological deficits and improve clinical outcomes. There is varied clinical presentation of CSM based on severity and cooccurring conditions that can complicate the outcomes.[2] Cervical deformities (CDs) are an increasingly recognized combination of clinical and radiographic entities. While CD can occur in the absence of neurological dysfunction, its presence has been shown to be strongly associated with CSM, as malalignment of the cervical spine itself causes the spinal cord to be compressed or altered in contour in ways to accommodate the deformity, leading to similar neurologic symptoms.

20.2 Pathophysiology of Cervical Spondylotic Myelopathy

CSM is the most common cause of cervical myelopathy. It is a degenerative, age-related condition that involves direct compression and ischemic dysfunction of the spinal cord. CSM is more common in males than in females and presently mostly in patients older than 55 years.[5] The demographic of CSM patients varies by geographical region, with the average age of CSM patients being the highest in North America and lowest in Asia.[5] Spinal cord compression can arise from anterior degenerative changes, including osteophytes and disc osteophyte complexes, as well as posterior changes and can span multiple levels of the cervical spine.[6,7] Most commonly, degenerative changes occur at the C5–C6 and C6–C7 levels, though degeneration can occur anywhere in the spine. Congenital narrowing of the cervical spinal canal (congenital stenosis) can predispose individuals to myelopathic symptoms in combination with degenerative changes over time.[8] Intramedullary hyperintensity on T2-weighted MRI of the cervical spinal cord can detect spinal cord edema which can ultimately lead to myelomalacia and demyelination associated with spinal canal volume loss caused by long-term compression.[9,10]

CSM is also associated with cervical kyphosis, in which curve progression can compress and/or flatten the spinal cord and cause symptoms. Cervical malalignment can cause the anterior and posterior margins of the spinal cord compress and the lateral margins expand. When the spinal cord becomes tethered and bends around the kyphotic regions of the spine, it causes increased intramedullary pressure and neuronal loss and potential demyelination of the spinal cord.[11] Individuals with kyphotic cervical spinal deformities display shifts in the spinal cord to the anterior region of the spinal canal and presses against the vertebral bodies posteriorly at the apex of the deformity.[12,13] As the kyphosis of the cervical spine progresses and becomes more severe, there is additional mechanical stress applied to the spinal cord and the cord is stretched out on the posterior side of the vertebra.[14] When the spinal cord experiences increased elongation as a result of dynamic motion, including flexion of the spine and increased stretching as a result of the deformity, the strain becomes heightened and can lead to myelopathy.[11]

20.3 Natural History of Cervical Spondylotic Myelopathy

The natural history of CSM is based on studies with inconsistent findings and clinical evaluations.[3] CSM generally presents later in life and can have periods of asymptomatic presentation and also progresses slowly.[15,16] One study reported that 95% of CSM patients had a slow, stepwise decline in neurological function with only 5% of patients experiencing rapid, dramatic deterioration.[17] Other studies have reported mixed patterns as well, with some patients deteriorating quickly in neurological function and others experiencing a slow decline.[18,19]

Given that CSM is a progressive disease, there are estimates that between 20 and 60% of symptomatic CSM patients will have their symptoms deteriorate without surgical intervention.[20,21] Consistent recommendations for treatment for CSM have been difficult to establish, given that the course of CSM progression is widely varied and differs between individuals.[21,22] In assessing neurological outcomes by means of Japanese Orthopedic Association (JOA) score, one prospective study showed that 15% of patients either worsened or remained unchanged at or below a score of 14 on the JOA at 1-year follow-up, and 27% by 3 years.[23,24,25,26] In the same prospective study, they reported a mean JOA score of 15 at 1-year and a median JOA score of 15 at 10-year follow-up. Retrospective studies reported that 31% of patients deteriorated in JOA score at 3-year and 37% at 4-year follow-up.[27,28]

Worsening neurologic or functional symptoms lead to some patients undergoing surgical treatment. The rate of conversion from nonoperative to surgical treatment for CSM ranged from 4 to 40% in studies with 3- to 7-year follow-up.[19,27,28,29,30,31,32,33] One study reported that cervical hypermobility, segmental kyphosis, and instability were factors for conversion to surgical treatment.[30] Deterioration is also associated with a long duration of symptoms, and rigorous conservative treatment showed higher improvement rates than less intense methods of conservative treatment.[32] The circumferential spinal cord compression in the segment with the maximum compression on an axial MRI was a significant prognostic factor for surgical treatment in a subset of CSM patients.[33] Another study reported that surgery for CSM was associated with improvements in functional, disability-related, and quality-of-life outcomes, regardless of baseline severity of the disease.[34]

20.4 Clinical Presentation of Cervical Spondylotic Myelopathy

Given that the spinal cord involves nerves that carry signals to diffuse regions of the body, patients with CSM can experience a wide range of symptoms. Commonly, patients present with upper extremity symptoms such as hand weakness and numbness, and motor dysfunction characterized by the inability to perform fine motor skills, difficultly buttoning a shirt, and tendency to drop objects.[15,35] Patients with CSM also commonly present with balance problems and unsteady gait. Less than 50% of CSM patients present with neck pain, though this rate becomes much higher for patients with CD. Lhermitte sign and sphincter dysfunction can also present in CSM patients, though at lower rates. More severe CSM progression may present at paraparesis and hand numbness. Most commonly, CSM involves cervical levels C5–C6, C6–C7, followed by C4–C5 and C3–C4. Early recognition of symptoms and treatment prior to spinal cord damage or deterioration of symptoms is critical for optimal clinical outcomes.

20.5 Other Cervical Spondylotic Myelopathy Etiologies Associated with Cervical Deformities

20.5.1 Ossification of the Posterior Longitudinal Ligament

Ossification of the posterior longitudinal ligament (OPLL) can elicit cervical spinal canal stenosis.[36,37] OPLL is one of the most common causes of cervical myelopathy particularly in the Asian population, with the highest prevalence found in Japan (1.9–4.3% incidence), with lower rates found in Korea, the United States, and Germany.[5,37,38,39] As OPLL progresses, it eventually causes compression of the spinal cord and myelopathy.[40,41,42] Postlaminectomy kyphosis after treatment for OPLL has been reported in the literature and cervical malalignment is a crucial consideration when treating OPLL.[43] Cervical lordosis (CL) is important in performing a laminoplasty for OPLL with an occupying ratio greater than 60%, as suggested by findings that patients who underwent a laminoplasty and achieved a good outcome had a greater degree of CL even though they also had a larger ossification-occupying ratio.[44] The K-line was developed to assess cervical alignment and OPLL size using only one parameter that aids surgeons in decisions regarding the surgical approach for patients with cervical OPLL while taking into account cervical malalignment.[45] The K-line is drawn from the midpoints of the spinal canal at C2 to the midpoint at C7 and then OPLL cases can be divided into two cases: K-line (+) where the OPLL does not exceed the K-line and K-line (-) where OPLL extends beyond the K-line.[45]

20.6 Atlantoaxial Dislocations

Atlantoaxial dislocations are a loss of stability between the atlas and the axis that causes a loss of normal articulation between the joints, caused by traumatic, inflammatory, idiopathic, or congenital abnormalities.[46,47] Myelopathy is one clinical presentation of atlantoaxial dislocations that can lead to more severe clinical presentation and increased morbidity and mortality associated with the atlantoaxial dislocation.[46,48,49,50] Though rare, atlantoaxial dislocations are associated with complex CDs that often require surgical intervention. It has been shown that the subaxial cervical spinal alignment is in part determined by the direction of the dislocation, with anterior dislocations causing hyperlordosis of the subaxial cervical spine and posterior dislocations causing straightening or kyphosis, all in an effort to maintain overall balance.[47]

Swan neck deformities of the cervical spine have been documented first in patients after multilevel cervical laminectomies, tumor resections, and osteomyelitis and then after upper cervical procedures.[51,52,53,54] More recently, studies have looked at the preoperative development of swan neck deformities in patients with chronic atlantoaxial dislocations with abnormal kyphosis at the occipitoaxial segment and subaxial hyperlordosis.[55] Another study investigated whether abnormalities in subaxial alignment could be reversed following surgical correction of occipitoaxial malalignment for patients with swan neck deformities secondary to chronic atlantoaxial dislocation, defining a swan neck deformity as lordosis of the subaxial spine greater than 30 degrees with upper cervical kyphosis (less than 0 degrees). The authors found that these swan neck deformities can be reversed following correction of the primary upper CD.[56]

20.7 Chiari Malformations

Chiari malformations, most commonly type 1, present with the cerebellar tonsils below the foramen magnum, giving rise to brainstem and spinal cord compression and disruptions of cerebrospinal fluid.[57,58,59] A case report of a 51-year-old patient with previous intradural surgery for Chiari malformation presented with recurrent cervical myelopathy and progressive kyphotic CD and spinal cord tethering.[60] Spinal malalignment is frequently associated with Chiari 1 malformations, though the presentation varies significantly.[61,62]

20.8 Cervical Spondylotic Myelopathy and Cervical Deformity

20.8.1 Cooccurrence of Cervical Deformity and Cervical Spondylotic Myelopathy

CSM with associated cervical kyphosis results from the progressive subluxation of the apophyseal joints from facet joints and discs degeneration.[12] The cooccurrence of CD and CSM has been previously reported for patients mostly older than 60 years, with the majority of patients being male.[12,63] The operative treatment for patients with concurrent CD and CSM can be higher than for a patient with isolated CD or CSM, given that progression of the kyphotic deformity can lead to worsening and possibly irreversible spinal cord compression and myelopathic symptoms. Surgical correction of both the malalignment and the spinal cord compression from the CSM can help mitigate further neurologic deficit and help improve patients' overall quality of life. Given the known natural history of CSM and its often rapid progression once symptoms present, early surgical intervention for these CD patients with CSM can help optimize outcomes.

CD is a complex group of disorders with etiologies including spondylosis, inflammatory arthropathy, posttraumatic, postsurgical, and others.[64,65] CDs occur in both the coronal and sagittal planes; however, sagittal plane deformities are more frequent.[66] Deformities can either be primary (often congenital) or secondary (iatrogenic cause or ankylosing spondylitis).[67,68] Cervical kyphosis is the most common cervical spine deformity and is often the result of iatrogenic causes, including postlaminectomy kyphosis. When the deformity begins, it leads to postural shifts including the head and neck shifting forward and the change in load on the spine can influence further spinal deformities. Additionally, dropped head syndrome leading to a flexible chin-on-chest kyphotic deformity has been reported in conjunction with CSM and, while rare, leads to debilitating consequences for patients' quality of life.[69] These clinical presentations highlight the similar and interconnected degenerative processes of CD and CSM, as the compressive effect of multilevel disc degeneration is exacerbated by the kyphosis of the vertebrae.

The relationship between alignment of the upper cervical and subaxial spine has been documented in previous reports.[70,71,72] Studies have shown that changes in subaxial alignment can result following upper cervical fusion procedures, primarily in atlantoaxial dislocation patients. One study showed that when the atlantoaxial joint was surgically fixed in a hyperlordotic position, the subaxial spine responded with kyphotic sagittal alignment.[73] Another study showed that for complex swan neck deformity patients involving alignment changes of the upper cervical and subaxial spine, the sagittal alignment of the subaxial spine can still be reversed when the alignment in the upper cervical spine is treated.[56] They also found that age was a significant and independent predictor that was related to the amount of change in alignment of the subaxial spine after surgical correction of the occipitoaxial malalignment, suggesting that younger and more flexible spines can better compensate in order to maintain proper horizontal gaze. One case report described a patient with acute kyphotic swan neck CD that caused spinal canal narrowing and spinal cord compression after cervical laminectomy.[74]

20.8.2 Common Classification for CD Incorporating CSM and Radiographic Components

Recent advances in CD correction techniques and improved understanding of regional sagittal alignment of the cervical spine have led to the development of a new classification system for CD.[2] This classification system developed by Ames-ISSG et al primarily characterizes CD according to the apex of the deformity whether in the cervical, thoracic, or the cervicothoracic junction with added modifiers in the form of cervical sagittal vertical axis (cSVA), T1 slope minus cervical lordosis (TS–CL), chin–brow vertical angle (CBVA), SRS–Schwab modifier, and modified JOA (mJOA). The incorporation of a myelopathy modifier was found to be vital. Progressive cervical kyphosis has been associated with development of myelopathy, through draping and tensioning of the spinal cord over anterior pathology. This results in direct neural injury and ischemic changes.[3,4,5,6,7] Surgical correction for CD has led to improvement in radiographic alignment and patient-reported outcomes related to pain, disability, and neurologic and myelopathic improvement.[8]

20.8.3 Relevant Radiographic Parameters

The most common radiographic parameters to assess cervical alignment include CL, cSVA, TS–CL, and CBVA. Normative values for CL range from 15 degrees ± 10 degrees in young adults and 25 degrees ± 16 degrees in patients older than 60 years.[75] While normative values for cSVA have been reported as 1.5 cm ± 1 cm, reports suggest that a cSVA greater than 4 cm is correlated to inferior health-related quality-of-life (HRQOL) scores.[76] TS–CL takes into account both the CL and T1 slope and studies have shown that the parameter should be less than 17 degrees and higher TS–CL values are associated with worse clinical outcomes.[77] CBVA values ranging from 1 to 10 degrees have been used in the CD classification system of Ames and this parameter is useful especially in the management of severe, rigid, kyphotic CDs, since the loss of horizontal gaze significantly impacts quality of life and daily activities.[78,79]

20.8.4 Correlation of Cervical Deformity and Cervical Spondylotic Myelopathy Improvement with Outcomes

Multiple studies have examined the relationship between radiographic parameters and HRQOL scores, both in asymptomatic and spinal deformity patients, and correlations between the two measures have been well established.[80] Tang et al concluded that a C2–C7 SVA greater than 4 cm was associated with worse Neck Disability Index (NDI) scores at 6 months postoperative interval following correction of CDs.[80] One of the limitations of their study was the inability to comment on the preoperative cervical alignment and HRQOL outcomes due to lack of available data. Recently, Iyer et al studied the relationships between neck disability and preoperative cervical alignment in patients with degenerative cervical spine disease. They concluded that increased CL and T1 slope correlated with decreased NDI. Increasing cSVA was found to be an independent predictor of high preoperative NDI.[81] Both these studies prove the importance of restoring a cSVA less than 4 cm as an alignment goal while treating cervical sagittal malalignment. It is important to note, however, that restoration of cervical alignment is not the only factor contributing to improved patient outcomes following CD-corrective surgery. Postoperative myelopathy improvement may also contribute to improved patient-reported outcome measures, but the extent of this influence is ill characterized in the literature.[80,82]

In addition, recent work focusing on prospectively collected severe CD patients has shown that improvements in myelopathy symptoms and mJOA functional scores were significantly associated with superior 1-year postoperative outcomes in comparison to patients who improved only in alignment parameters.[83] This work, along with other preliminary investigations, indicates a strong connection between CD alignment correction and improvement and patient-reported outcomes, with myelopathy improvement as a key driver of patient-reported outcomes for patients undergoing CD surgical correction.

20.9 Spinal Cord Symptoms Resulting from Cervical Deformity

Progressive cervical kyphosis is associated with myelopathy. Deformity of the spine causes the spinal cord to bend and elongate against the vertebral bodies, which increases spinal cord tension.[13,84,85] With curve progression, the spinal cord becomes compressed and flattens,[86] as described previously. Spinal cord tethering leads to increased intramedullary pressure and neuronal loss and demyelination of the cord. Additionally, when the blood vessels on the spinal cord flatten, blood supply is reduced, which causes an abnormal blood supply network. One study found a significant correlation between the degree of kyphosis and the amount that the spinal cord was flattened in a population of small game fowls.[86] Further study using angiography showed that the anterior portion of the cord displays decreased vascular supply. Sagittal alignment of the cervical spine and cervical myelopathy are closely linked. When degenerative changes in the spine occur and osteophytes form, in addition to ligamentous and facet hypertrophy, cervical spinal stenosis develops and can compress the spinal cord. Stenosis and compression on a long-term scale can lead to demyelination and necrosis of gray and white matter due to hypovascularization of the cord.[87] Changes in the spinal cord can first be detected by high signal intensity of the cord at the level of the compression and then by the "snake-eyes" appearance of myelomalacia or necrotic changes.[88]

20.10 Surgical Management of Cervical Deformity and Cervical Spondylotic Myelopathy

20.10.1 Technical Goals for Patients with Cervical Deformity and Cervical Spondylotic Myelopathy

Cervical deformity without compression of the neurologic elements may be treated without central decompression. The addition of myelopathy requires that central decompression be performed in addition to reduction of deformity and stabilization if adequate decompression of the spinal cord is not achieved with realignment alone. The intrinsic damage to the spinal cord causing myelopathy may be as a result of direct compression or it may be a result of traction placed on the cord by malalignment. The surgeon has two interrelated considerations prior to deciding the most appropriate surgical approach. The first is deciding the method for correcting the deformity, and the second consideration is the approach to neural element decompression. In selected patients, cervical realignment alone may be sufficient to decompress the neural elements. Presented but yet unpublished data show that for patients with CD and myelopathy symptoms, realignment alone improves symptoms in a subset of patients.[83] Other variables requiring consideration include age and medical comorbidities, global sagittal alignment, cervical sagittal alignment, rigid or flexible CD, smoking status, body mass index, prior cervical spine surgical approaches, the combined presence of a thoracolumbar deformity, ventral versus dorsal compression, focal or diffuse compression, and etiology of the compressive component. Approaches to the cervical spine can be ventral, dorsal, or a combination of both.

The general options for posterior central neural decompression include standalone laminectomy, laminoplasty, and fusion. Cervical alignment and lordosis is an important factor when deciding on an operative approach. Isolated laminectomy is the least invasive procedure but is associated with increased incidence of postoperative kyphosis, even in patients with straight (30%) and lordotic (14%) preoperative alignments.[43] Standalone laminectomy is even less palatable in the setting of cervical spinal deformity.

A literature review published in 2013 noted the overall evidence for effectiveness of laminoplasty compared to laminectomy and fusion for treatment of CSM is insufficient to recommend one procedure over the other.[89] Moreover, only two articles examined the development of kyphotic deformity between the two procedures. One article looking at patients with multilevel CSM found laminectomy and fusion to have a higher rate of kyphotic deformity development than laminoplasty (0 vs. 15%).[90] This study also found significantly increased loss of lordosis in laminectomy and fusion group versus the laminoplasty group. In CSM patients with preoperative CL, laminoplasty has shown to increase lordosis slightly (1.8 degrees) relative to preoperative lordosis as well as maintain 87.9% of preoperative flexion/extension range of motion.[91] Perhaps more intuitively, a recent large case series comparing laminoplasty versus laminectomy and fusion found no difference in postoperative sagittal cervical Cobb angle, despite the fusion group having significantly less preoperative lordosis (5.8 vs. 10.9 degrees).[92] Fusion was also associated with improved neurologic outcome as measured by the Nurick score; however, it had significantly longer operative time and blood loss. Neck pain was similar between groups. This study underscores the bias preventing matched comparison between these two procedures in the setting of CD. Specifically, in patients with worse preoperative sagittal balance, surgeons are unlikely to randomize between the two posterior options and will choose laminectomy and fusion over laminoplasty.

The general options for anterior neural decompression include anterior cervical discectomy and fusion, anterior disc replacement, corpectomy, combination of anterior cervical discectomy and fusion, and corpectomy. It has been recommended that patients with CSM without dorsal compression will have superior neurological recovery, less neck pain, and superior correction of sagittal alignment if multiple anterior discectomies are performed instead of corpectomy or combined discectomy–corpectomy approaches.[93]

20.10.2 Surgical Goals for Patients with Cervical Deformity and Cervical Spondylotic Myelopathy

There is a paucity of literature comparing the effect of anterior versus posterior surgical approach on operative outcomes in patients with sagittal CD and CSM. Uchida et al compared anterior decompression and fusion with posterior open door laminoplasty in patients with CSM who also had cervical kyphosis of at least 10 degrees on lateral radiograph in the neutral position (average: 15.9 degrees ± 5.9 degrees). Their results showed a significantly smaller kyphotic angle in neutral and flexion positions in the anterior spondylectomy approach compared with the laminoplasty approach.[12] A more general review comparing anterior versus posterior approach for CSM (not restricted to those with deformity) found no clear advantage to either approach. Neurological outcome based on mJOA was similar, rates of C5 palsy were

similar, canal diameter was larger with posterior surgery, infection rate was lower with anterior surgery, and dysphagia was lower with posterior approach.[94]

Ideal degree of deformity correction is not established. An analysis of 56 operative CSM cases found no correlation between cervical sagittal balance (C2–C7) and myelopathy severity as measured by mJOA.[95] However, this was not a cohort specifically with deformity. In patients undergoing posterior cervical spine fusion, sagittal CD as measured by C2 SVA has been shown by Tang et al to correlate with worse postoperative HRQOL. They proposed C2–C7 SVA greater than 40 mm as the threshold beyond which HRQOL will be negatively affected.[76] This suggests reducing C2–C7 SVA to less than 40 mm as a minimal threshold for CD correction; however, further study is necessary to confirm this. Other radiographic parameters to assess when correcting CD include T1S–C2–C7 lordosis less than 15 degrees and CBVA between -10 and +20 degrees. Patients with a CBVA less than -10 degrees have significantly lower scores on horizontal gaze testing.[78] An upper CBVA limit of 20 degrees has been proposed, but perhaps an upper limit of 10 degrees may be a superior goal.[96] The mismatch between T1 slope and CL (T1S–C2–C7 lordosis) attempts to account for the increasing lordotic requirements as the T1 slope increases. It has been proposed by expert opinion that less than 15 degrees is a reasonable goal.[79] It should again be noted that the earlier-mentioned alignment parameters are established in the literature as generally accepted values, but each patient must be evaluated and treated based on their particular needs and deformity. From a functional deformity perspective, operative goals should be to restore forward gaze, reduce muscle strain, and minimize axial neck pain. Lastly, it has been shown that dynamic spinal cord compression increases in extension more so than flexion in all kyphotic deformity subtypes.[97] This suggests that it would be prudent to perform decompression of the spinal cord prior to attempted reduction of deformity, particularly if the reduction of the deformity involves extension.

In summary, in the setting of CSM and cervical spinal deformity, the operative goals are twofold, neural decompression and reduction and stabilization of the CD. There is a paucity of evidence to recommend specific surgical approaches. The surgeon must individualize the approach to the patient based on the location of compression, the curvature of the deformity, and their comfort with various approaches.

20.10.3 Case Examples of Patients with Concurrent Cervical Deformity and Cervical Spondylotic Myelopathy

We present three case examples of patients with concurrent CD and CSM. In ▶ Fig. 20.1, the patient improves in cervical alignment only postoperatively. In ▶ Fig. 20.3, the patient improves only in myelopathy, with cSVA worsening postoperatively. ▶ Fig. 20.2 displays a CD patient with CSM who improves in both cervical alignment and myelopathy symptoms after surgical correction.

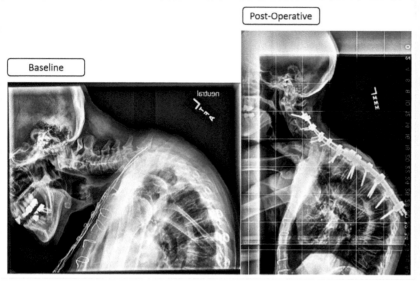

Fig. 20.1 Cervical deformity patients with myelopathy who improved only in alignment. Pre- and postoperative radiographs of a cervical deformity patient with baseline myelopathy symptoms. This is a 73-year-old female patient with a TS–CL of 77 degrees and cSVA of 90 degrees. The baseline NDI score was 42 and mJOA was 13. She underwent a C2–T7 posterior fusion, with a three-column osteotomy at T2. Postoperative improvement was seen in alignment, with TS–CL decreasing to 34 degrees and cSVA to 54 degrees, though myelopathy symptoms remained the same (post-op mJOA score of 14). cSVA, cervical sagittal vertical axis; mJOA, modified Japanese Orthopedic Association; NDI, Neck Disability Index; TS–CL, T1 slope minus cervical lordosis.

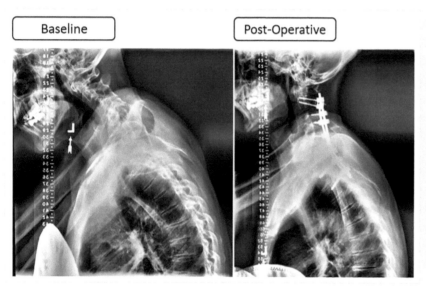

Fig. 20.2 Cervical deformity patients with myelopathy who improved both in alignment and myelopathy symptoms. Pre- and postoperative radiographs of a cervical deformity patient with baseline myelopathy symptoms. This is a 58-year-old female patient with a TS–CL of 72 degrees and cSVA of 40 degrees. The baseline NDI score was 66 and mJOA was 7. She underwent a C2–T3 posterior fusion, with decompression and Smith–Peterson osteotomies at C2–C4 and C6–C7. Postoperative improvement was seen for cervical alignment, with TS–CL decreasing to 33 degrees and cSVA to 25 degrees. She also improved in myelopathy, with her mJOA score increasing from a 7 (severe) to 14 (moderate). cSVA, cervical sagittal vertical axis; mJOA, modified Japanese Orthopedic Association; NDI, Neck Disability Index; TS–CL, T1 slope minus cervical lordosis.

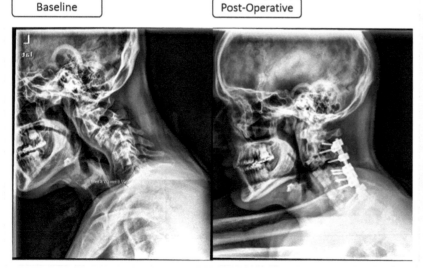

Fig. 20.3 Cervical deformity patients with myelopathy who improved only in myelopathy. Pre- and postoperative radiographs of a cervical deformity patient with baseline myelopathy symptoms. This is a 40-year-old male patient with a TS–CL of 40 degrees and cSVA of 46 degrees. The baseline NDI score was 54 and mJOA was 11. He underwent a C2–T2 posterior fusion with decompression. Postoperative cSVA worsened (46–50 degrees). Myelopathy symptoms significantly improved (mJOA score increased from 11 to 17), as well as NDI improved from 54 to 4. cSVA, cervical sagittal vertical axis; mJOA, modified Japanese Orthopedic Association; NDI, Neck Disability Index; TS–CL, T1 slope minus cervical lordosis.

References

[1] Lebl DR, Hughes A, Cammisa FP, Jr, O'Leary PF. Cervical spondylotic myelopathy: pathophysiology, clinical presentation, and treatment. HSS J. 2011; 7 (2):170–178

[2] Yarbrough CK, Murphy RKJ, Ray WZ, Stewart TJ. The natural history and clinical presentation of cervical spondylotic myelopathy. Adv Orthop. 2012; 2012:480643

[3] Klineberg E. Cervical spondylotic myelopathy: a review of the evidence. Orthop Clin North Am. 2010; 41(2):193–202

[4] Montgomery DM, Brower RS. Cervical spondylotic myelopathy. Clinical syndrome and natural history. Orthop Clin North Am. 1992; 23(3):487–493

[5] Fehlings MG, Kopjar B, Ibrahim A, et al. Geographic variations in clinical presentation and outcomes of decompressive surgery in patients with symptomatic degenerative cervical myelopathy: analysis of a prospective, international multicenter cohort study of 757 patients. Spine J. 2018; 18(4):593–605

[6] Payne EE, Spillane JD. The cervical spine; an anatomico-pathological study of 70 specimens (using a special technique) with particular reference to the problem of cervical spondylosis. Brain. 1957; 80(4):571–596

[7] Ahn JS, Lee JK, Kim BK. Prognostic factors that affect the surgical outcome of the laminoplasty in cervical spondylotic myelopathy. Clin Orthop Surg. 2010; 2(2):98–104

[8] Breig A, Turnbull I, Hassler O. Effects of mechanical stresses on the spinal cord in cervical spondylosis. A study on fresh cadaver material. J Neurosurg. 1966; 25(1):45–56

[9] Lee J, Koyanagi I, Hida K, Seki T, Iwasaki Y, Mitsumori K. Spinal cord edema: unusual magnetic resonance imaging findings in cervical spondylosis. J Neurosurg. 2003; 99(1) Suppl:8–13

[10] Tetreault LA, Dettori JR, Wilson JR, et al. Systematic review of magnetic resonance imaging characteristics that affect treatment decision making and predict clinical outcome in patients with cervical spondylotic myelopathy. Spine. 2013; 38(22) Suppl 1:S89–S110

[11] Dickson RA. The aetiology of spinal deformities. Lancet. 1988; 1(8595):1151–1155

[12] Uchida K, Nakajima H, Sato R, et al. Cervical spondylotic myelopathy associated with kyphosis or sagittal sigmoid alignment: outcome after anterior or posterior decompression. J Neurosurg Spine. 2009; 11(5):521–528

[13] Albert TJ, Vacarro A. Postlaminectomy kyphosis. Spine. 1998; 23(24):2738–2745

[14] Masini M, Maranhão V. Experimental determination of the effect of progressive sharp-angle spinal deformity on the spinal cord. Eur Spine J. 1997; 6 (2):89–92

[15] Cuellar J, Passias P. Cervical spondylotic myelopathy: a review of clinical diagnosis and treatment. Bull Hosp Jt Dis (2013). 2017; 75(1):21–29

[16] Matz PG, Anderson PA, Holly LT, et al. Joint Section on Disorders of the Spine and Peripheral Nerves of the American Association of Neurological Surgeons and Congress of Neurological Surgeons. The natural history of cervical spondylotic myelopathy. J Neurosurg Spine. 2009; 11(2):104–111

[17] Clarke E, Robinson PK. Cervical myelopathy: a complication of cervical spondylosis. Brain. 1956; 79(3):483–510

[18] Nurick S. The pathogenesis of the spinal cord disorder associated with cervical spondylosis. Brain. 1972; 95(1):87–100

[19] Lees F, Turner JW. Natural history and prognosis of cervical spondylosis. BMJ. 1963; 2(5373):1607–1610

[20] Tetreault LA, Côté P, Kopjar B, Arnold P, Fehlings MG, AOSpine North America and International Clinical Trial Research Network. A clinical prediction model to assess surgical outcome in patients with cervical spondylotic myelopathy: internal and external validations using the prospective multicenter AOSpine North American and international datasets of 743 patients. Spine J. 2015; 15 (3):388–397

[21] Karadimas SK, Erwin WM, Ely CG, Dettori JR, Fehlings MG. Pathophysiology and natural history of cervical spondylotic myelopathy. Spine. 2013; 38(22) Suppl 1:S21–S36

[22] Kalsi-Ryan S, Karadimas SK, Fehlings MG. Cervical spondylotic myelopathy: the clinical phenomenon and the current pathobiology of an increasingly prevalent and devastating disorder. Neuroscientist. 2013; 19(4):409–421

[23] Kadaňka Z, Bednařík J, Novotný O, Urbánek I, Dušek L. Cervical spondylotic myelopathy: conservative versus surgical treatment after 10 years. Eur Spine J. 2011; 20(9):1533–1538

[24] Kadanka Z, Mares M, Bednaník J, et al. Approaches to spondylotic cervical myelopathy: conservative versus surgical results in a 3-year follow-up study. Spine. 2002; 27(20):2205–2210, discussion 2210–2211

[25] Kadanka Z, Mares M, Bednarík J, et al. Predictive factors for spondylotic cervical myelopathy treated conservatively or surgically. Eur J Neurol. 2005; 12 (1):55–63

[26] Kadanka Z, Bednarík J, Vohánka S, et al. Conservative treatment versus surgery in spondylotic cervical myelopathy: a prospective randomised study. Eur Spine J. 2000; 9(6):538–544

[27] Matsumoto M, Chiba K, Ishikawa M, Maruiwa H, Fujimura Y, Toyama Y. Relationships between outcomes of conservative treatment and magnetic resonance imaging findings in patients with mild cervical myelopathy caused by soft disc herniations. Spine. 2001; 26(14):1592–1598

[28] Matsumoto M, Toyama Y, Ishikawa M, Chiba K, Suzuki N, Fujimura Y. Increased signal intensity of the spinal cord on magnetic resonance images in cervical compressive myelopathy. Does it predict the outcome of conservative treatment? Spine. 2000; 25(6):677–682

[29] Nakamura K, Kurokawa T, Hoshino Y, Saita K, Takeshita K, Kawaguchi H. Conservative treatment for cervical spondylotic myelopathy: achievement and sustainability of a level of "no disability". J Spinal Disord. 1998; 11(2):175–179

[30] Oshima Y, Seichi A, Takeshita K, et al. Natural course and prognostic factors in patients with mild cervical spondylotic myelopathy with increased signal intensity on T2-weighted magnetic resonance imaging. Spine. 2012; 37 (22):1909–1913

[31] Sumi M, Miyamoto H, Suzuki T, Kaneyama S, Kanatani T, Uno K. Prospective cohort study of mild cervical spondylotic myelopathy without surgical treatment. J Neurosurg Spine. 2012; 16(1):8–14

[32] Yoshimatsu H, Nagata K, Goto H, et al. Conservative treatment for cervical spondylotic myelopathy. prediction of treatment effects by multivariate analysis. Spine J. 2001; 1(4):269–273

[33] Shimomura T, Sumi M, Nishida K, et al. Prognostic factors for deterioration of patients with cervical spondylotic myelopathy after nonsurgical treatment. Spine. 2007; 32(22):2474–2479

[34] Fehlings MG, Wilson JR, Kopjar B, et al. Efficacy and safety of surgical decompression in patients with cervical spondylotic myelopathy: results of the AOSpine North America prospective multi-center study. J Bone Joint Surg Am. 2013; 95(18):1651–1658

[35] Geck MJ, Eismont FJ. Surgical options for the treatment of cervical spondylotic myelopathy. Orthop Clin North Am. 2002; 33(2):329–348

[36] Li H, Wang J, Chen G, Li F, Zhu J, Chen Q. Combined upper cervical canal stenosis and cervical ossification of the posterior longitudinal ligament resulting in myelopathy: A case series and literature review. J Clin Neurosci. 2017; 45:270–275

[37] Matsunaga S, Sakou T. Ossification of the posterior longitudinal ligament of the cervical spine: etiology and natural history. Spine. 2012; 37(5):E309–E314

[38] Kim TJ, Bae KW, Uhm WS, Kim TH, Joo KB, Jun JB. Prevalence of ossification of the posterior longitudinal ligament of the cervical spine. Joint Bone Spine. 2008; 75(4):471–474

[39] Ikegawa S. Genetics of ossification of the posterior longitudinal ligament of the spine: a mini review. J Bone Metab. 2014; 21(2):127–132

[40] Harsh GR, IV, Sypert GW, Weinstein PR, Ross DA, Wilson CB. Cervical spine stenosis secondary to ossification of the posterior longitudinal ligament. J Neurosurg. 1987; 67(3):349–357

[41] Lin D, Ding Z, Lian K, Hong J, Zhai W. Cervical ossification of the posterior longitudinal ligament: Anterior versus posterior approach. Indian J Orthop. 2012; 46(1):92–98

[42] Kim B, Yoon DH, Shin HC, et al. Surgical outcome and prognostic factors of anterior decompression and fusion for cervical compressive myelopathy due to ossification of the posterior longitudinal ligament. Spine J. 2015; 15 (5):875–884

[43] Kaptain GJ, Simmons NE, Replogle RE, Pobereskin L. Incidence and outcome of kyphotic deformity following laminectomy for cervical spondylotic myelopathy. J Neurosurg. 2000; 93(2) Suppl:199–204

[44] Fujimori T, Iwasaki M, Okuda S, et al. Long-term results of cervical myelopathy due to ossification of the posterior longitudinal ligament with an occupying ratio of 60% or more. Spine. 2014; 39(1):58–67

[45] Fujiyoshi T, Yamazaki M, Kawabe J, et al. A new concept for making decisions regarding the surgical approach for cervical ossification of the posterior longitudinal ligament: the K-line. Spine. 2008; 33(26):E990–E993

[46] Yang SY, Boniello AJ, Poorman CE, Chang AL, Wang S, Passias PG. A review of the diagnosis and treatment of atlantoaxial dislocations. Global Spine J. 2014; 4(3):197–210

[47] Wang S, Passias PG, Cui L, et al. Does atlantoaxial dislocation influence the subaxial cervical spine? Eur Spine J. 2013; 22(7):1603–1607

[48] Wadia NH. Myelopathy complicating congenital atlanto-axial dislocation. (A study of 28 cases). Brain. 1967; 90(2):449–472

[49] Reddy KRM, Rao GSU, Devi BI, Prasad PVS, Ramesh VJ. Pulmonary function after surgery for congenital atlantoaxial dislocation: a comparison with surgery for compressive cervical myelopathy and craniotomy. J Neurosurg Anesthesiol. 2009; 21(3):196–201

[50] Papadopoulos SM, Dickman CA, Sonntag VK. Atlantoaxial stabilization in rheumatoid arthritis. J Neurosurg. 1991; 74(1):1–7

[51] Sim FH, Svien HJ, Bickel WH, Janes JM. Swan-neck deformity following extensive cervical laminectomy. A review of twenty-one cases. J Bone Joint Surg Am. 1974; 56(3):564–580

[52] Fassett DR, Clark R, Brockmeyer DL, Schmidt MH. Cervical spine deformity associated with resection of spinal cord tumors. Neurosurg Focus. 2006; 20(2):E2

[53] Malik GM, Crawford AH, Halter R. Swan-neck deformity secondary to osteomyelitis of the posterior elements of the cervical spine. Case report. J Neurosurg. 1979; 50(3):388–390

[54] Toyama Y, Matsumoto M, Chiba K, et al. Realignment of postoperative cervical kyphosis in children by vertebral remodeling. Spine. 1994; 19(22):2565–2570

[55] Passias PG, Wang S, Kozanek M, Wang S, Wang C. Relationship between the alignment of the occipitoaxial and subaxial cervical spine in patients with congenital atlantoaxial dislocations. J Spinal Disord Tech. 2013; 26(1):15–21

[56] Passias PG, Wang S, Zhao D, Wang S, Kozanek M, Wang C. The reversibility of swan neck deformity in chronic atlantoaxial dislocations. Spine. 2013; 38(7): E379–E385

[57] Speer MC, Enterline DS, Mehltretter L, et al. Review article: Chiari Type I malformation with or without syringomyelia: prevalence and genetics. J Genet Couns. 2003; 12(4):297–311

[58] McVige JW, Leonardo J. Neuroimaging and the clinical manifestations of Chiari malformation Type I (CMI). Curr Pain Headache Rep. 2015; 19(6):18

[59] Akar E, Kara S, Akdemir H, Kırış A. 3D structural complexity analysis of cerebellum in Chiari malformation type I. Med Biol Eng Comput. 2017; 55 (12):2169–2182

[60] Heller RS, Hwang SW, Riesenburger RI. Dorsal cervical spinal cord herniation precipitated by kyphosis deformity correction for spinal cord tethering. World Neurosurg. 2017; 100:709.e1–709.e4

[61] Kelly MP, Guillaume TJ, Lenke LG. Spinal deformity associated with Chiari malformation. Neurosurg Clin N Am. 2015; 26(4):579–585

[62] Eule JM, Erickson MA, O'Brien MF, Handler M. Chiari I malformation associated with syringomyelia and scoliosis: a twenty-year review of surgical and nonsurgical treatment in a pediatric population. Spine. 2002; 27(13): 1451–1455

[63] Smith JS, Ramchandran S, Lafage V, et al. Prospective multicenter assessment of early complication rates associated with adult cervical deformity surgery in 78 patients. Neurosurgery. 2016; 79(3):378–388

[64] Smith JS, Lafage V, Schwab FJ, et al. International Spine Study Group. Prevalence and type of cervical deformity among 470 adults with thoracolumbar deformity. Spine. 2014; 39(17):E1001–E1009

[65] Scheer JK, Tang JA, Smith JS, et al. International Spine Study Group. Cervical spine alignment, sagittal deformity, and clinical implications: a review. J Neurosurg Spine. 2013; 19(2):141–159

[66] Steinmetz MP, Stewart TJ, Kager CD, Benzel EC, Vaccaro AR. Cervical deformity correction. Neurosurgery. 2007; 60(1, Suppl 1):S90–S97

[67] Belanger TA, Milam RA, IV, Roh JS, Bohlman HH. Cervicothoracic extension osteotomy for chin-on-chest deformity in ankylosing spondylitis. J Bone Joint Surg Am. 2005; 87(8):1732–1738

[68] Zdeblick TA, Bohlman HH. Cervical kyphosis and myelopathy. Treatment by anterior corpectomy and strut-grafting. J Bone Joint Surg Am. 1989; 71 (2):170–182

[69] Rahimizadeh A, Soufiani HF, Rahimizadeh S. Cervical spondylotic myelopathy secondary to dropped head syndrome: report of a case and review of the literature. Case Rep Orthop. 2016; 2016:5247102

[70] Kraus DR, Peppelman WC, Agarwal AK, DeLeeuw HW, Donaldson WF, III. Incidence of subaxial subluxation in patients with generalized rheumatoid arthritis who have had previous occipital cervical fusions. Spine. 1991; 16(10) Suppl:S486–S489

[71] Agarwal AK, Peppelman WC, Kraus DR, et al. Recurrence of cervical spine instability in rheumatoid arthritis following previous fusion: can disease progression be prevented by early surgery? J Rheumatol. 1992; 19(9):1364–1370

[72] Zygmunt SC, Christensson D, Säveland H, Rydholm U, Alund M. Occipito-cervical fixation in rheumatoid arthritis–an analysis of surgical risk factors in 163 patients. Acta Neurochir (Wien). 1995; 135(1–2):25–31

[73] Yoshimoto H, Ito M, Abumi K, et al. A retrospective radiographic analysis of subaxial sagittal alignment after posterior C1-C2 fusion. Spine. 2004; 29 (2):175–181

[74] Rahme R, Boubez G, Bouthillier A, Moumdjian R. Acute swan-neck deformity and spinal cord compression after cervical laminectomy. Can J Neurol Sci. 2009; 36(4):504–506

[75] Gore DR, Sepic SB, Gardner GM. Roentgenographic findings of the cervical spine in asymptomatic people. Spine. 1986; 11(6):521–524

[76] Tang JA, Scheer JK, Smith JS, ISSG. The impact of standing regional cervical sagittal alignment on outcomes in posterior cervical fusion surgery. Neurosurgery. 2015; 76 Suppl 1:S14–S21, discussion S21

[77] Protopsaltis TS, Terran J, Bronsard N, et al. T1 slope minus cervical lordosis (TS-CL), the cervical answer to PI-LL, defines cervical sagittal deformity in patients undergoing thoracolumbar osteotomy. Paper presented at: Cervical Spine Research Society (CSRS) Annual Meeting; December 5–7, 2013

[78] Suk KS, Kim KT, Lee S-HS, Kim JM. Significance of chin-brow vertical angle in correction of kyphotic deformity of ankylosing spondylitis patients. Spine. 2003; 28(17):2001–2005

[79] Ames CP, Smith JS, Eastlack R, et al. International Spine Study Group. Reliability assessment of a novel cervical spine deformity classification system. J Neurosurg Spine. 2015; 23(6):673–683

[80] Tang JA, Scheer JK, Smith JS, et al. ISSG. The impact of standing regional cervical sagittal alignment on outcomes in posterior cervical fusion surgery. Neurosurgery. 2012; 71(3):662–669, discussion 669

[81] Iyer S, Nemani VM, Nguyen J, et al. Impact of cervical sagittal alignment parameters on neck disability. Spine. 2016; 41(5):371–377

[82] Ames CP, Blondel B, Scheer JK, et al. Cervical radiographical alignment: comprehensive assessment techniques and potential importance in cervical myelopathy. Spine. 2013; 38(22) Suppl 1:S149–S160

[83] Passias PG, Lavery J, Ramchandran S, et al. The relationship between improvements in myelopathy and sagittal realignment in cervical deformity surgery. Spine J. 2017; 17(10) Suppl:S137–S138

[84] Deutsch H, Haid RW, Rodts GE, Mummaneni PV. Postlaminectomy cervical deformity. Neurosurg Focus. 2003; 15(3):E5

[85] Scheer JK, Ames CP, Deviren V. Assessment and treatment of cervical deformity. Neurosurg Clin N Am. 2013; 24(2):249–274

[86] Shimizu K, Nakamura M, Nishikawa Y, Hijikata S, Chiba K, Toyama Y. Spinal kyphosis causes demyelination and neuronal loss in the spinal cord: a new model of kyphotic deformity using juvenile Japanese small game fowls. Spine. 2005; 30(21):2388–2392

[87] Matz PG, Anderson PA, Holly LT, et al. Joint Section on Disorders of the Spine and Peripheral Nerves of the American Association of Neurological Surgeons and Congress of Neurological Surgeons. The natural history of cervical spondylotic myelopathy. J Neurosurg Spine. 2009; 11(2):104–111

[88] Al-Mefty O, Harkey LH, Middleton TH, Smith RR, Fox JL. Myelopathic cervical spondylotic lesions demonstrated by magnetic resonance imaging. J Neurosurg. 1988; 68(2):217–222

[89] Yoon ST, Hashimoto RE, Raich A, Shaffrey CI, Rhee JM, Riew KD. Outcomes after laminoplasty compared with laminectomy and fusion in patients with cervical myelopathy: a systematic review. Spine. 2013; 38(22) Suppl 1:S183–S194

[90] Woods BI, Hohl J, Lee J, Donaldson W, III, Kang J. Laminoplasty versus laminectomy and fusion for multilevel cervical spondylotic myelopathy. Clin Orthop Relat Res. 2011; 469(3):688–695

[91] Machino M, Yukawa Y, Hida T, et al. Cervical alignment and range of motion after laminoplasty: radiographical data from more than 500 cases with cervical spondylotic myelopathy and a review of the literature. Spine. 2012; 37 (20):E1243–E1250

[92] Lau D, Winkler EA, Than KD, Chou D, Mummaneni PV. Laminoplasty versus laminectomy with posterior spinal fusion for multilevel cervical spondylotic myelopathy: influence of cervical alignment on outcomes. J Neurosurg Spine. 2017; 27(5):508–517

[93] Lawrence BD, Shamji MF, Traynelis VC, et al. Surgical management of degenerative cervical myelopathy: a consensus statement. Spine. 2013; 38(22) Suppl 1:S171–S172

[94] Lawrence BD, Jacobs WB, Norvell DC, Hermsmeyer JT, Chapman JR, Brodke DS. Anterior versus posterior approach for treatment of cervical spondylotic myelopathy: a systematic review. Spine. 2013; 38(22) Suppl 1:S173–S182

[95] Smith JS, Lafage V, Ryan DJ, et al. Association of myelopathy scores with cervical sagittal balance and normalized spinal cord volume: analysis of 56 preoperative cases from the AOSpine North America Myelopathy study. Spine. 2013; 38(22) Suppl 1:S161–S170

[96] Song K, Su X, Zhang Y, et al. Optimal chin-brow vertical angle for sagittal visual fields in ankylosing spondylitis kyphosis. Eur Spine J. 2016; 25(8):2596–2604

[97] Ruangchainikom M, Daubs MD, Suzuki A, et al. Effect of cervical kyphotic deformity type on the motion characteristics and dynamic spinal cord compression. Spine. 2014; 39(12):932–938

21 C1–C2 Joint Osteotomy and Reduction of Craniovertebral Junction Deformity

Jae Taek Hong

Abstract

Craniovertebral junction (CVJ) deformity is a rare and challenging pathology that can result in progressive deformity, myelopathy, severe neck pain, and functional disability, such as difficulty swallowing. The most common causes of CVJ deformity include rheumatoid arthritis, trauma, neoplasm, infection, and congenital bony malformation. This deformity may alter the quality of life because of the neck pain, disabling headache, dysphagia, and myelopathy. Surgical management of CVJ deformity is complex for anatomical reasons; given the sensitive relationships involved in the surrounding neurovascular structures and intricate biomechanical issues, access to this region is relatively difficult. Evaluation of the reducibility of the upper cervical spine, CVJ alignment, and direction of the mechanical compression may determine surgical strategy. If CVJ deformity is reducible, posterior in situ fixation may be a viable solution. If the deformity is rigid and C1–C2 facet is fixed, osteotomy may be necessary to make the C1–C2 facet joint reducible. C1–C2 facet release with vertical reduction technique could be useful especially when the C1–C2 facet joint is the main pathology of CVJ kyphotic deformity or basilar invagination (BI). The indications for transoral surgery as a treatment for CVJ deformity are decreasing. However, transoral decompression and subsequent posterior fixation are still available surgical options when CVJ deformity is irreducible and ventral bony compression is prominent. In this chapter, we review several cases of CVJ deformity, including BI, fixed atlantoaxial dislocation, and fixed CVJ kyphosis. Moreover, we also present a discussion of CVJ alignment and various strategies for the management of this complex disease entity, as well as possible ways to prevent complications and improve surgical outcomes.

Keywords: craniovertebral junction, cervicomedullary junction, alignment, basilar invagination, fixed deformity, atlantoaxial dislocation, osteotomy, joint distraction, vertical reduction

21.1 Introduction

Craniovertebral junction (CVJ) is the region around the skull base and the upper cervical spine (atlas and axis), along with its neurovascular components, including the brain stem, spinal cord, vertebral artery (VA), and venous plexus.[1,2,3] The stability of CVJ is dependent on a strong ligamentous complex and the shape of the bony structures, which are also responsible for much of the axial rotation (C1–C2 joint) and flexion–extension movements (C0–C1 and C1–C2 joint).[4,5,6]

CVJ deformity has various etiologies, such as congenital anomaly, tumor, infection, rheumatoid arthritis, and trauma.[7] One of the most common CVJ anomalies is basilar invagination (BI), either congenital or degenerative, as represented by the upward migration of the odontoid process into an already limited space of the foramen magnum causing compressive myelopathy around the cervicomedullary junction.[8,9] Many bony anomalies are associated with BI, such as clivus and condyle hypoplasia, occipital assimilation, os odontoideum, bifid C1 arch, and Klippel–Feil syndrome.[10,11] It is widely believed that the hypoplastic effect of normal bony structures results in BI, as seen in achondroplasia, clival hypoplasia, atlas hypoplasia, occipital condyle hypoplasia, or atlantooccipital assimilation.[12]

Rheumatoid arthritis is the leading cause of secondary BI, which is also called basilar impression, atlantoaxial impaction, vertical settling, and cranial settling.[13] Symmetrical rheumatoid destruction of the C0–C1 and C1–C2 joints allows for the cranium to settle on the cervical spine and for the dens to enter the foramen magnum. However, an involvement of only one lateral mass may result in a fixed rotational tilt of the head. Secondary BI often results in a reduction of atlantodental interval (ADI) due to the conical shape of dens and reduced motion, producing a false impression of anatomic improvement known as "pseudostabilization."[14]

CVJ deformity results in sagittal and coronal imbalances, which causes significant pain due to arthritis, instability, and C2 foraminal stenosis. Moreover, malalignment can be a potentially life-threatening instability or cervicomedullary compressive myelopathy.

Patients presenting with intractable pain related to CVJ instability or myelopathy caused by the CVJ deformity usually require surgical treatment. Decompression of neural structures, sagittal and coronal spinal realignment, and stabilization are the primary goals of surgical intervention.

21.2 Craniovertebral Junction Alignment

During fetal development, the spine assumes the shape of the letter "C", with the curved side facing toward the back, while the open side faces the front of the fetus. This C-shaped curve is the primary curve of the spine and is well suited to the cramped confines of the womb. Newborn infants retain this primary curve and, with growth and maturity, develop secondary curves, first in the neck and later in the lower back. Of the two secondary spinal curves, the cervical curve in the neck region develops first. Within the first few months of life, with sufficient development of strength and coordination to bear his or her own head, the cervical lordotic curvature begins to develop. This curve develops in the opposite direction from the primary spinal curvature. This important milestone allows the infant to have visual access to his surroundings. The enhanced visual perspective contributes to additional developments, such as reaching, grasping objects, and intentional crawling. Although there are so many factors affecting the normal cervical curvature, the aforementioned reason is why most people have lordotic cervical spine curvature.[15,16]

This secondary cervical curvature is also found in quadrupedal animals as well as in humans. However, there is a significant difference between humans and animals with respect to this curvature: the upper cervical alignment compared to the cranium. It is because the location of the human foramen magnum is quite different from any other kind of animal.

In humans, the foramen magnum is anteriorly positioned, with its anterior portion lying on the bitympanic line (a line that connects the inferolateral points of the right and left tympanic plates) and is inferiorly oriented (opening directly downward). The occipital condyle that lies anterior to the foramen magnum (the basioccipital or basiocciput) is relatively short in humans. Contrastingly, in apes, the foramen magnum lies well behind the bitympanic line, posterior to a relatively long basiocciput. In addition to being more posteriorly positioned, the foramen magnum in apes is more vertically oriented (opening backward and downward, rather than directly downward).[17,18]

Most researchers explained the anterior position of the human foramen magnum as an adaptation to maintain balance of the head atop the cervical vertebral column during bipedalism.[18,19,20,21]

Hence, the human head is naturally in equilibrium upon the vertebral column in a standing position, without any strenuous effort. However, quadrupeds with posteriorly positioned foramina magna require well-developed nuchal musculature and ligaments to bear the weight of the head to maintain horizontal gaze. Therefore, the demands on the neck musculature differ between humans and quadrupedal mammals. Volume of the rectus capitis muscle is also quite different between humans and quadrupeds. In quadrupeds, the surface area of C1 posterior arch is quite broad for the rectus capitis muscle attachment, and V3 segment of VA is covered by the broad bony roof (▶ Fig. 21.1a), but in humans, the C1 arch is narrow and VA is not covered by the bony structure above the C1 arch in the general human population (▶ Fig. 21.1b). Posterior ponticulus is the bony bridge formed between the posterior portion of the superior articular process and the posterolateral portion of the C1 posterior arch (▶ Fig. 21.1b), which mimics the broad C1 arch of quadrupeds.[22,23,24] Its prevalence has been reported to be between 5.14 and 37.83%.[25,26,27,28,29,30] It could be a vestigial structure as humans have evolved, as upper cervical spine

locates down below the head and strenuous rectus muscles become unnecessary to hold up the head.

Positional difference of the foramen magnum causes a difference in CVJ alignment between humans and other quadrupeds with respect to the C0–C1 segment.

When humans are at rest, the C0–C1 articulation is held rather flexibly, whereas the C1–C2 joints are held slightly in an extended position. This is because the human cervical spine is located inferior to the foramen magnum, and these characteristics ensure an energy-saving balance of the head and neck when at rest, allowing humans to maintain horizontal vision effectively without significant effort of the neck extensor muscle.

Radiographically, the C1 slope is backwardly slanted and kyphotic angulation of the C0–C1 segment allows some degree of freedom for neck extension as the space between the occiput and C1 posterior arch allows for upper cervical extension (▶ Fig. 21.2a).

When patients have kyphotic deformity in the lower cervical spine or thoracolumbar spine, C0–C1 segment can hold up the head to compensate for distal kyphosis, maintaining the sagittal balance and horizontal gaze (▶ Fig. 21.2b, c). Therefore, a normal kyphotic angulation of C0–C1 segment could be referred to as a "tertiary curvature" to characterize human CVJ alignment, to differentiate between upper cervical spine alignment and primary/secondary curvature of the human spine, as well as to differentiate between the cervical spine curvature of humans and that of quadrupeds.

Although asymptomatic population may have different types of cervical alignment, such as "straight" or "kyphotic" cervical spines ranging from 7 to 40%, it has been well accepted that cervical lordosis is a physiological posture in asymptomatic subjects, and a large percentage (about 75–80%) of cervical lordosis is localized to the C1–C2 segment. Only a small percentage (15%) of cervical lordosis exists in the lower cervical levels. On average, the C0–C1 segment is kyphotic.[31,32,33,34,35,36] The loss of subaxial lordosis has been reported in CVJ fixation in which excessive hyperlordosis is created at the C0–C2 segment.[37] Moreover, craniometric studies revealed that an excessive CVJ kyphosis can cause subaxial compensatory lordosis (▶ Fig. 21.2d).[38,39,40] The anatomy of the cervicothoracic

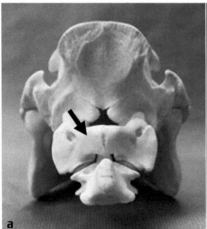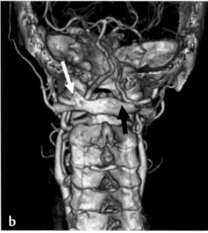

Fig. 21.1 **(a)** Posterior view of dried quadruped's specimen shows the craniovertebral junction and broad C1 posterior arch (*arrow*). **(b)** 3D reconstruction CTA shows normal C1 arch (*black arrow*) on the right side and posterior ponticulus (*white arrow*) covering the V3 segment of VA on the left side.

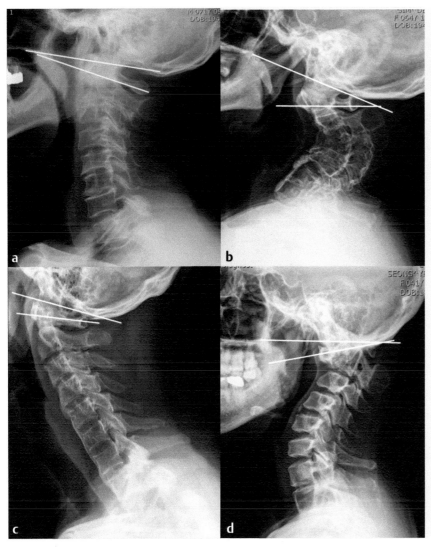

Fig. 21.2 Lateral X-ray shows normal alignment of the cervical spine. In most occasions, cervical lordosis occurs at the C1–C2 segment. C0–C1 segment is kyphotic and C1 slope is posteriorly slanted (**a**). C1 slope is reversely slanted and C0–C1 segment is hyperlordotic to maintain horizontal gaze in subaxial cervical kyphotic deformity patient (**b**) and ankylosing spondylitis patient (**c**). Lateral X-ray of CVJ deformity patient shows a kyphotic CVJ alignment and hyperlordotic compensation in the C0–C1 segment (reversed C1 slope) and subaxial cervical spine (**d**).

junction (CTJ) has been shown to be the main determining factor for cervical lordosis. However, the angle of CVJ has also been shown to be significantly related to the angle of subaxial cervical spine. These findings suggest that reciprocal interaction may likely affect not only global balance but also regional balance.[41]

Another interesting finding is that neck flexion and extension movement are initiated primarily by motions between the head and C1.[42] As the head approaches full flexion and extension, contribution from the upper cervical segments decreases, whereas contribution from the lower cervical segments increases. Understanding the normal CVJ alignment and segmental motion is paramount to better understand CVJ deformity and to decide on a more appropriate surgical strategy according to the pathologies of CVJ.

21.3 Clinical Symptom and Sign

There are various presentations for CVJ deformity, with many of them being a direct result of compression, and it may be associated with Chiari malformation. The degree of upward migration of the dens determines the neurologic sequelae, as this creates significant crowding at the foramen magnum and at the

medulla oblongata. Moreover, this crowding could obstruct cerebrospinal fluid (CSF) flow leading to syringomyelia. In the cases with cervicomedullary dysfunction, patients may have ataxia, dysmetria, nystagmus, dysphagia, or cranial nerve palsies, and report weakness, loss of endurance, loss of dexterity, gait disturbance, and paresthesia.[43,44]

Neck pain is the most common complaint of CVJ deformity. It is usually associated with occipital headache. Occipital neuralgia, facial pain, and periauricular pain can occur from compression of the greater occipital nerve (C2 root), nucleus of the spinal trigeminal tract, and greater auricular nerve, respectively. Exertional cough headache is a well-documented symptom in cases with syringomyelia.[44]

Difficulty swallowing may be associated with CVJ deformity, especially in cases of CVJ kyphosis.[45,46] In cases with severe-degree CVJ kyphosis, dysphagia may be inevitable, not only because the oropharyngeal space becomes narrow but also because the angle change and movement of C0–C1 segment are not possible to compensate for the mechanical restriction in fixed kyphosis.[46,47] Hence, it is important to correct CVJ kyphosis to relieve dysphagia. In addition, sparing C0–C1 segment could provide a certain degree of freedom as a compensatory movement and angle change to avoid dysphagia when treating

CVJ pathologies if C0–C1 segment is not the primary pathology for treatment.

21.4 Preoperative Radiologic Assessment

Irreducibility was defined as a nonalignment of C1–C2 after neck extension (determined on lateral X-ray) or after cervical traction. Lateral radiography with dynamic study is necessary to evaluate ADI, degree of vertical subluxation, and reducibility. Furthermore, bony abnormalities, such as atlas occipitalization, os odontoideum, bifid C1 arch, and C2–C3 fusion can be evaluated on lateral radiography.

Traction can be a useful tool in evaluating the reducibility and predicting intraoperative neurological worsening by surgical position. Preoperative cervical traction may correct the atlantoaxial dislocation (AAD) and vertical subluxation in some reducible deformity cases. This could especially be important for the management of fragile patients because they can be treated with only a stabilization procedure postreduction, reducing the level of fixation. Gardner cervical traction was applied, depending on age and weight, starting with 2 to 5 kg for 1 or 2 days. The head of the bed was elevated to provide a countertraction. Serial radiographs were assessed for reduction. These patients who demonstrated a reduction were classified as reducible AAD or BI.

MRI is critical to evaluate cord compression, T2 signal change, Chiari malformation, and syringomyelia. CT scans can confirm bony abnormalities, exact location of the dens, C1–C2 joint destruction, and abnormal C1–C2 facet angle. CT scans are also used to determine the extent of facet fusion and osteophytic bridging to assess the need for C1–C2 osteotomy.

CTA screening is a useful tool for getting a three-dimensional information of complex deformity and for identifying VA anomaly around CVJ.[26,48] The incidence of V3 segment anomalies has been reported to be as high as 10% (▶ Fig. 21.3).[26,49] In V3 segment anomalies, since the VA or its major branch courses inferiorly to the C1 arch, these anomalies pose a surgical challenge.

These anomalous vessels may likely be injured during drilling, tapping, and insertion of the lateral mass screws. Therefore, when a V3 segment anomaly is detected, a more optimal entry point for C1 fixation should be selected to avoid significant morbidities associated with VA injury. In these cases, five alternative techniques can be utilized to avoid V3 segment injury. The first technique is to choose the superior lateral mass as an alternative starting point for C1 posterior screw placement. It could be useful especially in cases of persistent first intersegmental artery, which is the most common anomalous V3 segment. The second is to choose the C1 dorsal arch as the entry point for C1 screw placement. The C1 dorsal arch might be the best entry point in cases with fenestrated VA or posterior inferior cerebellar artery early branch. The third method involves C1–C2 transarticular screw fixation to avoid causing an injury to the abnormal VA below the C1 arch. The fourth technique is to skip the C1 screw fixation and extend the level of fixation proximally or distally. The last technique is to mobilize the VA inferiorly together with the C2 nerve root before screw placement at the C1 inferior lateral mass. Although there could be a racial difference in the incidence of V3 segment anomaly, existing literature indicates that V3 segment anomaly is more common in the group with congenital bony anomaly. Therefore, we suggest that preoperative CTA might be informative for deciding on a surgical technique, especially in high-risk group of the V3 segment anomaly, such as Asians and those with CVJ deformity with congenital bony anomaly.[49]

21.5 Treatment of Craniovertebral Junction Deformity

A surgical treatment of CVJ abnormalities was first proposed in 1977.[50] It was further advanced by the introduction of posterior segmental fixation. Factors that influence specific treatment of CVJ deformity are as follows: (1) the reducibility of deformity (i.e., restoring anatomic alignment, thereby relieving neural compression); (2) the direction of mechanical compression; (3) the presence of abnormal craniocervical angle and alignment;

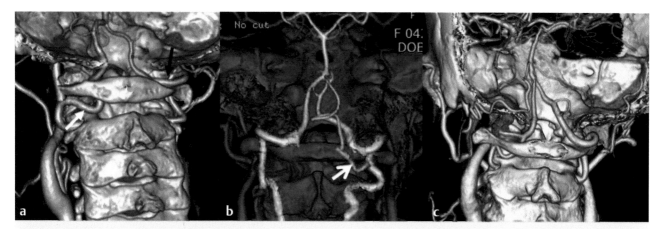

Fig. 21.3 3D CTA images show three different types of V3 segment anomaly. **(a)** 3D CTA demonstrates the persistent intersegmental artery on the left side (*white arrow*), the VA course abnormally below the C1 arch after leaving the transverse foramen of the C2 and enter the spinal canal not passing through the C1 transverse foramen. Right side V3 segment (*black arrow*) is normal. **(b)** 3D CTA demonstrates the main V3 segment was normal, but the right side posterior inferior cerebellar artery (*white arrow*) originated from the VA between C1 and C2. **(c)** 3D CTA shows the fenestrated VA on the left side; one courses as usual, while the other entered spinal canal below the C1 arch and joins the former above the C1 arch.

and (4) the presence of hindbrain herniation, syrinx, and vascular abnormalities.

The primary goal of treatment is to relieve compression at the cervicomedullary junction. Stabilization is critical to treat reducible deformity and to maintain neural decompression. Irreducible lesions may require decompression at the site of compression or may require an osteotomy procedure to make the lesion reducible and relieve neural compression.[41]

Irreducible lesions can be divided into two types: the ventral compressive lesion and the dorsal compressive lesion. Dorsal compression cases need either a posterior or posterolateral decompression procedure, and if there is instability after decompression, posterior fixation is mandatory to gain stability.

Transoral surgery is a procedure carried out through the oral cavity to gain access to ventral compressive lesion of CVJ. Under normal conditions, surgeons should be able to expose the area from the lower rim of clivus cranially to the level of C23 disc space caudally. Transoral surgery is often necessary in case of irreducible CVJ deformity, where ventral compression to neutral structures is present.[51] Other indications for transoral surgery include CVJ tumor and infection, in which the anterior compression cannot be decompressed by a simple posterior reduction.[52] Although the combined anterior-posterior approach may provide satisfactory neural decompression and fusion, it poses several disadvantages, such as higher risk of surgical morbidities, prolonged postoperative intubation/nasogastric feeding, phonation difficulty, and potential infection.[53,54,55] The risk of infection is a big concern particularly in cases where the subarachnoid space had to be opened, which may cause catastrophic sequelae. Another issue is that transoral decompression can induce significant instability of CVJ, inevitably requiring a subsequent posterior stabilization procedure. These issues are reasons why the initial enthusiasm vanished and indication of transoral decompression has become less clear in recent literature.

A C1–C2 joint distraction technique, as introduced by Goel, has been gaining popularity recently as a possible treatment modality for selected cases of AAD and BI.[56,57,58] This technique seems to have several advantages over conventional transoral surgery and occipitocervical (OC) fixation. First, direct reduction and fixation are possible posteriorly for cervicomedullary decompression. Hence, a transoral surgery and its related complications could be avoided. Second, the dimension of the fusion bed could substantially be increased because C1–C2 facet surface is rather large. Third, it can avoid occipital fixation and conserve C0–C1 segmental motion. Fourth, C1–C2 joint manipulation can make a fixed subluxation or deformity reducible, minimizing the need for a head traction, before and during surgery.

However, despite these advantages, some concerns have also been expressed in the literature regarding this joint distraction technique. First, there is a debate regarding the C2 neuropathic pain after C2 root resection. Although C2 root resection is not mandatory for C1–C2 facet opening, it is useful to make a wide exposure for the C1–C2 facet surface, especially when C1–C2 interlaminar space is narrow and venous plexus is prominent.[58,59] Thus, C2 root resection is one of the key parts of the C1–C2 joint distraction procedure. In the literature, most authors have reported that the incidence of C2 neuropathic pain is quite low after C2 root resection.[58,59] However, C2 neuropathic pain could be troublesome for some patients. Therefore, surgeons should be aware of both the benefits and risks associated with C2 root

resection. Second, we do not fully know the adequate amount of distraction required for the best neurological recovery and prevention of neurological complications related to the overstretching of the spinal cord and VA. Moreover, the long-term fate of adjacent C0–C1 segment has rarely been reported in patients after receiving C1–C2 vertical distraction procedure with respect to the segmental motion and adjacent segmental degeneration. Yoshida et al reported that C1–C2 rigid fixation can provide prophylactic benefits against vertical subluxation and subaxial subluxation in RA patients.[60] Werle et al reported that C0–C1 degeneration is very low after C1–C2 fusion in RA patients.[61] Therefore, C0–C1 segment sparing monosegmental C1–C2 fusion should be the preferred treatment of choice, especially for RA patients.

21.5.1 Preoperative Planning

▶ Fig. 21.4 provides decision-making pathways to treat CVJ deformity.

Preoperative cervical traction may correct AAD and vertical subluxation in some patients with reducible deformity. This could especially be important for the management of fragile patients because they can be treated with only a stabilization procedure after reduction and decreasing the numbers of fixation level.

The direction of the mechanical compression was the key factor in deciding a surgical approach. With recent advancements in surgical techniques and instruments, the results of posterior C1–C2 release and reduction have been satisfactory. However, difficult or insufficient reduction and loss of reduction have been observed after posterior reduction and fixation.[51] Thus, anterior release reduction and posterior fixation could still be available options for irreducible BI with AAD, especially in patients with severely deformed bony mass anteriorly compressing the cervicomedullary junction.

CVJ alignment is another key factor to decide surgical strategy. Clivus–canal angle and cervicomedullary angle are tended to be kyphotic in congenital CVJ anomaly which is caused by the short clivus, platybasia, or abnormal angulation of deformed odontoid process.[38,39,40] Craniocervical realignment through screws and rod system may be a safe and efficacious surgical technique for the treatment of congenital craniocervical anomaly with abnormal angulation of the clivus. However, craniocervical realignment procedure including distraction, compression, and skull extension need additional fixation up to the cranium and it should be cautiously performed, especially in cases with deformed bony anomalies and severe canal stenosis.

21.5.2 Surgical Techniques

Rheumatoid Basilar Invagination

Rheumatoid arthritis (RA) causes a gradual degeneration of all ligaments in the C1–C2 joint complex, compromising mechanical instability. The failure in regions of fibrocartilage through autoimmune response in C1–C2 facet joint and transverse ligament subsequently leads to C1–C2 joint mutilation and BI. Most rheumatoid BI is caused by C1–C2 joint destruction and subsequent upward migration of odontoid process. These findings suggest that the main pathology of rheumatoid BI is C1–C2 joint, not

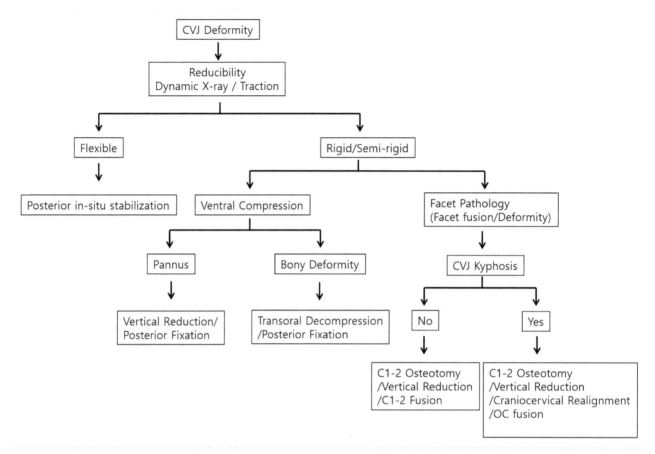

Fig. 21.4 Algorithm shows decision-making pathways for the treatment of the CVJ deformity.

C0–C1 joint. Hence, spine surgeons should focus on C1–C2 joint reduction to treat rheumatoid BI in efforts to spare the innocent C0–C1 segmental motion. Rheumatoid destruction of the C1–C2 joint could easily be confused with spontaneous fusion mass on CT scan due to the narrowing of the joint space and destruction of joint cartilage. However, C1–C2 joint of rheumatoid BI is unstable and easily reducible in vertical distraction that preoperative traction or osteotomy is not necessary to reduce it.

Following general anesthesia, patients were placed in the prone position with the head fixed using a Mayfield head holder. The neck was positioned in a slightly flexed posture, allowing for better surgical exposure of the CVJ. However, in the case of severe degree of cervicomedullary compression, neutral position is recommended. Using a fluoroscopic C-arm, proper alignment of the atlantoaxial bony structures is confirmed. If necessary, adjustment can be made while patients are still in the Mayfield head holder to obtain upper cervical reduction.

Intraoperative electrophysiologic neuromonitoring (IONM) system was performed during surgery, including MEP, SSEP, and EMG. Through a midline skin incision, the posterior edge of the foramen magnum, posterior arch of C1, and the C2–C3 lamina were exposed. For patients with posterior compressive lesion around the foramen magnum, the posterior margin of the foramen magnum and C1 arch were removed. Intentional sacrifice of bilateral C2 ganglions was performed to obtain enough space for C1 screw entry point, joint manipulation, and bone fusion (▶ Fig. 21.5). Subsequently, by the application of Harms

technique, polyaxial screws were inserted to the bilateral C1 lateral masses and the C2 pedicle. The C1 and C2 screw were partially loosened. Distraction between the C1 and C2 screws was performed using a distractor to achieve vertical reduction; the nuts were then subsequently locked. Vertical reduction results in the migration of the odontoid process inferiorly, reducing the neural compression around the ventral cervicomedullary junction. The C1–C2 articular cartilages were removed widely using a curette and a high-speed burr. The facet cage or tricortical iliac bone autograft was inserted bilaterally as joint spacers to maintain the location of the odontoid process in a down-migrated position. The Mayfield head holder was adjusted to fix the neck in a slight extension position, which will help the process of reduction and realignment. Then compression between the C1 and C2 screw head increases the graft contact inside the C1–C2 joint, creating adequate C1–C2 lordosis. Subsequently, interlaminar fusion could be performed using autograft iliac bone blocks and cables.

In cases of rheumatoid BI, C2 root resection almost always requires for vertical reduction. Given that C1–C2 joint mutilation is so severe, the height of C2 foramen becomes too narrow for the manipulation of C1–C2 facet joint and insertion of screw without damaging the C2 nerve root.

A substantial number of rheumatoid BI cases involve the compression of the spinal cord ventrally by the retro-odontoid pannus, which needs transoral decompression. However, posterior atlantoaxial fixation with vertical reduction technique has

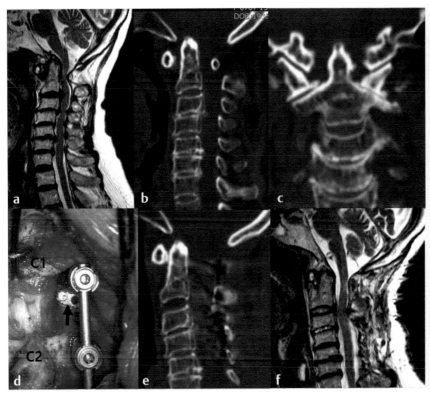

Fig. 21.5 Illustrative case. RA basilar invagination. **(a,b)** Sagittal T2 MRI and sagittal reconstruction CT image show odontoid compression over the brain stem and upper cervical cord. Odontoid tip is located above the foramen magnum. **(c)** Coronal reconstruction CT scan shows narrow C1–C2 facet joint space bilaterally and joint mutilation on the left side. **(d)** Intraoperative photograph shows the panoramic view of the C1–C2 facet joint after C2 root resection and facet cage insertion (*arrow*). **(e,f)** Postoperative CT and MRI scan show the decompression of the cervicomedullary junction and odontoid tip is pulled down below the foramen magnum.

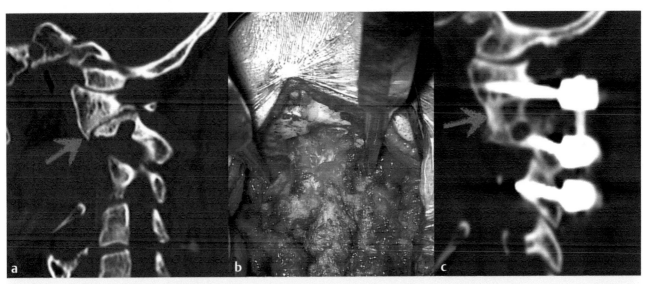

Fig. 21.6 Illustrative case. Fixed C1–C2 subluxation. **(a)** Sagittal reconstructed CT scan showing the osteophyte (*arrow*) and oblique orientation of C1–C2 facet joint. **(b)** Intraoperative photograph demonstrates small osteotomes inside the C1–C2 joint space bilaterally for release. **(c)** Sagittal reconstructed CT scan showing remodeling and flattening of the C1–C2 facet joint (*arrow*).

been reported to provide early reduction of retro-odontoid rheumatoid pannus, as well as a reduction of BI and AAD.[62,63,64,65,66] This suggests that rheumatoid pannus could be a buckling of ligamentous complex around CVJ caused by BI rather than granulation tissue caused by the inflammation.

Fixed Atlantoaxial Rotatory Fixation

Reducible AAD can be defined as C1–C2 alignment on extension or cervical traction. If the dislocation cannot be reduced on extension position and preoperative traction, it is labeled as an irreducible or fixed AAD and rotatory subluxation. Management

becomes difficult with this type of fixed deformity. Since the introduction of C1–C2 distraction method by Goel, the focus in the treatment of CVJ pathology has shifted to the dislocated C1–C2 facets rather than the C2 dens, and C1–C2 joint manipulation has been the preferred method of treatment for irreducible AAD.[14,57] This is because the cause of irreducibility is in the C1–C2 facets. In cases of irreducible AAD or rotatory fixation, C1–C2 joint mutilation or osteophyte formation is so severe that dislocation cannot be reduced despite cervical traction. Therefore, C1–C2 facet mobilization is necessary to make this fixed deformity reducible using facet osteotomies (▶ Fig. 21.6).

After the release of C1–C2 facet joint capsule and removal of osteophytes, the mobility between C1 and C2 is usually identifiable intraoperatively. The cartilage endplate was curetted and drilled to further increase the mobility and to remodel the C1–C2 facet joint plane. The rotated C1–C2 facet joint could be mobilized and reduced in neutral position after releasing the C1–C2 facet joint.

In the cases with horizontal subluxation, surgical assistant pressed down firmly on the C2 spinous process or pulled the C1 arch using cables to reduce horizontal subluxation. Adjusting the patient's neck to allow for slight extension should help the process of reduction. Bone block or cage filled with cancellous bone can be placed inside the decorticated C1–C2 joint.

Congenital Basilar Invagination

Congenital BI is usually irreducible. Irreducibility results from the combined bony malformation, as well as the oblique orientation of the C1–C2 facet joint.

In severe subluxation with oblique C1–C2 facet joint orientation, the joint space was not visible even after C2 root resection. The drilling of the posterior superior corner of the C2 facet allowed the visibility of the C1–C2 joint space. Then the small

osteotome was inserted into the joint space to open it. Then drilling, reaming, and curettage were continued to release the fixed C1–C2 joint space. Drilling and osteotome were focused on the anterior-inferior corner of the C1 facet to make the C1–C2 joint flat and reducible. Osteotome was used as a lever arm with the posterior edge of the C1 facet as a fulcrum to open the joint space and reduce the subluxation both for the vertical and horizontal translation. Reduction was then maintained using the C1–C2 spacers (bone block or PEEK cage filled with bone), and C1–C2 was fixed using the polyaxial screw system. In those who needed C1 laminectomy for the posterior decompression, C1 laminectomy bone could also be used as the C1–C2 facet spacer.

If BI and CVJ kyphosis are not severe, C1–C2 facet joint distraction and C1–C2 joint remodeling may be sufficient to reduce and decompress the cervicomedullary compression. However, in cases with a severe degree of CVJ kyphotic angulation and ventral cord compression, C1–C2 joint vertical reduction and fixation may not be sufficient to obtain good CVJ alignment and decompression. Therefore, occipital fixation, distraction, compression, and head extension are mandatory to obtain craniocervical realignment in the case of severe CVJ kyphotic deformity (▶ Fig. 21.7).

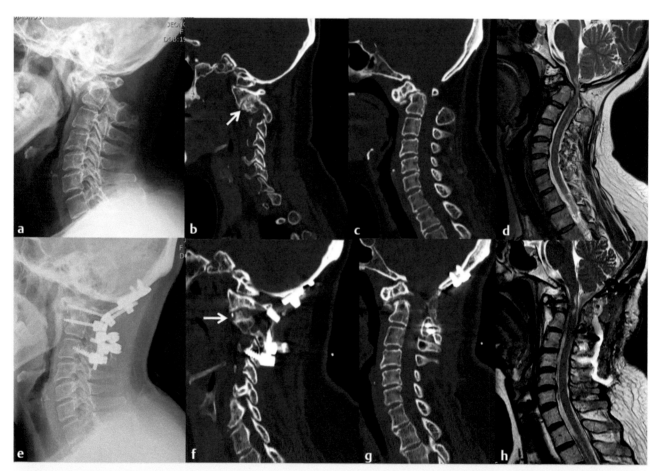

Fig. 21.7 Congenital basilar invagination and CVJ kyphosis. **(a)** Preoperative X-ray shows the atlantoaxial dislocation (AAD) and severe kyphotic CVJ deformity caused by the os odontoideum. **(b)** Sagittal reconstructed CT scan reveals the abnormal oblique C1–C2 facet angle (*arrow*). **(c)** Os odontoideum is fused to the anterior tubercle of C1. Clival angle is relatively blunt and clivus–canal angle is kyphotic. **(d)** MRI scan shows the cord signal change and severe compression around the cervicomedullary junction. **(e)** Postoperative X-ray shows a reduction of AAD. **(f)** Sagittal reconstructed CT scan reveals postoperative remodeling and flattening of the C1–C2 facet joint and PEEK cage inside the joint (*arrow*). **(g,h)** Postoperative CT and MRI show the adequate reduction of AAD and complete cord decompression around the foramen magnum. CVJ angle becomes extended and clivus–canal angle is increased.

After placement of the screw for occiput, C1 lateral mass, and C2 pedicle, C2 screw heads were tightened to ensure that the screws, C2 body, and the odontoid process became an integrated unit. The C1 and occipital screw heads were not tightened yet. The C1 screw placement was not mandatory in cases with occipital assimilation and in cases where the space was not sufficient for C1 screw placement or rod application. The rod bent more than the patient's CVJ alignment and head was extended using Mayfield head holder to approximate the rod to occipital screw head. The occipital screw and C1 screw head were only tightened loosely at this stage. Then, the vertical distraction between the screws pulled the odontoid process downward and anteriorly. Once the joint space was distracted, facet cages or bone blocks were placed bilaterally and the occipital screws and C1 screws were tightened after head

extension using Mayfield skull pin, which reduced the AAD and CVJ kyphosis. For patients who needed more horizontal reduction for AAD and forward movement of odontoid process, the C2 pedicle screws were loosened, and vertical compression was performed between C1 and C2 screw heads after placement of facet spacers (▸ Fig. 21.8). Excessive vertical reduction and CVJ realignment may pose a higher risk of postoperative neurological impairment. Therefore, the C1–C2 distraction and craniocervical realignment should be performed very carefully under IONM to avoid overdistraction and subsequent stretching injury of the spinal cord or VA. After satisfactory reduction and a confirmation was provided by fluoroscopy, the posterior bony surface was decorticated to prepare for fusion bed. The bone grafts were placed over the decorticated fusion surface.

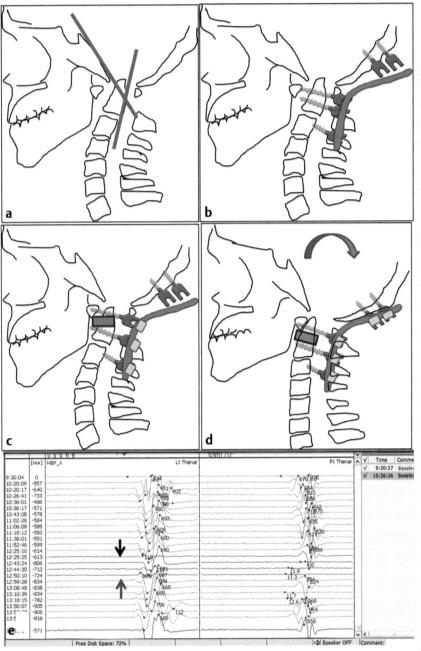

Fig. 21.8 Sequence of craniocervical realignment. **(a)** Illustration shows preoperative clivus–canal angle (*angle between red lines*) is kyphotic in congenital CVJ deformity. **(b)** Illustration shows the posterior instrumentation including occipital screw, cervical screw from C1 to C3. The rod bending is more than the patient's CVJ angle for further craniocervical realignment by head extension. **(c)** Vertical reduction technique down migrates the tip of odontoid process using C1–C2 facet cage (*rectangle*). **(d)** Distraction, compression, head extension, and craniocervical realignment reduce the CVJ kyphosis and atlantoaxial dislocation. **(e)** Intraoperative MEP monitoring shows a sudden loss of tcMEP signal during the vertical reduction technique (*black arrow*), and a recovery of transcranial MEP (tcMEP) wave just after the reduction in amount of C1–C2 joint distraction and size of the facet cage (*red arrow*).

In cases with platybasia or a very high BI with a significant thecal compression, even the maximal C1–C2 facet distraction will still be unable to bring about complete C1–C2 reduction as well as odontoid descent from its invaginated position within the foramen magnum and achieve an adequate spinal decompression. When clivus–canal angle and cervicomedullary angle are kyphotic in those cases, both vertical reduction and head extension are mandatory to reduce three-dimensional deformities such as horizontal, vertical, and angular deformity. Although suboccipital craniectomy and C1 laminectomy provide some degree of indirect decompression for cervicomedullary compression, prominent ventral bony mass and kyphotic angulation could stretch the spinal cord and cause myelopathy. Moreover, contracted muscle, complete C1–C2 facet dislocation, stiff ligament, and joint capsule may hinder the reduction from posterior. There is still requirement of the anterior decompression of the odontoid. Anterior decompression with posterior fixation and fusion can effectively treat the ventral compressive bony lesion, releasing the irreducibility in such cases (▶ Fig. 21.9).

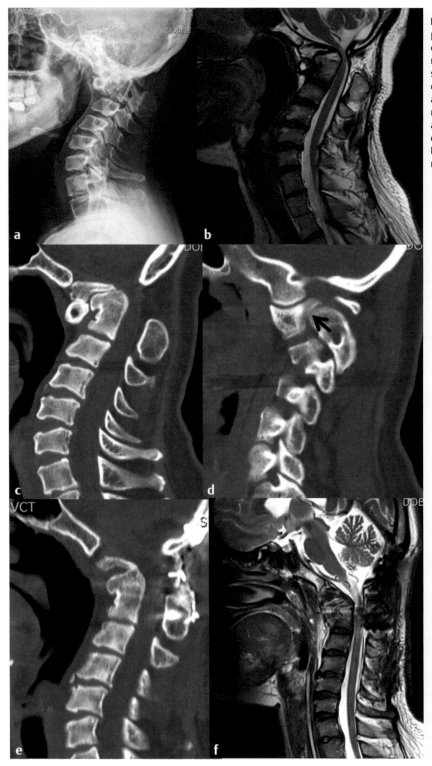

Fig. 21.9 Congenital basilar invagination and prominent ventral bony compression. **(a)** Preoperative X-ray shows severe CVJ kyphosis and reactive subaxial lordosis. **(b)** MRI scan shows severe ventral cord compression by the atypical os odontoideum and the cord signal change and around cervicomedullary junction. **(c,d)** Sagittal reconstructed CT scan reveals the bony deformity and C1–C2 facet dislocation (*arrow*). **(e,f)** Postoperative CT scan and MRI show the reduction of BI and cord decompression around the foramen magnum.

Postsurgical Fixed CVJ Kyphosis

Postoperative CVJ kyphosis induced recurrent compressive myelopathy and evoked swallowing difficulty postoperatively. For patients with evidence of previous bony union inside the C1–C2 facet joints or irreducible C1–C2 facet joint, anterior odontoidectomy or C1–C2 facet osteotomy should be performed prior to posterior reduction and fixation. However, when patients have a severe degree of fixed CVJ kyphosis, optimal surgical position and trajectory cannot be obtained for transoral surgery. Posterior C1–C2 facet release and reduction could be the only available treatment option in this situation (▶ Fig. 21.10).

After midline exposure of the occiput and cervical spine, C1–C2 facet fusion was released using a drill and osteotome. Releasing the C1–C2 facet joint allowed kyphotic angulation of the upper cervical alignment flexible and reducible.

C1–C2 vertical distraction decompressed the ventral cervicomedullary compression caused by odontoid kinking into the foramen magnum. Subsequent facet cage insertion and posterior fixation maintained the position of the down-migrated odontoid tip. C1–C2 screw head compression, posterior shortening of the segment, and head extension reversed CVJ kyphosis and obtained neutral craniocervical alignment. Correction of CVJ kyphosis relieved the mechanical constriction of oropharyngeal space and improve the swallowing difficulty immediately after the surgery.

Osteotome and high-speed drill are useful tools for C1–C2 facet joint osteotomy. However, the proximity of the critical neurovascular structures, such as VA, spinal cord, and nerve, may result in iatrogenic injury despite the advancement of high-speed drills. The Misonix bone scalpel (MBS) has recently been developed and is designed for precise removal of the rigid bone, while minimizing trauma to the surrounding soft tissues. The clinical advantages of these characteristics include reduced incidence of iatrogenic neurovascular injury.

21.5.3 Complication and Prevention

Mechanical failure, various kinds of neurovascular complications, and postoperative swallowing difficulty can occur after the surgery in patients with CVJ deformity.

Nonunion and Instrument Failure

Despite recent advancements in posterior cervical instrument, high biomechanical loading around this special junctional area poses a risk for instrument failure or nonunion. Fusion bed preparation and graft material selection are important for increasing the fusion rate. We usually use an iliac autograft as much as possible. Although posterior surface of occipital bone and C1–C2 interlaminar space are popular fusion bed, C1–C2 facet joint is the critical area for higher fusion rate as well as malalignment correction for CVJ kyphosis patients.

Neurological Worsening

Postoperative neurological worsening is a possible complication in this area. Even though several reports of vertical reduction technique showed excellent clinical and radiological results without neurological complication,[14,51,57,58] we experienced a significant change in IONM using the vertical reduction technique. To date, we are not sure whether it is related to spinal cord stretch or spinal cord ischemia due to the VA stretch. However, we found that IONM change is usually recovered after we reduce the amount of C1–C2 joint distraction and size of the facet graft (▶ Fig. 21.8e). This finding shows the efficacy of IONM during craniocervical realignment surgery for congenital craniocervical segmentation anomaly. IONM change is more common in CVJ surgery than in any other level of cervical spine. Preoperative T2 signal change on MRI, lower preoperative JOA score, and congenital anomaly/tumor pathologies are risk factors that are significantly related to IONM change in our CVJ

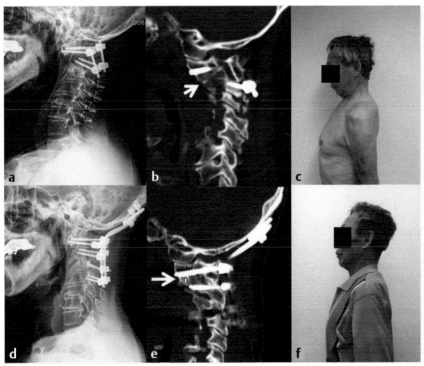

Fig. 21.10 Postsurgical fixed CVJ kyphosis.
(a) Preoperative X-ray shows the CVJ kyphosis following C1–C2 fusion. **(b)** Sagittal reconstructed CT scan reveals the oblique C1–C2 facet angle (*arrow*), C1–C2 fusion mass inside the facet joint, and C1–C2 interlaminar space (*black arrow*). **(c)** Clinical photograph shows the fixed upper cervical kyphosis in military tuck posture. **(d)** Postoperative X-ray reveals the correction of upper cervical kyphosis. **(e)** Sagittal reconstructed CT scan reveals the horizontal C1–C2 facet angle and fusion mass around the PEEK cage (*arrow*). **(f)** Postoperatively clinical photography reveals the comfortable neck posture and horizontal vision.

surgery case series. We suggest that IONM may help in preventing unexpected neurological deterioration during posterior craniocervical distraction and realignment.

Dysphagia

A "military tuck" posture (neutral head posture, extension of the lower cervical spine, posterior translation of the occiput–C1 complex) usually reduces C1–C2 subluxation, while optimizing the surgical exposure and allowing for a favorable screw trajectory.[46] It is a commonly used posture for posterior instrumentation in the upper cervical spine.

However, previous studies have shown that a decrease in the CO–2 angle in the retraction position causes a reduction in the oropharyngeal airway space and postoperative dysphagia.[67,68]

Dysphagia is not an uncommon complication after posterior cervical surgeries, as well as anterior cervical spine surgeries.[69,70,71] Moreover, dysphagia after posterior OC fusion has been recognized as a serious postoperative complication. Miyata el al reported that dysphagia after OC fusion is caused by glossoptosis, which is the downward displacement of the tongue root, resulting in the narrowing of the oropharynx and the impairment of the ability of the epiglottis to move sufficiently.[67] They emphasized that a decrease in the cO–2 angle may likely induce a reduction in the pharyngeal space and can be a predictor of postoperative dysphagia, which is not compensated by the middle or lower cervical spine. We reported that the movement of the upper cervical segments could be an important compensation mechanism for swallowing, and the fixation of the upper cervical spine could be one of the risk factors for postoperative dysphagia. Moreover, C0–C1 angle change and movement during swallowing is significantly higher in the retraction posture than in the neutral posture, and C0–C1 segment is the dominant level of compensatory motion that occurs when subjects experience dysphagia in the retraction position.[47] Therefore, if we fix up to the cranium in the retraction position, the major segment of compensatory movement cannot function properly to allow swallowing, leading to postoperative dysphagia. Therefore, avoiding OC fixation during retraction posture and sparing C0–C1 segment are important technical tips for preventing postoperative dysphagia.

21.6 Conclusion

CVJ alignment is unique, both for the segmental motion and biomechanical perspective. CVJ deformities are complex and can result in severe pain, myelopathy, and difficulty with swallowing. The treatment goal of CVJ deformity must be to restore normal alignment, relieve neural compression, and stabilization without neurological complication. To date, there are many known etiologies for CVJ deformity, with each having its own characteristics and treatment challenges. Regardless of the underlying cause, however, this complex disease entity can be divided into two types—reducible deformity and irreducible deformity—based on whether the dislocation is reduced after dynamic X-ray and traction. Simple posterior fixation and fusion are effective for reducible CVJ deformity, and any type of reduction procedure is necessary for irreducible CVJ deformity. Congenital CVJ deformity associated with malalignment of the odontoid process is usually irreducible, causing progressive

ventral compression of the spinal cord and medulla oblongata with subsequent neurological deficits. A reduction of irreducible deformity can be achieved using anterior transoral surgery or posterior C1–C2 vertical reduction technique, depending on the primary focus of pathology. With recent advancements in surgical techniques and internal fixation devices, ventral decompression and craniocervical realignment can be achieved by posterior-only surgery. Craniocervical realignment through the screws and rod system may be a safe and efficacious surgical technique to treat congenital craniocervical anomaly with abnormal CVJ kyphosis. The principle of the posterior reduction procedure is to pull down the odontoid process, away from the cervicomedullary junction and craniocervical realignment without neurological injury. To avoid neurological complication around this complicated junctional area, preoperative radiological assessment is critical to detect structural anomaly and decide optimal surgical plan. IONM may help in preventing any unexpected neurological deterioration during posterior craniocervical distraction and realignment.

By understanding the nature of CVJ alignment, recent advancements in posterior cervical instrumentation, all available treatment options, and decision-making process, physicians can improve quality of life of patients with CVJ deformity.

References

[1] Visocchi M, Mattogno PP, Signorelli F, Zhong J, Iacopino G, Barbagallo G. Complications in craniovertebral junction instrumentation: hardware removal can be associated with long-lasting stability. Personal experience. Acta Neurochir Suppl (Wien). 2017; 124:187–194

[2] Morota N. Pediatric craniovertebral junction surgery. Neurol Med Chir (Tokyo). 2017; 57(9):435–460

[3] Goel A, Sathe P, Shah A. Atlantoaxial fixation for basilar invagination without obvious atlantoaxial instability (Group B Basilar Invagination): outcome analysis of 63 surgically treated cases. World Neurosurg. 2017; 99:164–170

[4] Dlouhy BJ, Policeni BA, Menezes AH. Reduction of atlantoaxial dislocation prevented by pathological position of the transverse ligament in fixed, irreducible os odontoideum: operative illustrations and radiographic correlates in 41 patients. J Neurosurg Spine. 2017; 27(1):20–28

[5] Deepak AN, Salunke P, Sahoo SK, Prasad PK, Khandelwal NK. Revisiting the differences between irreducible and reducible atlantoaxial dislocation in the era of direct posterior approach and C1–2 joint manipulation. J Neurosurg Spine. 2017; 26(3):331–340

[6] Yin YH, Tong HY, Qiao GY, Yu XG. Posterior reduction of fixed atlantoaxial dislocation and basilar invagination by atlantoaxial facet joint release and fixation: a modified technique with 174 cases. Neurosurgery. 2016; 78(3):391–400, discussion 400

[7] Kukreja S, Ambekar S, Sin AH, Nanda A. Occipitocervical fusion surgery: review of operative techniques and results. J Neurol Surg B Skull Base. 2015; 76(5):331–339

[8] Salunke P, Sahoo S, Deepak AN. Different facets in the management of congenital atlantoaxial dislocation and basilar invagination. Neurosurgery. 2015; 77(6):E985–E987

[9] Salunke P, Sahoo SK, Deepak AN, Ghuman MS, Khandelwal NK. Comprehensive drilling of the C1–2 facets to achieve direct posterior reduction in irreducible atlantoaxial dislocation. J Neurosurg Spine. 2015; 23(3):294–302

[10] Goel A, Nadkarni T, Shah A, Ramdasi R, Patni N. Bifid anterior and posterior arches of atlas: surgical implication and analysis of 70 cases. Neurosurgery. 2015; 77(2):296–305, discussion 305–306

[11] Debernardi A, D'Aliberti G, Talamonti G, Villa F, Piparo M, Collice M. The craniovertebral junction area and the role of the ligaments and membranes. Neurosurgery. 2015; 76 Suppl 1:S22–S32

[12] Reina V, Baujat G, Fauroux B, et al. Craniovertebral junction anomalies in achondroplastic children. Adv Tech Stand Neurosurg. 2014; 40:295–312

[13] Krauss WE, Bledsoe JM, Clarke MJ, Nottmeier EW, Pichelmann MA. Rheumatoid arthritis of the craniovertebral junction. Neurosurgery. 2010; 66(3) Suppl:83–95

[14] Goel A, Pareikh S, Sharma P. Atlantoaxial joint distraction for treatment of basilar invagination secondary to rheumatoid arthritis. Neurol India. 2005; 53 (2):238–240

[15] Been E, Gómez-Olivencia A, Shefi S, Soudack M, Bastir M, Barash A. Evolution of spinopelvic alignment in hominins. Anat Rec (Hoboken). 2017; 300 (5):900–911

[16] Cil A, Yazici M, Uzumcugil A, et al. The evolution of sagittal segmental alignment of the spine during childhood. Spine. 2005; 30(1):93–100

[17] Russo GA, Kirk EC. Foramen magnum position in bipedal mammals. J Hum Evol. 2013; 65(5):656–670

[18] Richards GD, Jabbour RS. Foramen magnum ontogeny in Homo sapiens: a functional matrix perspective. Anat Rec (Hoboken). 2011; 294(2):199–216

[19] Kimbel WH, Rak Y. The cranial base of Australopithecus afarensis: new insights from the female skull. Philos Trans R Soc Lond B Biol Sci. 2010; 365 (1556):3365–3376

[20] Russo GA, Kirk EC. Another look at the foramen magnum in bipedal mammals. J Hum Evol. 2017; 105:24–40

[21] Stock MK, Reynolds DG, Masters AJ, Bromage TG, Enlow DH. Line of sight in hominoids. J Clin Pediatr Dent. 2016; 40(3):251–258

[22] Vaněk P, Bradáč O, de Lacy P, Konopková R, Lacman J, Beneš V. Vertebral artery and osseous anomalies characteristic at the craniocervical junction diagnosed by CT and 3D CT angiography in normal Czech population: analysis of 511 consecutive patients. Neurosurg Rev. 2017; 40(3):369–376

[23] Pękala PA, Henry BM, Pękala JR, et al. Prevalence of foramen arcuale and its clinical significance: a meta-analysis of 55,985 subjects. J Neurosurg Spine. 2017; 27(3):276–290

[24] Gibelli D, Cappella A, Cerutti E, Spagnoli L, Dolci C, Sforza C. Prevalence of ponticulus posticus in a Northern Italian orthodontic population: a lateral cephalometric study. Surg Radiol Anat. 2016; 38(3):309–312

[25] Krishnamurthy A, Nayak SR, Khan S, et al. Arcuate foramen of atlas: incidence, phylogenetic and clinical significance. Rom J Morphol Embryol. 2007; 48 (3):263–266

[26] Hong JT, Lee SW, Son BC, et al. Analysis of anatomical variations of bone and vascular structures around the posterior atlantal arch using three-dimensional computed tomography angiography. J Neurosurg Spine. 2008; 8(3):230–236

[27] Lee MJ, Cassinelli E, Riew KD. The feasibility of inserting atlas lateral mass screws via the posterior arch. Spine. 2006; 31(24):2798–2801

[28] Son DJ, Jung YY, Park MH, et al. Activated natural killer cells mediate the suppressive effect of interleukin-4 on tumor development via STAT6 activation in an atopic condition melanoma model. Neoplasia. 2017; 19(7):537–548

[29] Elliott RE, Tanweer O. The prevalence of the ponticulus posticus (arcuate foramen) and its importance in the Goel-Harms procedure: meta-analysis and review of the literature. World Neurosurg. 2014; 82(1–2):e335–e343

[30] Buna M, Coghlan W, deGruchy M, Williams D, Zmiywsky O. Ponticles of the atlas: a review and clinical perspective. J Manipulative Physiol Ther. 1984; 7 (4):261–266

[31] Mizutani J, Verma K, Endo K, et al. Global spinal alignment in cervical kyphotic deformity: the importance of head position and thoracolumbar alignment in the compensatory mechanism. Neurosurgery. 2018; 82(5): 686–694

[32] Karabag H, Iplikcioglu AC. The assessment of upright cervical spinal alignment using supine MRI studies. Clin Spine Surg. 2017; 30(7):E892–E895

[33] Sharan AD, Krystal JD, Singla A, Nassr A, Kang JD, Riew KD. Advances in the understanding of cervical spine deformity. Instr Course Lect. 2015; 64:417–426

[34] Joaquim AF, Riew KD. Management of cervical spine deformity after intradural tumor resection. Neurosurg Focus. 2015; 39(2):E13

[35] Kim HJ, Lenke LG, Oshima Y, et al. Cervical lordosis actually increases with aging and progressive degeneration in spinal deformity patients. Spine Deform. 2014; 2(5):410–414

[36] Scheer JK, Tang JA, Smith JS, et al. International Spine Study Group. Cervical spine alignment, sagittal deformity, and clinical implications: a review. J Neurosurg Spine. 2013; 19(2):141–159

[37] Miyamoto H, Hashimoto K, Ikeda T, Akagi M. Effect of correction surgery for cervical kyphosis on compensatory mechanisms in overall spinopelvic sagittal alignment. Eur Spine J. 2017; 26(9):2380–2385

[38] Botelho RV, Ferreira ED. Angular craniometry in craniocervical junction malformation. Neurosurg Rev. 2013; 36(4):603–610, discussion 610

[39] Ferreira JA, Botelho RV. The odontoid process invagination in normal subjects, Chiari malformation and Basilar invagination patients: pathophysiologic correlations with angular craniometry. Surg Neurol Int. 2015; 6:118

[40] Xu S, Gong R. Clivodens angle: a new diagnostic method for basilar invagination at computed tomography. Spine. 2016; 41(17):1365–1371

[41] Chandra PS, Goyal N, Chauhan A, Ansari A, Sharma BS, Garg A. The severity of basilar invagination and atlantoaxial dislocation correlates with sagittal joint inclination, coronal joint inclination, and craniocervical tilt: a description of new indexes for the craniovertebral junction. Neurosurgery. 2014; 10 Suppl 4:621–629, discussion 629–630

[42] Anderst WJ, Donaldson WF, III, Lee JY, Kang JD. Cervical motion segment contributions to head motion during flexion, lateral bending, and axial rotation. Spine J. 2015; 15(12):2538–2543

[43] Zong R, Yin Y, Qiao G, Jin Y, Yu X. Quantitative measurements of the skull base and craniovertebral junction in congenital occipitalization of the atlas: a computed tomography-based anatomic study. World Neurosurg. 2017; 99:96–103

[44] Goldstein HE, Anderson RC. Craniovertebral junction instability in the setting of Chiari I malformation. Neurosurg Clin N Am. 2015; 26(4):561–569

[45] Tian W, Yu J. The role of C2-C7 and O-C2 angle in the development of dysphagia after cervical spine surgery. Dysphagia. 2013; 28(2):131–138

[46] Hong J, Lim S. Dysphagia after occipitocervical fusion. N Engl J Med. 2017; 376(22):e46

[47] Kim JY, Hong JT, Oh JS, et al. Influence of neck postural changes on cervical spine motion and angle during swallowing. Medicine (Baltimore). 2017; 96 (45):e8566

[48] Song MS, Lee HJ, Kim JT, Kim JH, Hong JT. Ponticulus posticus: morphometric analysis and its anatomical implications for occipito-cervical fusion. Clin Neurol Neurosurg. 2017; 157:76–81

[49] Hong JT, Kim IS, Kim JY, et al. Risk factor analysis and decision-making of surgical strategy for V3 segment anomaly: significance of preoperative CT angiography for posterior C1 instrumentation. Spine. 2016; 16(9):1055–1061

[50] Epstein BS, Epstein JA, Jones MD. Cervical spinal stenosis. Radiol Clin North Am. 1977; 15(2):215–226

[51] Liao Y, Pu L, Guo H, et al. Selection of surgical procedures for basilar invagination with atlantoaxial dislocation. Spine J. 2016; 16(10):1184–1193

[52] Menezes AH, Traynelis VC, Gantz BJ. Surgical approaches to the craniovertebral junction. Clin Neurosurg. 1994; 41:187–203

[53] Menezes AH. Surgical approaches: postoperative care and complications "transoral-transpalatopharyngeal approach to the craniocervical junction". Childs Nerv Syst. 2008; 24(10):1187–1193

[54] Perrini P, Benedetto N, Di Lorenzo N. Transoral approach to extradural nonneoplastic lesions of the craniovertebral junction. Acta Neurochir (Wien). 2014; 156(6):1231–1236

[55] Jain VK, Behari S, Banerji D, Bhargava V, Chhabra DK. Transoral decompression for craniovertebral osseous anomalies: perioperative management dilemmas. Neurol India. 1999; 47(3):188–195

[56] Goel A, Phalke U, Cacciola F, Muzumdar D. Surgical management of high cervical disc prolapse associated with basilar invagination–two case reports. Neurol Med Chir (Tokyo). 2004; 44(3):142–145

[57] Goel A, Shah A. Atlantoaxial joint distraction as a treatment for basilar invagination: a report of an experience with 11 cases. Neurol India. 2008; 56(2):144–150

[58] Chandra PS, Prabhu M, Goyal N, Garg A, Chauhan A, Sharma BS. Distraction, compression, extension, and reduction combined with joint remodeling and extra-articular distraction: description of 2 new modifications for its application in basilar invagination and atlantoaxial dislocation: prospective study in 79 cases. Neurosurgery. 2015; 77(1):67–80, discussion 80

[59] Goel A, Bhatjiwale M, Desai K. Basilar invagination: a study based on 190 surgically treated patients. J Neurosurg. 1998; 88(6):962–968

[60] Yoshida G, Kamiya M, Yukawa Y, et al. Rheumatoid vertical and subaxial subluxation can be prevented by atlantoaxial posterior screw fixation. Eur Spine J. 2012; 21(12):2498–2505

[61] Werle S, Ezzati A, ElSaghir H, Boehm H. Is inclusion of the occiput necessary in fusion for C1-2 instability in rheumatoid arthritis? J Neurosurg Spine. 2013; 18(1):50–56

[62] Bydon M, Macki M, Qadi M, et al. Regression of an atlantoaxial rheumatoid pannus following posterior instrumented fusion. Clin Neurol Neurosurg. 2015; 137:28–33

[63] Yonezawa I, Okuda T, Won J, et al. Retrodental mass in rheumatoid arthritis. J Spinal Disord Tech. 2013; 26(2):E65–E69

[64] Landi A, Marotta N, Morselli C, Marongiu A, Delfini R. Pannus regression after posterior decompression and occipito-cervical fixation in occipito-atlantoaxial instability due to rheumatoid arthritis: case report and literature review. Clin Neurol Neurosurg. 2013; 115(2):111–116

[65] Goel A, Dange N. Immediate postoperative regression of retroodontoid pannus after lateral mass reconstruction in a patient with rheumatoid disease of the craniovertebral junction. Case report. J Neurosurg Spine. 2008; 9(3):273–276

[66] Lagares A, Arrese I, Pascual B, Gòmez PA, Ramos A, Lobato RD. Pannus resolution after occipitocervical fusion in a non-rheumatoid atlanto-axial instability. Eur Spine J. 2006; 15(3):366–369

[67] Miyata M, Neo M, Fujibayashi S, Ito H, Takemoto M, Nakamura T. O-C2 angle as a predictor of dyspnea and/or dysphagia after occipitocervical fusion. Spine. 2009; 34(2):184–188

[68] Maulucci CM, Ghobrial GM, Sharan AD, et al. Correlation of posterior occipitocervical angle and surgical outcomes for occipitocervical fusion. Evid Based Spine Care J. 2014; 5(2):163–165

[69] Hong JT, Lee SW, Son BC, Sung JH, Kim IS, Park CK. Hypoglossal nerve palsy after posterior screw placement on the C-1 lateral mass. Case report. J Neurosurg Spine. 2006; 5(1):83–85

[70] Hsu WK. Advanced techniques in cervical spine surgery. Instr Course Lect. 2012; 61:441–450

[71] Kim SW, Jang C, Yang MH, et al. The natural course of prevertebral soft tissue swelling after anterior cervical spine surgery: how long will it last? Spine J. 2017; 17(9):1297–1309

22 Cervical Deformity Classification

Jeffrey P. Mullin, Davis G. Taylor, Justin S. Smith, Christopher I. Shaffrey, and Christopher P. Ames

Abstract

In spinal deformity research, there has been growing use and study of various deformity classification systems. Recently, a cervical deformity classification system has been proposed. This system has great potential to increase our knowledge and understanding of cervical deformity. We review each descriptor and the five modifiers of this classification system.

Keywords: cervical deformity classification, C2–C7 sagittal vertical axis, horizontal gaze, cervical lordosis, T1 slope, chin–brow vertical angle

22.1 Introduction

The cervical spine is a complex bony and ligamentous region divided anatomically into the subaxial spine (C3–C7) and the occipitocervical junction (occiput to C2).[1] Deformities that affect the cervical spine include a broad range of etiologies, including spondylosis, inflammatory arthropathy, trauma, infection, iatrogenic, congenital, and neuromuscular pathologies. Kyphosis, the most common cervical deformity, can have an apex within the cervical spine, at the cervicothoracic junction, or extending into the thoracic spine.

Although there are a number of classification systems for injury of the cervical spine, only one comprehensive classification system of cervical spine deformity has been reported.[2,3] Without a cogent classification system, studies comparing management and outcome of disease may suffer from heterogeneity and poor communication. To bring uniformity to the classification and reporting of surgical literature and to help facilitate communication among those who care for these patients, a cervical deformity classification system was developed based on expert opinion and existing literature. The resulting cervical deformity classification system classifies cervical deformity based on five primary deformity "descriptors" and five clinically relevant modifiers.[2,4] The minimum imaging and assessments required for classification of a cervical deformity with the proposed classification are summarized in ▶ Table 22.1.

Table 22.1 Minimum studies and assessments required for classification

- Standing lateral and PA cervical spine radiographs
- Full-length standing lateral and PA spine radiographs
- Clinical photograph or radiographic imaging to allow measurement of the CBVA
- Completed and scored mJOA questionnaire

Abbreviations: CBVA, chin–brow vertical angle; mJOA, modified Japanese Orthopedic Association; PA, posteroanterior.

22.2 Case Discussion

A 50-year-old woman is referred to your clinic with a primary complaint of chronic neck pain and complaints of mild decrease in sensation of her hands. She brings with her a cervical MRI obtained by her primary care physician (▶ Fig. 22.1).

How would you classify her deformity? What are the next steps of your outpatient evaluation?

22.3 Descriptors

The five primary deformity descriptors were developed to identify the principal deformity type (sagittal vs. coronal vs. craniovertebral junction) and in order to quickly segregate deformity types based on the major deformity present (▶ Fig. 22.2). Sagittal deformities make up the first three descriptors and are based on the apex of the deformity. Type C deformities have an apex within the cervical spine. Type CT deformities have an apex at the cervicothoracic junction, and type T deformities have an apex within the thoracic spine. The remaining two deformity descriptors reflect primary coronal deformity, designated as type S (scoliosis), and primary deformities of the craniovertebral junction, designated as type CVJ (▶ Fig. 22.3).

22.4 Modifiers

Following determination and designation of the primary deformity descriptor, a number of modifiers are then considered. These

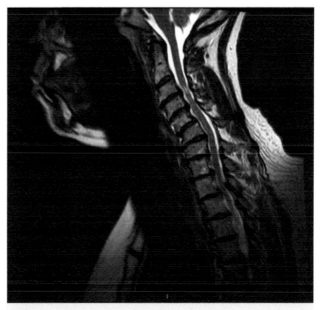

Fig. 22.1 MRI demonstrating cervical deformity.

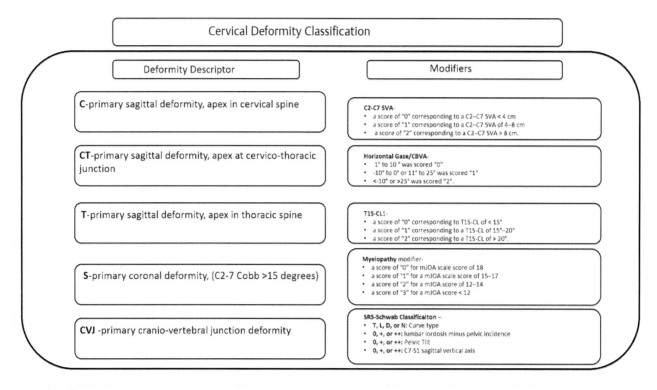

Fig. 22.2 Cervical deformity classification. Modified from original.[1]

modifiers were selected based on available literature and expert opinion as factors that may impact disease morbidity (e.g., pain, disability, and myelopathy) and that may have implications for surgical planning. These modifiers are C2–C7 sagittal vertical axis (SVA), horizontal gaze assessed by the chin–brow vertical angle (CBVA), T1 slope minus C2–C7 lordosis (T1S–CL), myelopathy as assessed by the modified Japanese Orthopedic Association (mJOA) score, and the Scoliosis Research Society (SRS)–Schwab adult thoracolumbar deformity classification.

22.4.1 C2–C7 Sagittal Vertical Axis

Global sagittal alignment has recently become appreciated as a significant source of disability, increased pain, and worsened quality of life among patients with spinal deformity.[5,6,7] The C2–C7 SVA is a measure of the overall sagittal alignment across the cervical spine. The C2–C7 SVA is assessed on an upright radiograph of the cervical spine's visualization from at least the C2–C7 vertebral bodies. The measurement reflects the offset of a plumb line dropped from the center of the C2 vertebral body relative to the posterosuperior corner of the C7 vertebral body (▶ Fig. 22.4). Tang et al reported that an increased C2–C7 SVA correlates with worse Neck Disability Index (NDI) scores and that a threshold of 4 cm correlated with moderate to severe disability.[8] In addition, Smith et al reported a significant correlation between C2–C7 SVA and severity of myelopathy based on the mJOA score.[9] Thus, three scores were proposed for the C2–C7 SVA modifier:

1. A score of "0" corresponding to a C2–C7 SVA < 4 cm.
2. A score of "1" corresponding to a C2–C7 SVA of 4–8 cm.
3. A score of "2" corresponding to a C2–C7 SVA > 8 cm.[2]

22.4.2 Horizontal Gaze/Chin–Brow Vertical Angle

The CBVA is a measure of a patient's horizontal gaze, which has been previously reported to correlate with quality of life and postoperative satisfaction.[10,11,12,13,14,15] CBVA is measured as the angle between a line from patient's chin to brow and a vertical line (▶ Fig. 22.5 and ▶ Fig. 22.6). The CBVA can be measured using a clinical photograph or a radiograph of the skull. Regardless of the imaging modality, it is important for the patient to be standing with their neck in a neutral positon with their hips and knees extended. A limitation of the CBVA that has limited its use is that the necessary anatomic landmarks are often not visualized on classic lateral radiographs.[16] To overcome this limitation, Lafage et al correlated two more readily available measurements: the slope of the line of sight (SLS) and the slope of McGregor's line (McGS). They found a strong correlation between these two measurements and the CBVA. They concluded that the SLS or McGS could be used as surrogates for the CBVA in routine clinical practice.[16] The SLS is measured as the angle between a line from the inferior margin of the orbit to the top of the external auditory meatus and a horizontal line. McGS is defined as the angle between a line from the posterior margin of the hard palate to the most caudal portion of the occiput and a horizontal line.

Owing to the potential for significant impact of altered horizontal gaze on functional activities, particularly in postsurgical patients with a rigid or fused cervical spine, the CBVA was selected as a modifier for cervical deformity classification. A patient with a fixed negative CBVA (upward gaze) may have increased difficulty with activities requiring downward gaze,

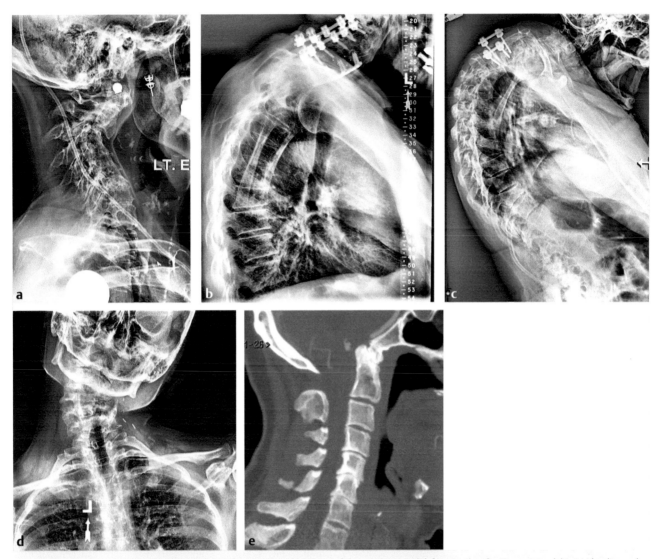

Fig. 22.3 Example cases demonstrating the five deformity descriptor types of the Ames cervical deformity classification system. (a) Lateral radiograph demonstrating deformity apex in cervical spine; C classification. (b) Lateral radiograph demonstrating deformity apex in cervicothoracic junction, CT classification. (c) Lateral radiograph demonstrating deformity apex in thoracic spine, T classification. (d) AP radiograph demonstrating coronal deformity, S classification. (e) Sagittal CT demonstrating deformity of craniovertebral junction, CVJ classification.

such as walking down stairs, due to the increased effort or inability to look downward. Numerous studies have reported an association between a physiologic CBVA and favorable outcomes following surgery for spinal deformity, based on improved gaze, ambulation, and activities of daily living.[10,11,12,13,14,15] There are no clearly defined normal value ranges for CBVA; however, Scheer et al reported favorable surgical outcomes if CBVA is greater than -10, with varying opinion on the maximum positive value associated with favorable outcomes (from -10 to +10 degrees to +10 to +20 degrees).[14] Additionally, Suk et al reported the negative impact of overcorrecting CBVA to greater than -10 degrees.[15] Song et al recently published that in ankylosing spondylitis patients, CBVA of 10 to 20 degrees was optimal.[17] It should be noted that in general patients can better tolerate a downward facing horizontal gaze than a fixed upward gaze (referred to as a "birdwatcher's gaze") since the inability to see the ground for safe ambulation and walking

down steps can compromise safety. The expert opinion of Ames and colleagues established three scores for the modifier CBVA[2]:
1. CBVA from 1 to 10 degrees was scored "0."
2. CBVA from -10 to 0 degrees or 11 to 25 degrees was scored "1."
3. CBVA less than -10 or greater than 25 degrees was scored "2."

22.4.3 T1 Slope minus C2–C7 Lordosis (T1S–CL)

Recent work has demonstrated a significant relationship between lumbar lordosis (LL) and pelvic incidence (PI) with respect to global spinal alignment and quality of life. A pragmatic estimate has been proposed that the ideal LL for an individual should be within 10 degrees of that individual's PI (i.e., LL = PI ± 10 degrees).[7,18] Thus, a patient with a high PI (more horizontal

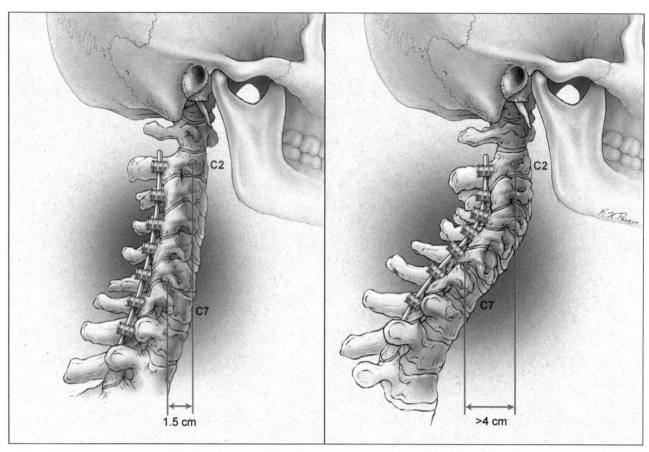

Fig. 22.4 Diagrams demonstrating calculation of C2–C7 sagittal vertical axis. In these scenarios, the figure on the left would receive a modifier of 0. The image on the right would receive a modifier of 1. (Reprinted with permission from Xavier Studios.)

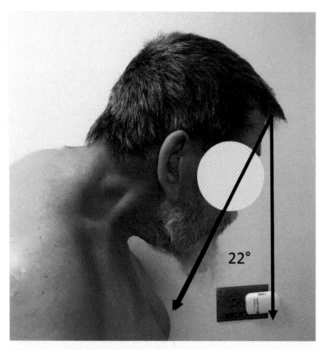

Fig. 22.5 CBVA photograph.

sacrum) will require more LL than an individual with a low PI (more vertical sacrum).[2] A PI–LL mismatch that falls outside of the normal range has been shown to be correlated with significantly worse health-related quality of life (HRQOL) outcome scores in patients with thoracolumbar deformity, including specific measures of pain and disability.[7,19,20]

In contrast to the progress that has been made in determining normal values for LL, the normal ranges of CL are not well defined, and what is normal CL for an individual is even less well defined.[21] Additionally, whether and to what degree CL correlates with HRQOL remains controversial, as several studies have failed to demonstrate similar significant correlations as those identified for LL.[22,23,24] However, loss of CL has been shown to be associated with worsened neck pain in the settings of trauma or postoperative fusion.[25,26,27] Furthermore, in myelopathic patients, cervical kyphosis has a negative prognosis with respect to postoperative neurological recovery.[27] Given that cervical kyphosis is the most common cervical deformity, Ames and colleagues selected a parameter reflective of CL as a modifier for their classification system (▶ Fig. 22.6).[2] Similar in principal to the measure and assessment of LL in the context of PI, Lee and colleagues proposed assessment of the CL in relationship with the T1S.[14,28] Just as the pelvis serves as the base for the lumbar spine and helps set the amount of required LL,

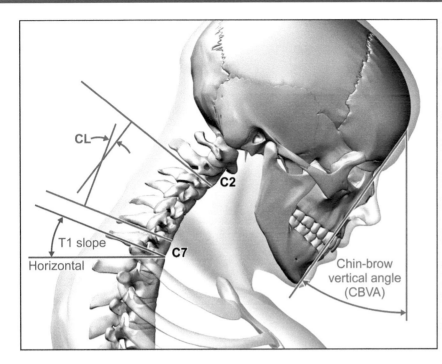

Fig. 22.6 Chin–brow vertical angle is the angle between a line connecting a patient's chin and brow and a vertical line (*red lines*). Cervical lordosis (CL) is obtained measuring angle between inferior endplate of C2 and superior endplate of C7 (*green lines*). T1 slope is the degree of the angle between the T1 superior endplate and the horizon (*purple lines*). (Reprinted with permission from Xavier Studios.)

the T1 vertebral body is the base of the cervical spine and the slope of the T1 body helps set the harmonious amount of CL required for physiologic positioning of the head. Hyun and colleagues assessed the correlation between T1S–CL and NDI and suggested that CL should be within 22 degrees of T1S.[29] Based on these findings and the rising appreciation of the importance of sagittal alignment, Ames and colleagues included the T1S–CL modifier in the cervical deformity classification system[2]:

1. A score of "0" corresponding to T1S–CL of < 15 degrees.
2. A score of "1" corresponding to a T1S–CL of 15 to 20 degrees.
3. A score of "2" corresponding to a T1S–CL of greater than 20 degrees.

22.4.4 Myelopathy Modifier

Cervical deformity, and notably cervical kyphosis, has been associated with the development of cervical myelopathy due to local pressure, stretch, and ischemic changes at the area of deformity (▶ Fig. 22.7).[21,30,31,32,33,34,35] Two cadaveric studies demonstrated the significant rise in intramedullary pressure with increasing cervical kyphosis.[36,37] Winestone et al demonstrated that performing a posterior decompression was able to reduce the kyphosis-induced increase in intramedullary pressure by 25%. However, when correcting the deformity, the increase in intramedullary pressure was reduced to 0.[37] There is a demonstrated association between kyphosis and the severity of myelopathy, but myelopathy may also occur due to associated degenerative changes such as osteophytes, local discoligamentous changes, and facet hypertrophy.[9] Due to the profound impact myelopathy can have on a patient's life and that the cervical deformity may be a causative factor, a measure of myelopathy was included in the cervical spinal deformity classification. The mJOA score was selected, since it is the most widely accepted and applied quantitative functional assessment of myelopathy severity.[38] The mJOA assigns a score ranging from 0 to 18, with a lower score associated with more severe

myelopathy. Thus, the expert panel devised a categorization system for myelopathy that is consistent with previous publications[39]:

1. A score of "0" corresponding to an mJOA scale score of 18 (no myelopathy).
2. A score of "1" corresponding to an mJOA scale score of 15 to 17 (mild myelopathy).
3. A score of "2" corresponding to an mJOA score of 12 to 14 (moderate myelopathy).
4. A score of "3" corresponding to an mJOA score of less than 12 (severe myelopathy).[2]

22.4.5 SRS–Schwab Classification

As our understanding of global spinal alignment continues to increase, it has become increasingly apparent that deformity or malalignment in one region of the spine can impact other spinal regions. For example, a cervical deformity may result from or be exacerbated by a primary thoracolumbar deformity and vice versa.[14] Ames and colleagues reported a correlation between sagittal pelvic parameters and the cervical spine,[21] while Smith and colleagues demonstrated that patients with positive global sagittal malalignment tended to have a compensatory increase in cervical lordosis in an effort to maintain horizontal gaze and that surgical correction of the spinopelvic mismatch resulted in improvement of the compensatory hyperlordosis.[40,41] Collectively, these findings support the need to obtain full-length spine standing radiographs and to assess not only cervical parameters but also thoracolumbar pelvic parameters when assessing a patient with cervical deformity. Thus, inclusion of the SRS–Schwab adult thoracolumbar deformity classification as a modifier for the cervical deformity classification was deemed necessary. The SRS–Schwab classification has been validated and shown to correlate with HRQOL measures in patients with spinal deformity.[18,42,43] This classification system consists of defining deformities based on five thoracolumbar coronal curve types and includes three sagittal modifiers (▶ Fig. 22.8).

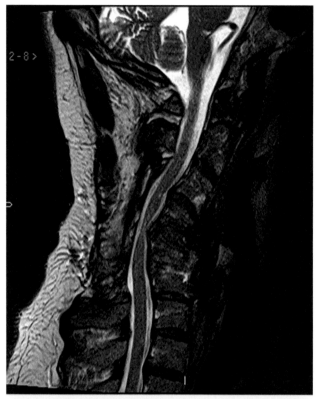

Fig. 22.7 Sagittal MRI (T2) demonstrating neural compression of the spinal cord due to cervical kyphotic deformity, despite posterior decompression.

22.5 Case Example Discussion

As a part of your outpatient workup for the case shown in ▶ Fig. 22.1, you obtained cervical and full-length standing spine radiographs (posteroanterior and lateral). These radiographs allow you to measure the parameters to define the patient's cervical deformity. The patient has a kyphotic deformity with an apex in the cervical spine (type C). She has relatively good global cervical sagittal alignment (C2–C7 SVA = 3.5 mm) and a T1S–CL mismatch of 5 degrees (Grade 0; ▶ Fig. 22.9). Her CBVA was measured at 3 degrees (Grade 0). Upon questioning, her mJOA score was found to be 15, reflecting a mild myelopathy (Grade 1). With regard to her SRS–Schwab classification, she has a curve type N, PI–LL mismatch of 12 degrees (Grade +), C7–S1 SVA of 10 mm (Grade 0), and a pelvic tilt of 14 degrees (Grade 0). Thus, her overall cervical deformity would be classified as type C/0/0/1/1; N + 00.

22.6 Discussion

Although this new classification system may require some physicians to obtain additional studies in order to fully apply all measurements, these further studies may provide clinically useful information and some degree of uniformity among practitioners and may further improve the ability to appreciate results and better enable comparison across practitioners and techniques. We recommend full-length standing lateral and posteroanterior (PA) spine radiographs (these must include the femoral heads and at least visualize C7), standing lateral and PA cervical spine radiographs, clinical photograph radiographic imaging to allow measurement of the CBVA, and a completed and scored mJOA questionnaire as a minimum for initial assessment of cervical deformity.

While this is a newly proposed classification system, it has been a well-received addition to the spine literature.[44,45,46,47,48,49] Many authors have noted the lack of previous cervical deformity

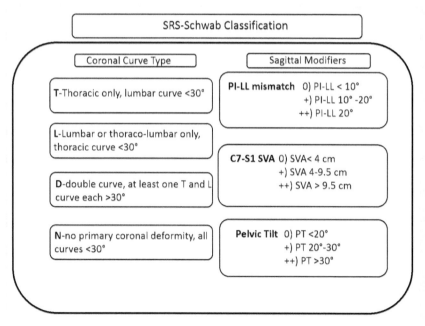

Fig. 22.8 SRS–Schwab classification system. Modified from original.[5,16]

SRS-Schwab Classification

Coronal Curve Type

T-Thoracic only, lumbar curve <30°

L-Lumbar or thoraco-lumbar only, thoracic curve <30°

D-double curve, at least one T and L curve each >30°

N-no primary coronal deformity, all curves <30°

Sagittal Modifiers

PI-LL mismatch 0) PI-LL < 10°
+) PI-LL 10° -20°
++) PI-LL 20°

C7-S1 SVA 0) SVA< 4 cm
+) SVA 4-9.5 cm
++) SVA > 9.5 cm

Pelvic Tilt 0) PT <20°
+) PT 20°-30°
++) PT >30°

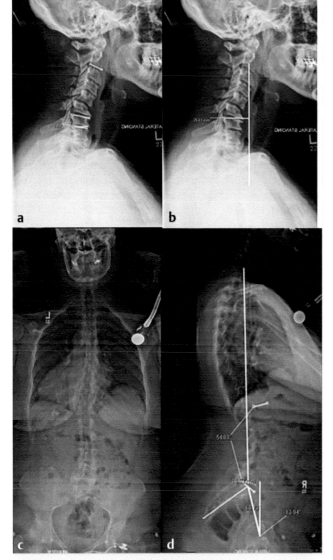

Fig. 22.9 Case example radiographs. **(a)** Lateral radiograph demonstrating C2–C7 lordosis and T1 slope. **(b)** Lateral radiograph demonstrating CVA measurement. **(c,d)** AP and lateral long cassette radiographs used to evaluate global alignment and determine SRS–Schwab classification.

patients from a multicenter patient registry. They found C and CT descriptors to be the most prevalent: 58 and 24%, respectively. They also found significant differences between T1S–CL grades and C2–C7 SVA grades across the various deformity descriptor categories. Furthermore, CT and S deformities and the horizontal gaze modifier imparted the most significant disability impact on preoperative NDI score and mJOA score.[4] One of the additional findings from the study of Passias and colleagues was the important interplay between the cervical deformity measures and the SRS–Schwab spinal deformity classifications as related to pre- and postoperative disability.[4] Another study correlated improvement in the modifier scores of the classification system to be associated improved 1-year outcomes.[50] Horn et al retrospectively reported the results from a multicenter study; in this study, they reviewed 73 patients with cervical deformity who underwent surgery. They found, at 1 year, that improvements in cervical deformity classification modifiers was associated with a minimal clinically important difference in mJOA, NDI, and EQ-5D outcome measures.[50] While the proposed cervical deformity classification system has shown reliability, additional studies are needed to examine its applicability, especially with regard to patient management decisions and correlations with long-term clinical follow-up.

References

[1] Kuntz C. Evaluation of Spinal Alignment. Youmans and Winn Neurological Surgery; 312:2565–2569

[2] Ames CP, Smith JS, Eastlack R, et al. International Spine Study Group. Reliability assessment of a novel cervical spine deformity classification system. J Neurosurg Spine. 2015; 23(6):673–683

[3] Vialle LRG. AOSpine Masters Series. Volume 5: Cervical Spine Trauma. New York: Thieme; 2015

[4] Passias PG, Jalai CM, Smith JS, et al. Characterizing adult cervical deformity and disability based on existing cervical and adult deformity classification schemes at presentation and following correction. Neurosurgery. 2018; 82 (2):192–201

[5] Glassman SD, Berven S, Bridwell K, Horton W, Dimar JR. Correlation of radiographic parameters and clinical symptoms in adult scoliosis. Spine. 2005; 30 (6):682–688

[6] Glassman SD, Bridwell K, Dimar JR, Horton W, Berven S, Schwab F. The impact of positive sagittal balance in adult spinal deformity. Spine. 2005; 30 (18):2024–2029

[7] Schwab FJ, Blondel B, Bess S, et al. International Spine Study Group (ISSG). Radiographical spinopelvic parameters and disability in the setting of adult spinal deformity: a prospective multicenter analysis. Spine. 2013; 38(13): E803–E812

[8] Tang JA, Scheer JK, Deviren V, et al. Positive Cervical Sagittal Alignment Negatively Impacts Outcomes Following Adult Cervical Fusion Procedures: Poster no. 4. Spine Journal Meeting Abstracts; 2011: 228

[9] Smith JS, Lafage V, Ryan DJ, et al. Association of myelopathy scores with cervical sagittal balance and normalized spinal cord volume: analysis of 56 preoperative cases from the AOSpine North America Myelopathy study. Spine. 2013; 38(22) Suppl 1:S161–S170

[10] Deviren V, Scheer JK, Ames CP. Technique of cervicothoracic junction pedicle subtraction osteotomy for cervical sagittal imbalance: report of 11 cases. J Neurosurg Spine. 2011; 15(2):174–181

[11] Etame AB, Than KD, Wang AC, La Marca F, Park P. Surgical management of symptomatic cervical or cervicothoracic kyphosis due to ankylosing spondylitis. Spine. 2008; 33(16):E559–E564

[12] Kim K-T, Lee S-H, Son E-S, Kwack Y-H, Chun Y-S, Lee J-H. Surgical treatment of "chin-on-pubis" deformity in a patient with ankylosing spondylitis: a case report of consecutive cervical, thoracic, and lumbar corrective osteotomies. Spine. 2012; 37(16):E1017–E1021

[13] Pigge RR, Scheerder FJ, Smit TH, Mullender MG, van Royen BJ. Effectiveness of preoperative planning in the restoration of balance and view in ankylosing spondylitis. Neurosurg Focus. 2008; 24(1):E7

classification systems. The authors of the classification system acknowledge that cervical deformity classification is in its infancy and there may be changes to the current system as further research occurs, which may result in further revisions and additions to either major descriptors or modifiers.[2] This possible evolution of the classification system would be similar to the SRS–Schwab classification system which underwent several changes as it matured in the literature before reaching its current form. One of the crucial components of classification systems is their reproducibility. The proposed classification system has been shown to have significant interuser and intrauser reproducibility.[2]

Another crucial aspect of classification systems is applicability. Currently, one study has prospectively reviewed the cervical deformity classification system.[4] The authors reviewed 84

[14] Scheer JK, Tang JA, Smith JS, et al. International Spine Study Group. Cervical spine alignment, sagittal deformity, and clinical implications: a review. J Neurosurg Spine. 2013; 19(2):141–159

[15] Suk K-S, Kim K-T, Lee S-H, Kim J-M. Significance of chin-brow vertical angle in correction of kyphotic deformity of ankylosing spondylitis patients. Spine. 2003; 28(17):2001–2005

[16] Lafage R, Challier V, Liabaud B, et al. Natural head posture in the setting of sagittal spinal deformity: validation of chin-brow vertical angle, slope of line of sight, and McGregor's slope with health-related quality of life. Neurosurgery. 2016; 79(1):108–115

[17] Song K, Su X, Zhang Y, et al. Optimal chin-brow vertical angle for sagittal visual fields in ankylosing spondylitis kyphosis. Eur Spine J. 2016; 25(8): 2596–2604

[18] Schwab F, Ungar B, Blondel B, et al. Scoliosis Research Society-Schwab adult spinal deformity classification: a validation study. Spine. 2012; 37(12): 1077–1082

[19] Smith JS, Shaffrey CI, Fu K-MG, et al. Clinical and radiographic evaluation of the adult spinal deformity patient. Neurosurg Clin N Am. 2013; 24(2): 143–156

[20] Smith JS, Singh M, Klineberg E, et al. International Spine Study Group. Surgical treatment of pathological loss of lumbar lordosis (flatback) in patients with normal sagittal vertical axis achieves similar clinical improvement as surgical treatment of elevated sagittal vertical axis: clinical article. J Neurosurg Spine. 2014; 21(2):160–170

[21] Ames CP, Blondel B, Scheer JK, et al. Cervical radiographical alignment: comprehensive assessment techniques and potential importance in cervical myelopathy. Spine. 2013; 38(22) Suppl 1:S149–S160

[22] Guérin P, Obeid I, Gille O, et al. Sagittal alignment after single cervical disc arthroplasty. J Spinal Disord Tech. 2012; 25(1):10–16

[23] Jagannathan J, Shaffrey CI, Oskouian RJ, et al. Radiographic and clinical outcomes following single-level anterior cervical discectomy and allograft fusion without plate placement or cervical collar. J Neurosurg Spine. 2008; 8 (5):420–428

[24] Villavicencio AT, Babuska JM, Ashton A, et al. Prospective, randomized, double-blind clinical study evaluating the correlation of clinical outcomes and cervical sagittal alignment. Neurosurgery. 2011; 68(5):1309–1316, discussion –1316

[25] Jenkins LA, Capen DA, Zigler JE, Nelson RW, Nagelberg S. Cervical spine fusions for trauma. A long-term radiographic and clinical evaluation. Orthop Rev. 1994 Suppl:13–19

[26] Kwon B, Kim DH, Marvin A, Jenis LG. Outcomes following anterior cervical discectomy and fusion: the role of interbody disc height, angulation, and spinous process distance. J Spinal Disord Tech. 2005; 18(4):304–308

[27] Naderi S, Özgen S, Pamir MN, Özek MM, Erzen C. Cervical spondylotic myelopathy: surgical results and factors affecting prognosis. Neurosurgery. 1998; 43(1):43–49, discussion 49–50

[28] Lee S-H, Kim K-T, Seo E-M, Suk K-S, Kwack Y-H, Son E-S. The influence of thoracic inlet alignment on the craniocervical sagittal balance in asymptomatic adults. J Spinal Disord Tech. 2012; 25(2):E41–E47

[29] Hyun SJ, Kim KJ, Jahng TA, Kim HJ. Clinical impact of T1 slope minus cervical lordosis after multilevel posterior cervical fusion surgery: a minimum 2-year follow-up data. Spine. 2017; 42(24):1859–1864

[30] Albert TJ, Vacarro A. Postlaminectomy kyphosis. Spine. 1998; 23(24): 2738–2745

[31] Deutsch H, Haid RW, Rodts GE, Mummaneni PV. Postlaminectomy cervical deformity. Neurosurg Focus. 2003; 15(3):E5

[32] Iida H, Tachibana S. Spinal cord intramedullary pressure: direct cord traction test. Neurol Med Chir (Tokyo). 1995; 35(2):75–77

[33] Jarzem PF, Quance DR, Doyle DJ, Begin LR, Kostuik JP. Spinal cord tissue pressure during spinal cord distraction in dogs. Spine. 1992; 17(8) Suppl: S227–S234

[34] Kitahara Y, Iida H, Tachibana S. Effect of spinal cord stretching due to head flexion on intramedullary pressure. Neurol Med Chir (Tokyo). 1995; 35 (5):285–288

[35] Tachibana S, Kitahara Y, Iida H, Yada K. Spinal cord intramedullary pressure. A possible factor in syrinx growth. Spine. 1994; 19(19):2174–2178, discussion 2178–2179

[36] Chavanne A, Pettigrew DB, Holtz JR, Dollin N, Kuntz C, IV. Spinal cord intramedullary pressure in cervical kyphotic deformity: a cadaveric study. Spine. 2011; 36(20):1619–1626

[37] Winestone JS, Farley CW, Curt BA, et al. Laminectomy, durotomy, and piotomy effects on spinal cord intramedullary pressure in severe cervical and thoracic kyphotic deformity: a cadaveric study. J Neurosurg Spine. 2012; 16 (2):195–200

[38] Benzel EC, Lancon J, Kesterson L, Hadden T. Cervical laminectomy and dentate ligament section for cervical spondylotic myelopathy. J Spinal Disord. 1991; 4 (3):286–295

[39] Fehlings MG, Wilson JR, Kopjar B, et al. Efficacy and safety of surgical decompression in patients with cervical spondylotic myelopathy: results of the AO-Spine North America prospective multi-center study. J Bone Joint Surg Am. 2013; 95(18):1651–1658

[40] Smith JS, Lafage V, Schwab FJ, et al. International Spine Study Group. Prevalence and type of cervical deformity among 470 adults with thoracolumbar deformity. Spine. 2014; 39(17):E1001–E1009

[41] Smith JS, Shaffrey CI, Lafage V, et al. International Spine Study Group. Spontaneous improvement of cervical alignment after correction of global sagittal balance following pedicle subtraction osteotomy. J Neurosurg Spine. 2012; 17 (4):300–307

[42] Smith JS, Klineberg E, Schwab F, et al. International Spine Study Group. Change in classification grade by the SRS-Schwab Adult Spinal Deformity Classification predicts impact on health-related quality of life measures: prospective analysis of operative and nonoperative treatment. Spine. 2013; 38 (19):1663–1671

[43] Terran J, Schwab F, Shaffrey CI, et al. International Spine Study Group. The SRS-Schwab adult spinal deformity classification: assessment and clinical correlations based on a prospective operative and nonoperative cohort. Neurosurgery. 2013; 73(4):559–568

[44] Jalai CM, Passias PG, Lafage V, et al. International Spine Study Group (ISSG). A comparative analysis of the prevalence and characteristics of cervical malalignment in adults presenting with thoracolumbar spine deformity based on variations in treatment approach over 2 years. Eur Spine J. 2016; 25(8): 2423–2432

[45] Smith JS, Shaffrey CI, Bess S, et al. Recent and emerging advances in spinal deformity. Neurosurgery. 2017; 80 3S:S70–S85

[46] Rosenthal BD, Maslak JP, Jenkins TJ, Hsu WK, Patel AA. Cervical deformity: a clinical approach to diagnosis and treatment. Contemporary Spine Surgery. 2017; 18:1–7

[47] Smith JS, Ramchandran S, Lafage V, et al. International Spine Study Group. Prospective multicenter assessment of early complication rates associated with adult cervical deformity surgery in 78 patients. Neurosurgery. 2016; 79(3):378–388

[48] Turner JD, Sonntag VK. Evolution of cervical spine deformity surgery and ongoing challenges. World Neurosurg. 2016; 93:469–470

[49] Tan LA, Riew KD, Traynelis VC. Cervical spine deformity-Part 1: Biomechanics, radiographic parameters, and classification. Neurosurgery. 2017; 81 (2):197–203

[50] Horn R, Passias P, Lafage R, et al. Improvement in Ames-ISSG Cervical Deformity Classification Modifier Grades Correlate with Clinical Improvement and Likelihood of Reaching MCID in Multiple Metrics: Series of 73 Patients with 1 year Follow-up. Cervical Spine Research Society 45th Annual Meeting; 2017 November 30 to December 2, 2017; Hollywood, FL

23 Distal Junctional Kyphosis and Fusion Level Selection

Tina Raman, Nicholas D. Stekas, and Themistocles S. Protopsaltis

Abstract

Junctional failure at the proximal and distal segments of a long construct continues to pose a significant challenge to achieving stable correction of cervical spine deformity. Distal junctional kyphosis can occur in up to 24% of patients postoperatively and can range from an asymptomatic radiographic finding to continuously progressive degeneration of the segments caudal to a long fusion. Proposed risk factors include inappropriate selection of the distal fusion level and patient factors including age and osteoporosis. Extension of instrumentation and thorough neural decompression at the problematic level is indicated for progressive symptoms, grossly unstable instrumentation, and neurologic injury. In the absence of these, close follow-up with serial radiographs is recommended to document progression and optimize timing for intervention.

Keywords: adult cervical deformity, distal junctional kyphosis, instrumentation failure, adjacent segment disease, sagittal alignment

23.1 Introduction

Although there have been a myriad of advances in adult spinal deformity techniques and instrumentation over the past decade, junctional failure at the proximal and distal segments of a long construct continues to pose a challenge to even the most experienced deformity surgeon. It is well known that proximal junctional kyphosis (PJK) and proximal junctional failure can occur in 5 to 46% of patients, and recent studies have sought to elucidate risk factors for this significant complication, as well as efficacy of various preventive strategies.[1,2,3,4,5,6,7] Historically, distal junctional kyphosis (DJK) has been a concern in long cervicothoracic fusions for Scheuermann's kyphosis and ankylosing spondylitis.[8,9,10,11] Recent work has demonstrated, however, the prevalence of this complication in cervical spinal deformity, as well as its impact on long-term postoperative clinical and radiographic outcomes.[12,13]

DJK is a complication that was first described in a series of patients who had undergone thoracic fusion for Scheuermann's kyphosis.[12,13] Patients with a history of a previous thoracic or thoracolumbar fusion may develop symptomatic degeneration of the segments caudal to the fusion. Radiographic breakdown of levels caudal to the long fusion may manifest as kyphosis, stenosis, or olisthesis. Distal junctional degeneration may be acute, seen within the first 6 months to 1 year after surgery, or may develop gradually over time. The incidence can range from 0 to 28% in the setting of Scheuermann's kyphosis and other etiologies of thoracic hyperkyphosis including posttraumatic and postlaminectomy, and patients may require revision surgery for realignment of the deformity, and extension of fusion with osteotomy or wide decompression.[8,14]

Efforts to understand this complication have focused on selection of vertebral levels for fusion, reduction techniques, instrumentation, and patient-related factors.[8,15,16] It is critical that surgeons have an understanding of the diagnosis and prevention of this complication, as it has the potential for neurologic deficit, and can entail complex revision reconstruction. In this regard, this chapter will seek to deal with the historical context and prevalence of this complication in cervical deformity surgery, strategies for prevention, and approaches for unanticipated revision surgery.

23.2 Historical Perspective of Distal Junctional Kyphosis

In 1920, Dr. Holger Scheuermann first described Scheuermann's kyphosis, noting it to be a thoracic hyperkyphosis in adolescents, with associated abnormalities of the vertebrae including a wedge shape, endplate irregularities, Schmorl nodes, and decreased disc spaces.[17] While bracing can be an effective nonsurgical option in terms of pain control, it is known that fusion is indicated for curves greater than 60 degrees, rapid curve progression, excessive pain or discomfort, or neurologic compromise from the kyphosis or a herniated thoracic disc.[18,19,20,21] In 1980, Bradford et al published results in a series of 24 patients who underwent deformity correction through an anterior/posterior approach.[10] Though there was significant improvement of pain and global alignment after surgery, 5 of the 24 patients developed a progressive kyphotic deformity distal to the fusion requiring extension of fusion.[10] In retrospection, the authors emphasized the importance of extending the fusion to include the end vertebrae of the kyphotic deformity, or the vertebra tilted maximally into the concavity of the curve.[10]

In 1990, Reinhardt and Bassett expanded on this concept in a series of 14 patients who underwent anterior/posterior fusion for Scheuermann's kyphosis.[11] In this series, 5 of the 14 patients developed DJK with progressive deformity.[11] Interestingly, only two patients had undergone fusion stopping short of the end vertebrae, whereas the other three had fusions incorporating the end vertebrae, although the end vertebrae demonstrated wedging greater than 5 degrees. None of the patients who developed DJK required revision surgery at the time of publication.[11]

23.3 Pathophysiology

Broadly, DJK is a term used to refer to an abnormal kyphotic deformity at the lower instrumented vertebra (LIV).[22,23] DJK can occur through the bony vertebrae caudal to the construct, or through the caudal disc spaces. It is generally accepted that junctional pathology, which includes proximal junctional kyphosis (PJK), DJK, and adjacent segment disease with resulting stenosis, results from the differential stiffness between native bone and soft tissues, and instrumentation.[24,25,26] To date, there are no studies with a specific definition of DJK in terms of degrees of kyphosis or time point of occurrence. The only study to date examining the incidence of DJK is in the pediatric scoliosis population at 2-year follow-up; a 6.8% incidence of DJK was found.[27]

Though clear evidence of risk factors for DJK is lacking, suggested mechanisms and modes of DJK have been described. A well-known complication of Harrington rod instrumentation is flat back syndrome, or progressive loss or physiologic lumbar lordosis, and loss of disc height due to degeneration.[28] This can be associated with spinal stenosis and development of coronal malalignment and exacerbation of a fractional lumbosacral curve. Kyphotic deformity of the unfused segments distal to the construct may occur in this setting. Kyphosis or wedging of the disc caudal to instrumentation is an indication of DJK, and can occur when the fusion does not extend to the first stable vertebra, or incorporate the first lordotic disc space. Fractures of the inferior endplate of the LIV and pedicle screw ploughing can lead to a segmental kyphotic deformity at the distal aspect of the construct. Other fractures denoting instability that can result in a segmental kyphosis include fractures of the pars of vertebrae below the fusion construct, or sacral insufficiency fractures below lumbar instrumentation. Failure of instrumentation at the distal levels of a construct including rod fracture or pedicle screw loosening can also result in acute and segmental kyphosis, and the potential for neurologic deficits.[8,22] Finally, retrolisthesis or anterolisthesis of the vertebrae below the fusion construct may also comprise a form of DJK.

23.4 Risk Factors

Although data are sparse, risk factors for DJK have been elucidated in a handful of studies.

The selection of the distal fusion level is eminently critical in minimizing the risk for DJK.[8,14,22] Ending a fusion construct proximal to the first lordotic disc space, or proximal to the stable vertebra, can lead to increased stresses borne at the distal end of the construct.[8,14,22] Most of our work and knowledge with regard to selecting a distal fusion level is derived from the pediatric scoliosis literature, but it stands to reason that the premise and underlying principles are applicable for adult spinal deformity surgical planning. In both cases, there is often a trade-off between correction of the curve and sparing motion segments. Stopping the fusion short of the appropriate level may result in under- or overcorrection of the major curve, exacerbation of a compensatory curve below the construct, coronal malalignment and trunk imbalance, and adjacent segment disease. This concept will be explored in depth later in the chapter, with a discussion of selection of the distal fusion level.

Ending a long fusion at L5 may also be related to pedicle screw loosening, pseudarthrosis, and vertebral fracture at the distal aspect of the construct that can contribute to DJK. Edwards et al demonstrated a 61% rate of L5–S1 degeneration in a series of 34 patients who had undergone thoracolumbar posterior fusion ending at L5.[29] Sears et al similarly found that fusions ending at L5 results in greater adjacent segment disease than those extending to the sacrum.[30] Distal fixation in the sacrum may constitute S1 pedicular screws (unicortical, bicortical, or tricortical), S2 screws, and sacral alar screws. However, long construct fixation ending at the sacrum, including S1 pedicle screws and sacral alar screws, demonstrates high failure rates.[31,32,33] S1 screw strain and the risk of sacral fracture are appreciably increased when S1 pedicle screws alone are used as distal fixation for a long construct.[31] Ending a long construct at S1 without supplementing with pelvic fixation places increased biomechanical stress at the lumbosacral junction.[31,32,33,34,35,36,37] The flexion extension moment on an S1 screw is decreased by the addition of pelvic fixation.[31,32,33,34,35,36,37] The most commonly used type of sacropelvic fixation now are S2-alar-iliac screws and iliac screws. Pelvic fixation has also been shown to provide greater biomechanical stability at the lumbosacral junction and decrease pseudarthrosis rates.[31,32,33,34,35,36,37]

While patient-specific risk factors for PJK have been demonstrated including increased body mass index, decreased bone mineral density, and older age, none of these have been explored or borne out in studies of DJK. However, it is reasonable to expect that decreased bone mineral density, or osteoporosis, would contribute to the development of DJK. Finite element analyses have demonstrated that osteoporosis can lead to endplate microfractures of vertebrae adjacent to a long construct, which can create abnormal stress distributions in the intervertebral disc, and lead to disc degeneration.[38,39,40]

23.5 Prevention

Characteristics of the instrumentation used also play a role in potentially contributing to DJK. Stiffer implants can lead to increased stress at the bone–implant interface, potentiating or exacerbating degeneration and instability of the adjacent unfused level.[24,25,26] However, there is a subtle balance to be found given that less stiff implants may be more prone to fracture, particularly in the setting of complex osteotomies. A possible solution for this problem may be stiffer implants crossing the lumbosacral junction, where pseudarthrosis and/or rod fracture are most likely to occur, and using connectors to connect to a less stiff implant spanning the thoracic region. Another potential solution is to not place pedicle screws at every level, with the goal of decreasing the overall stiffness of the construct without compromising the additional stability needed for correction at the apex of the curve.

Adapting the correction to the patient's preexisting alignment is also important to prevent unintended effects of over- or undercorrection. In patients with sagittal malalignment, restoring balance in the sagittal plane can involve increasing lumbar lordosis or decreasing thoracic kyphosis. The latter can lead to increased kyphosis of the segments above the fused construct, and ultimately PJK or failure, and therefore this latter option is used rarely, only in the setting of severe hyperkyphosis. More commonly, the approach consists of restoring lumbar lordosis to within 10 to 11 degrees of the pelvic incidence. Ghasemi et al demonstrated in a series of 40 patients who underwent surgical correction for Scheuermann's kyphosis that patients who developed DJK had significantly more correction of their thoracic kyphosis than those who did not, that is, they were left with less thoracic kyphosis.[9] Those who developed DJK were also found to have less lumbar lordosis, although it is possible this was compensatory alignment in the setting of thoracic hypokyphosis.

The choice of LIV is also critical in preventing progression of a deformity distal to the construct. In this regard, extending a long cervical fusion to the upper thoracic spine, rather than ending in the middle of the thoracic kyphosis, can help ensure a gradual transition of stress at the distal end of the construct. However, the criteria for selection of the distal fusion level has varied between studies of long thoracic or thoracolumbar fusion for Scheuermann's kyphosis.[41,42,43,44] Some propose that the distal fusion level should be the stable vertebra, or the vertebra bisected by the central sacral vertical line.[41,42,43,44] Others propose that it should be the level with the first lordotic disc space.[41,42,43,44] It is an important distinction, as the stable vertebra is generally more caudal to the first lordotic vertebra, and a fusion to the stable vertebra thereby spares less levels. Lonner et al looked at 78 patients with Scheuermann's kyphosis and found no difference in DJK incidence whether the fusion ended at the stable or the first lordotic vertebra.[45] Cho et al presented the sagittal stable vertebra concept in their series of 31 patients who underwent anterior release and posterior fusion for thoracic hyperkyphosis. The authors proposed that fusion to the first lordotic vertebra was insufficient to prevent DJK, and proposed fusion to the stable vertebra.[44] In order to maintain sagittal alignment after surgery, the authors proposed that the upper instrumented vertebra (UIV) and LIV should be placed within the center of gravity, or the upper end of the kyphosis for the UIV, and the stable vertebra for the LIV.[44] Lundine et al had similar findings in 22 patients, demonstrating that fusion to the first lordotic vertebra had a lower rate of DJK than fusing short of it, and that fusion to the stable vertebra had the lowest rate of DJK.[43] They further found that fusion to the first lordotic vertebra conferred a four times greater risk of developing PJK than fusing to the stable vertebra.[43] A caveat of these studies is that they were retrospective reviews, in which there may have been other confounding factors other than choice of distal vertebral level, and in which there was heterogeneity in surgeon's technique.

It is hypothesized the disruption of the capsuloligamentous complex at the UIV can result in PJK. Similarly, there is ample reason to believe that the same principle holds true for DJK.

Facet joints and the supra- and intraspinous ligaments at the level below the construct should be left as intact as possible. Although this can be challenging in terms of exposure, or in a revision setting, the posterior tension band is a critical element in preventing kyphotic deformity at adjacent levels.

23.6 Distal Junctional Kyphosis in Adult Cervical Deformity

In cervical deformity surgery, as fusions generally extend to the upper cervical spine, the potential for DJK exists due to the increased stresses at the caudal aspect of the construct. Protopsaltis et al demonstrated a 24% rate of DJK in 67 patients who underwent cervical deformity surgery.[12] Sixty-nine percent of the DJK occurred within 3 months postoperatively, and 31% of DJK occurred between 3 and 6 months.[12] Furthermore, patients who developed DJK had worse baseline and postoperative radiographic alignment, despite similar degrees of intraoperative deformity correction.

It is helpful to consider an example of a patient who developed DJK after surgery for cervical deformity, and the treatment algorithm and revision approach (▶ Fig. 23.1).

23.7 Treatment

Distal junctional kyphosis can range from an asymptomatic radiographic finding to a continuously progressive degeneration of the caudal segments. Currently, there are no evidence-based guidelines for management or intervention for DJK. If a patient demonstrates radiographic evidence of distal junctional degeneration, a thorough clinical exam is warranted to evaluate for symptoms of local pain and neurologic deficits. In the absence of these, surgical treatment is usually not indicated, unless there is grossly unstable instrumentation with the potential for neurologic injury. Close follow-up with serial

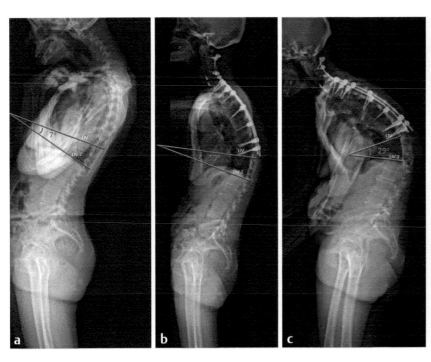

Fig. 23.1 Preoperative (**a**) and postoperative (**b,c**) radiographs of a patient with severe cervical deformity. (**b**) Postoperative radiograph at 3 months following cervical deformity correction demonstrating early distal junctional kyphosis (DJK). (**c**) Radiograph at 9-month follow-up showing progression of the DJK.

radiographs is critical to document any progression, and to optimize timing for intervention if needed.

One could propose that symptomatic DJK requiring revision surgery and distal junctional fracture represent a subtype of DJK, a distal junctional failure. For surgical treatment, a thorough neural decompression is required with extension of instrumentation in most cases to a stable distal level. Depending on the degree of kyphosis present at the distal junctional level, vertebrectomy may also be considered for global sagittal realignment.

23.8 Conclusion

Proximal and distal junctional kyphosis continue to be significant challenges within adult spinal deformity. To date, there is no definitive data for specific techniques or instrumentation configuration that consistently prevent the development of these complications. Importantly, for DJK, an understanding of the patient's overall sagittal alignment and selection of the appropriate distal fusion level can aid deformity surgeons in preoperative planning and in minimizing the risks for DJK.

References

[1] Watanabe K, Lenke LG, Bridwell KH, Kim YJ, Koester L, Hensley M. Proximal junctional vertebral fracture in adults after spinal deformity surgery using pedicle screw constructs: analysis of morphological features. Spine. 2010; 35 (2):138–145

[2] DeWald CJ, Stanley T. Instrumentation-related complications of multilevel fusions for adult spinal deformity patients over age 65: surgical considerations and treatment options in patients with poor bone quality. Spine. 2006; 31 (19) Suppl:S144–S151

[3] Cho KJ, Suk SI, Park SR, et al. Complications in posterior fusion and instrumentation for degenerative lumbar scoliosis. Spine. 2007; 32(20):2232–2237

[4] Kim HJ, Yagi M, Nyugen J, Cunningham ME, Boachie-Adjei O. Combined anterior-posterior surgery is the most important risk factor for developing proximal junctional kyphosis in idiopathic scoliosis. Clin Orthop Relat Res. 2012; 470(6):1633–1639

[5] O'Leary PT, Bridwell KH, Lenke LG, et al. Risk factors and outcomes for catastrophic failures at the top of long pedicle screw constructs: a matched cohort analysis performed at a single center. Spine. 2009; 34(20):2134–2139

[6] Smith MW, Annis P, Lawrence BD, Daubs MD, Brodke DS. Early proximal junctional failure in patients with preoperative sagittal imbalance. Evid Based Spine Care J. 2013; 4(2):163–164

[7] Hostin R, McCarthy I, O'Brien M, et al. International Spine Study Group. Incidence, mode, and location of acute proximal junctional failures after surgical treatment of adult spinal deformity. Spine. 2013; 38(12):1008–1015

[8] Denis F, Sun EC, Winter RB. Incidence and risk factors for proximal and distal junctional kyphosis following surgical treatment for Scheuermann kyphosis: minimum five-year follow-up. Spine. 2009; 34(20):E729–E734

[9] Ghasemi A, Stubig T, A Nasto L, Ahmed M, Mehdian H. Distal junctional kyphosis in patients with Scheuermann's disease: a retrospective radiographic analysis. Eur Spine J. 2017; 26(3):913–920

[10] Bradford DS, Ahmed KB, Moe JH, Winter RB, Lonstein JE. The surgical management of patients with Scheuermann's disease: a review of twenty-four cases managed by combined anterior and posterior spine fusion. J Bone Joint Surg Am. 1980; 62(5):705–712

[11] Reinhardt P, Bassett GS. Short segmental kyphosis following fusion for Scheuermann's disease. J Spinal Disord. 1990; 3(2):162–168

[12] Protopsaltis TS, Ramchandran S, Kim H, et al. International Spine Study Group. Analysis of early distal junctional kyphosis (DJK) after cervical deformity correction. Spine J. 2016; 16(10):S355–S356

[13] Passias PG, Vasquez-Montes D, Poorman GW, et al. ISSG. Predictive model for distal junctional kyphosis after cervical deformity surgery. Spine J. 2016; 10: S:244

[14] Cho KJ, Lenke LG, Bridwell KH, Kamiya M, Sides B. Selection of the optimal distal fusion level in posterior instrumentation and fusion for thoracic hyperkyphosis: the sagittal stable vertebra concept. Spine. 2009; 34(8):765–770

[15] Lowe TG, Lenke L, Betz R, et al. Distal junctional kyphosis of adolescent idiopathic thoracic curves following anterior or posterior instrumented fusion: incidence, risk factors, and prevention. Spine. 2006; 31(3):299–302

[16] Protopsaltis TS, Ramchandran S, Hamilton DK, et al. Analysis of successful versus failed radiographic outcomes following cervical deformity surgery. Spine (Phila Pa 1976). 2018; 43(13):E773–E781

[17] Scheuermann HW. Kyphosis dorsalis juvenilis. Ugeskr Laeger. 1920; 82:385

[18] Bradford DS, Garica A. Neurological complications in Scheuermann's disease. A case report and review of the literature. J Bone Joint Surg Am. 1969; 51 (3):567–572

[19] Bradford D, Lonstein J, Ogilvie JW, Winter RB. Scoliosis and Other SPINAL Deformities. Philadelphia, PA: W.B. Saunders; 1978

[20] Bradford DS, Moe JH, Montalvo FJ, Winter RB. Scheuermann's kyphosis and roundback deformity. Results of Milwaukee brace treatment. J Bone Joint Surg Am. 1974; 56(4):740–758

[21] Moe JH. Treatment of adolescent kyphosis by non-operative and operative methods. Manit Med Rev. 1965; 45(8):481–484

[22] Kwon BK, Elgafy H, Keynan O, et al. Progressive junctional kyphosis at the caudal end of lumbar instrumented fusion: etiology, predictors, and treatment. Spine. 2006; 31(17):1943–1951

[23] Arlet V, Aebi M. Junctional spinal disorders in operated adult spinal deformities: present understanding and future perspectives. Eur Spine J. 2013; 22 Suppl 2:S276–S295

[24] Han S, Hyun SJ, Kim KJ, Jahng TA, Lee S, Rhim SC. Rod stiffness as a risk factor of proximal junctional kyphosis after adult spinal deformity surgery: comparative study between cobalt chrome multiple-rod constructs and titanium alloy two-rod constructs. Spine J. 2017; 17(7):962–968

[25] Anderson AL, McIff TE, Asher MA, Burton DC, Glattes RC. The effect of posterior thoracic spine anatomical structures on motion segment flexion stiffness. Spine. 2009; 34(5):441–446

[26] Durrani A, Jain V, Desai R, et al. Could junctional problems at the end of a long construct be addressed by providing a graduated reduction in stiffness? A biomechanical investigation. Spine. 2012; 37(1):E16–E22

[27] Ameri E, Behtash H, Mobini B, Ghandhari H, Vahid Tari H, Khakinahad M. The prevalence of distal junctional kyphosis following posterior instrumentation and arthrodesis for adolescent idiopathic scoliosis. Acta Med Iran. 2011; 49 (6):357–363

[28] Miller DJ, Jameel O, Matsumoto H, et al. Factors affecting distal end & global decompensation in coronal/sagittal planes 2 years after fusion. Stud Health Technol Inform. 2010; 158:141–146

[29] Edwards CC, II, Bridwell KH, Patel A, et al. Thoracolumbar deformity arthrodesis to L5 in adults: the fate of the L5-S1 disc. Spine. 2003; 28(18):2122–2131

[30] Sears WR, Sergides IG, Kazemi N, Smith M, White GJ, Osburg B. Incidence and prevalence of surgery at segments adjacent to a previous posterior lumbar arthrodesis. Spine J. 2011; 11(1):11–20

[31] Lebwohl NH, Cunningham BW, Dmitriev A, et al. Biomechanical comparison of lumbosacral fixation techniques in a calf spine model. Spine. 2002; 27 (21):2312–2320

[32] Alegre GM, Gupta MC, Bay BK, Smith TS, Laubach JE. S1 screw bending moment with posterior spinal instrumentation across the lumbosacral junction after unilateral iliac crest harvest. Spine. 2001; 26(18):1950–1955

[33] Zindrick MR, Wiltse LL, Widell EH, et al. A biomechanical study of intrapeduncular screw fixation in the lumbosacral spine. Clin Orthop Relat Res. 1986 (203):99–112

[34] McCord DH, Cunningham BW, Shono Y, Myers JJ, McAfee PC. Biomechanical analysis of lumbosacral fixation. Spine. 1992; 17(8) Suppl:S235–S243

[35] Tsuchiya K, Bridwell KH, Kuklo TR, Lenke LG, Baldus C. Minimum 5-year analysis of L5-S1 fusion using sacropelvic fixation (bilateral S1 and iliac screws) for spinal deformity. Spine. 2006; 31(3):303–308

[36] Farcy JP, Rawlins BA, Glassman SD. Technique and results of fixation to the sacrum with iliosacral screws. Spine. 1992; 17(6) Suppl:S190–S195

[37] Camp JF, Caudle R, Ashmun RD, Roach J. Immediate complications of Cotrel-Dubousset instrumentation to the sacro-pelvis. A clinical and biomechanical study. Spine. 1990; 15(9):932–941

[38] Chen CS, Cheng CK, Liu CL, Lo WH. Stress analysis of the disc adjacent to interbody fusion in lumbar spine. Med Eng Phys. 2001; 23(7):483–491

[39] Goto K, Tajima N, Chosa E, et al. Effects of lumbar spinal fusion on the other lumbar intervertebral levels (three-dimensional finite element analysis). J Orthop Sci. 2003; 8(4):577–584

[40] Chosa E, Goto K, Totoribe K, Tajima N. Analysis of the effect of lumbar spine fusion on the superior adjacent intervertebral disk in the presence of disk degeneration, using the three-dimensional finite element method. J Spinal Disord Tech. 2004; 17(2):134–139

[41] Suk SI, Lee SM, Chung ER, Kim JH, Kim WJ, Sohn HM. Determination of distal fusion level with segmental pedicle screw fixation in single thoracic idiopathic scoliosis. Spine. 2003; 28(5):484–491

[42] Yanik HS, Ketenci IE, Coskun T, Ulusoy A, Erdem S. Selection of distal fusion level in posterior instrumentation and fusion of Scheuermann kyphosis: is fusion to sagittal stable vertebra necessary? Eur Spine J. 2016; 25(2):583–589

[43] Lundine K, Turner P, Johnson M. Thoracic hyperkyphosis: assessment of the distal fusion level. Global Spine J. 2012; 2(2):65–70

[44] Cho KJ, Lenke LG, Bridwell KH, Kamiya M, Sides B. Selection of the optimal distal fusion level in posterior instrumentation and fusion for thoracic hyperkyphosis: the sagittal stable vertebra concept. Spine. 2009; 34(8):765–770

[45] Lonner BS, Newton P, Betz R, et al. Operative management of Scheuermann's kyphosis in 78 patients: radiographic outcomes, complications, and technique. Spine. 2007; 32(24):2644–2652

24 Fusion Level Selection in Cervical Deformity

Anand H. Segar, Deeptee Jain, Peter G. Passias, and Themistocles S. Protopsaltis

Abstract

Adult cervical deformity is an expanding area of cervical spine research with vertebral level selection critical to ensuring satisfactory radiologic and clinical outcomes. Minimizing fusion levels has numerous benefits of motion preservation however may compromise the ultimate deformity correction and provide inadequate fixation. The primary driver of the cervical deformity must be identified and included. Recognition of reciprocal changes in the thoracic and lumbar spine is important. Finally, tailoring a surgical plan to the patient accounting for their comorbidities and tolerance to surgery is essential to minimize risks.

Keywords: cervical deformity, UIV, LIV, level selection, DJK, distal junctional kyphosis

24.1 Introduction

Adult cervical deformity (ACD) has a significant impact on patient's quality of life and presents a complex problem to the surgeon.[1] Vertebral level selection is seen as one of the most important surgical decisions to optimize radiographic outcomes and clinical improvement and prevent junctional failure.

The ideal surgical approach to ACD is often debated. A recent case-based survey of 14 spine deformity surgeons highlighted this with a marked variability in anterior (2–6) and posterior (2–16) fusion levels in ACD.[2] When considering fusion levels, the upper (UIV) and lower instrumented vertebrae (LIV) are usually the posterior levels included in the construct. Minimizing fusion levels may have the potential benefit of motion preservation, reduced operative time, and less surgical morbidity; however, a short fusion may compromise the ultimate deformity correction and provide inadequate fixation.

Currently, the literature to guide surgeons in level selection is limited without specific guidelines such as those used in adolescent idiopathic scoliosis or thoracolumbar adult sagittal deformity. Level selection in ACD can be broadly approached by considering radiographic, surgical, and medical factors.

24.2 Radiographic Considerations

It is paramount that assessment of the patient with ACD undergoes full-length standing radiographs. It is not uncommon to have concomitant thoracolumbar and cervical pathology with up to 53% of patients presenting with thoracolumbar deformity showing associated cervical kyphosis or increased cervical C2–C7 sagittal vertical axis (cSVA).[3]

The primary driver of the cervical deformity must be identified and included in the fusion to achieve appropriate radiological and clinical outcomes.[4] Passias et al showed that patients with a primary cervical apex sagittal deformity had the best radiological outcomes when the cervical driver of deformity was addressed.[4] On the other hand, patient improvement was limited if the cervical deformity was driven by a thoracic apex

sagittal deformity that was not addressed. This finding was similarly supported by Protopsaltis et al; 78% of patients who developed distal junctional kyphosis (DJK) did not have the thoracolumbar driver of the deformity addressed.[5]

Specific preoperative radiographic parameters suggestive of either a thoracic driver of deformity or a more severe cervical deformity have been shown to increase the risk of DJK, as defined by a change in kyphosis greater than 10 degrees between the LIV and LIV-2 from pre- to postoperatively. However, to date no studies have validated this distal kyphosis angle below the LIV in ACD unlike the proximal junctional kyphosis angle in in thoracolumbar deformity.[6]

A recent case–control study by Passias et al found that preoperative thoracic kyphosis (TK) greater than 50.6 degrees, C2–C7 lordosis less than -12 degrees, cervical lordosis/T1 slope mismatch (TS–CL) greater than 36 degrees, and cSVA greater than 56.3 mm were associated with DJK.[7] These scenarios suggest that the surgeon should consider extension of fusion further into the thoracic spine to prevent DJK; however, the exact LIV was not defined in this study.[7] Similarly, Protopsaltis et al demonstrated that TK greater than 50 degrees was also associated with DJK, and that 75% of patients with DJK had a LIV at or above T7, suggesting that extending the fusion distal to T7 might aid in preventing DJK.[5] ▶ Fig. 24.1 demonstrates balanced fusion to T10 in a case of severe cervical kyphosis and chin-on-chest deformity. ▶ Fig. 24.2 shows a case of DJK after C2 to T2 fusion. The patient has three surgical predictors of DJK which were specifically in the cervical spine. Ames and colleagues categorized ACD based on the location of the apex of the deformity.[8] In addressing a C-type deformity, a kyphotic angulation of greater than 10 degrees with a midcervical apex, the fusion should cross the cervicothoracic junction with a LIV of at least T1. In a retrospective cohort analysis, Schroeder et al showed that stopping a multilevel cervical construct at C7 was associated with a 2.3 times greater chance of revision surgery than if the construct was extended to T1.[9] These findings were supported by Osterhoff and colleagues who found a 31% incidence of distal junctional problems if the construct ended at C7 compared to 6.3% if terminated at T1.[10]

Ending the fusion at C7 is also associated with poorer postoperative sagittal alignment with Choi et al showing a greater cSVA, greater T1 slope (T1S), and greater TS–CL.[11] With regard to T1S, the authors hypothesize that with fusion T1, the surgeon can fix the angulation of T1. However, the increase in T1S seen with a LIV of C7 could simply be a reciprocal change due to an increase in postoperative C2–C7 lordosis.[12] ▶ Fig. 24.3 demonstrates balanced fusion to T2 in a case of mild cervical kyphosis.

In contrast, a multicenter retrospective study by Truumees et al found that extension to T1 was associated with greater intraoperative blood loss, length of surgery, and duration of inpatient stay albeit with a lower pseudoarthrosis rate, highlighting the negatives of crossing the cervicothoracic junction.[13] Not all patients in these studies had a kyphotic deformity; however, the benefits of crossing the C-T junction, namely, prevention of distal junctional problems and improved deformity correction, likely outweigh the costs of a slightly more invasive surgery in

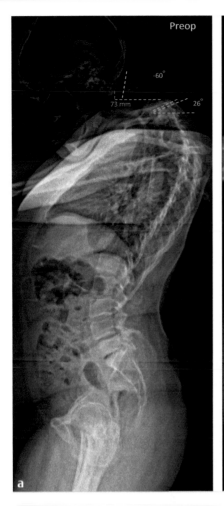
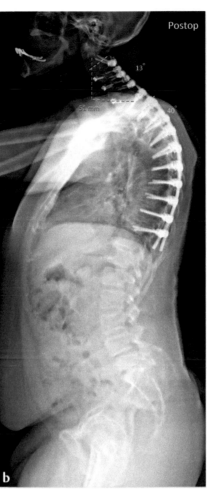

Fig. 24.1 A 64-year-old male who presented with a chin-on-chest deformity. His cervical deformity started in 2 years earlier. He denies any trouble swallowing and has minimal neck pain. He struggles to ambulate. He underwent anterior osteotomies for correction of kyphosis at C3/4, C4/5, and C6/7 and bilateral release of the sternocleidomastoid muscles. Posteriorly he underwent a Grade 2 posterior wedge osteotomy at C4/5 and posterior spinal fusion from C2 to T10. Pre- and postoperative X-rays show correction of the C2 SVA and marked improvement of cervical lordosis.

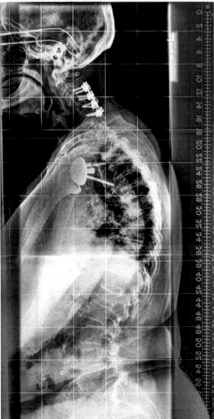
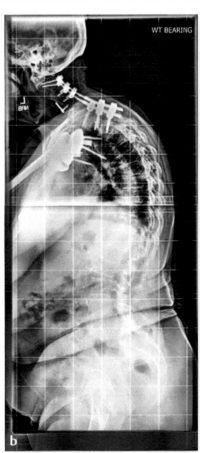

Fig. 24.2 A 76-year-old female who underwent a C3 to C6 posterior cervical decompression and fusion for myelopathy had ongoing neck pain and adjacent breakdown below. She had significant baseline deformity with TS–CL of 44.4 degrees, C2–C7 lordosis of 13.1 degrees, and cSVA of 50.9 mm. She underwent anterior discectomy and fusion at C4/5 and posterior fusion from C2 to T2, however, sustained distal junctional kyphosis at 3 months. Her risk factors for DJK were combined surgical approach, use of a transition rod, and multiple posterior osteotomies.

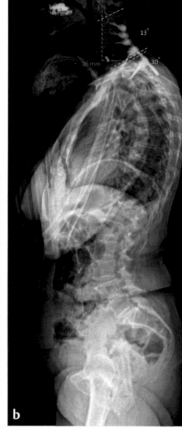
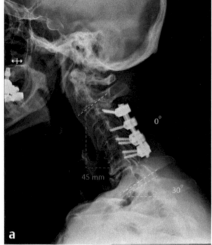

Fig. 24.3 A 71-year-old female presented with axial neck pain post a C3–C6 posterior decompression and fusion with instrumentation for cervical myelopathy. She had been experiencing pain in her mid-neck region associated with any movement. The pain radiated up the ears and into the head. The causes of her symptoms were likely kyphosis at C3–C6, the adjacent degeneration at C6–C7, the forward sagittal deformity from C2–C7, and the upper cervical compensatory hyperlordosis. She underwent anterior/posterior surgery with a discectomy and anterior uncovertebral osteotomy at C6–C7 followed by posterior C2–T2 fusion with Grade 2 posterior osteotomy at the cervicothoracic junction and C6/C7 and C7/T1 laminectomy for decompression of central canal and foramina. Pre- and postoperative X-rays show correction of the C2 SVA and improvement of cervical lordosis.

patients with midcervical kyphosis, suggesting that the LIV should extend into the thoracic spine.

Reciprocal changes in the thoracic and lumbar spine due to primary cervical pathology must be identified as well. Mizutani and colleagues showed that correction of severe cervical kyphotic deformity, defined as a cSVA greater than 40 mm, affects thoracolumbar decompensation down to the lumbar spine, whereas in midcervical kyphosis correction only leads to postoperative decompensation in thoracic segments.[14] In severe deformity, lumbar decompensation was evidenced by a decrease in lumbar lordosis (LL) and a corollary increase in the mismatch between pelvic incidence and LL. Unfortunately, the clinical relevance of this decompensation was not quantified. However, surgeons should be cognizant of these reciprocal changes and may consider a longer fusion into the lumbar spine especially in a patient with severe cervical deformity and pre-existing thoracolumbar deformity (▶ Table 24.1).

24.3 Surgical Considerations

Corroboration of clinical picture with the radiographic goals and tolerance to surgery is critical. Certainly, as patient frailty and surgical invasiveness increase, so does the risk of surgery and junctional failure. Hence, in addition to the driver of the deformity, the risk of surgery should be considered and tailored.

Certain surgical techniques may predispose a patient to junctional failure in ACD. Passias et al found that both combined

Table 24.1 Tips for level selection

Consider LIV below thoracic apex (T9 or below)

cSVA correction > 4 cm

T1 slope > 25–30 degrees

All cervicothoracic junction three-column osteotomy (except in ankylosing spondylitis)

Global SVA > 7–8 cm

Abbreviations: cSVA, cervical sagittal vertical axis; LIV, lower instrumented vertebra.

anterior-posterior approaches and the use of a Smith–Peterson osteotomy were associated with the development of DJK with an odds ratios of 2.67 and 2.55.[7] Similarly, Protopsaltis et al also found that a higher grade cervical osteotomy was associated with DJK.[5] It is important to note, however, that these associations were found with the use of binary analysis, and, thus, it is likely that these patients had more severe deformity preoperatively and underwent a greater deformity correction. It is likely that it is the amount of deformity correction that is the driving factor for DJK, a finding confirmed by Koller et al.[15]

Additionally, the interplay between cervical myelopathy and axial/postural symptomatology is a major factor. Primary myelopathic patients with mild to moderate regional deformity do well with focal decompression and realignment. However, those with severe ACD and concomitant myelopathy require more aggressive realignment to address draping of spinal cord over cervicothoracic junction, and hence the fusion should extend into the thoracic spine.

24.4 Medical Considerations

The surgeon must also be cognizant of the medical comorbidities, as these could adversely impact distal failure and consideration should be given to modifying the LIV.

Osteoporosis may present a substantial challenge in the management of cervical deformity. Prior to undergoing surgical intervention, a thorough workup to determine bone mineral density, including dual-energy X-ray absorptiometry, is indicated. Pharmacologic intervention with mineral supplementations or teriparatide might be indicated. Poor bone density might demand a lower LIV due to concern for adequate fixation. Interestingly, Passias et al were unable to demonstrate a relationship between osteoporosis and DJK, perhaps because this was a retrospective study and surgeons were performing longer fusions on patients with osteoporosis.[7]

Neurodegenerative diseases such as Parkinson disease, multiple sclerosis, myopathies, myositis, and amyotrophic lateral sclerosis present not only with bony deformity but also with motor dysfunction. These syndromes may present with isolated cervical deformities, such as anterocollis, or with sweeping deformities that include not only the cervical spine but also the thoracolumbar spine, such as Pisa syndrome. Surgical intervention must take into account the full pathophysiology of the disease when choosing fusion levels and given the distorted sensorimotor feedback mechanisms, consideration should be given to longer fusions. Furthermore, patients presenting with a neurological deficit as a result of the cervical deformity should also be approached in a similar fashion, as Passias el al showed increased odds of DJK.[7]

The mechanism of dropped head is thought to be secondary to either dystonia of the flexor neck muscles or weakness of the extensor neck muscles. It is this same pathophysiology that creates a constant drive for forward tilt and increased strain on the construct postoperatively. Bone anchorage is also of particular concern in this population; one study quoted an osteoporosis rate of 34% in patients with Parkinson disease.[16,17] For these reasons, the authors recommend longer fusions with a lower LIV in patients with neuromuscular disease, similar to what has been previously proposed for the thoracolumbar spine in the same population.[18] Full-length standing X-rays should be performed, and fusion should also be performed distally to the neutral level.[8]

In conclusion, while the optimal fusion levels in treating ACD remain not well understood, surgical evaluation requires a thorough understanding of the cervical deformity and careful preoperative surgical planning. Identification of the principal drivers of the deformity is key when determining whether to extend the fusion into the mid to lower thoracic spine, and in most cases of ACD, fusion should at least cross the C-T junction. In cases with osteoporosis or neuromuscular disease, surgeons should err with longer fixation. Unfortunately, there is a certain portion of patients with such severe frailty and deformity that the only durable option is extension to the pelvis. This is a burgeoning field of knowledge and we need to compile more prospective data to guide an evidence-based approach to choosing fusion levels in ACD.

References

[1] Smith JS, Line B, Bess S, et al. The health impact of adult cervical deformity in patients presenting for surgical treatment: comparison to United States population norms and chronic disease states based on the EuroQuol-5 Dimensions Questionnaire. Neurosurgery. 2017; 80(5):716–725

[2] Smith JS, Klineberg E, Shaffrey CI, et al. International Spine Study Group. Assessment of surgical treatment strategies for moderate to severe cervical spinal deformity reveals marked variation in approaches, osteotomies, and fusion levels. World Neurosurg. 2016; 91(C):228–237

[3] Smith JS, Lafage V, Schwab FJ, et al. International Spine Study Group. Prevalence and type of cervical deformity among 470 adults with thoracolumbar deformity. Spine. 2014; 39(17):E1001–E1009

[4] Passias PG, Bortz C, Horn S, et al. International Spine Study Group. Drivers of cervical deformity have a strong influence on achieving optimal radiographic and clinical outcomes at 1 year after cervical deformity surgery. World Neurosurg. 2018; 112:e61–e68

[5] Protopsaltis TS, Ramchandran S, Kim H-J, et al. Analysis of early distal junctional kyphosis (DJK) after cervical deformity correction. Spine J. 2016; 16 (10):S355–S356

[6] Bridwell KH, Lenke LG, Cho SK, et al. Proximal junctional kyphosis in primary adult deformity surgery: evaluation of 20 degrees as a critical angle. Neurosurgery. 2013; 72(6):899–906

[7] Passias PG, Vasquez-Montes D, Poorman GW, et al. ISSG. Predictive model for distal junctional kyphosis after cervical deformity surgery. Spine J. 2018; 18 (12):2187–2194

[8] Ames CP, Smith JS, Eastlack R, et al. International Spine Study Group. Reliability assessment of a novel cervical spine deformity classification system. J Neurosurg Spine. 2015; 23(6):673–683

[9] Schroeder GD, Kepler CK, Kurd MF, et al. Is it necessary to extend a multilevel posterior cervical decompression and fusion to the upper thoracic spine? Spine. 2016; 41(23):1845–1849

[10] Osterhoff G, Ryang Y-M, von Oelhafen J, Meyer B, Ringel F. Posterior multilevel instrumentation of the lower cervical spine: is bridging the cervicothoracic junction necessary? World Neurosurg. 2017; 103:419–423

[11] Choi S-J, Suk K-S, Yang J-H, et al. What is a right distal fusion level for prevention of sagittal imbalance in multilevel posterior cervical spine surgery: C7 or T1? Clin Spine Surg. 2018; 31(10):441–445

[12] Ames CP, Blondel B, Scheer JK, et al. Cervical radiographical alignment: comprehensive assessment techniques and potential importance in cervical myelopathy. Spine. 2013; 38(22) Suppl 1:S149–S160

[13] Truumees E, Singh D, Geck MJ, Stokes JK. Should long-segment cervical fusions be routinely carried into the thoracic spine? A multicenter analysis. Spine J. 2018; 18(5):782–787

[14] Mizutani J, Strom R, Abumi K, et al. How cervical reconstruction surgery affects global spinal alignment. Neurosurgery. 2018; 23(6):1177

[15] Koller H, Ames C, Mehdian H, et al. Characteristics of deformity surgery in patients with severe and rigid cervical kyphosis (CK): results of the CSRS-Europe multi-centre study project. Eur Spine J. 2018; 24 Suppl 1:S23

[16] Robin GC, Span Y, Steinberg R, Makin M, Menczel J. Scoliosis in the elderly: a follow-up study. Spine. 1982; 7(4):355–359

[17] Ha Y, Oh JK, Smith JS, et al. Impact of movement disorders on management of spinal deformity in the elderly. Neurosurgery. 2015; 77 Suppl 4:S173–S185

[18] Bourghli A, Guérin P, Vital J-M, et al. Posterior spinal fusion from T2 to the sacrum for the management of major deformities in patients with Parkinson disease: a retrospective review with analysis of complications. J Spinal Disord Tech. 2012; 25(3):E53–E60

Index